Gender and Self in Islam

Gender and Self in Islam examines the theological, cultural, and social roots of hierarchical gender system in the Muslim communities and its impact on the constitution of the self. It traces the historical and contemporary patterns of women's lives, including their oppressions and their resistance to what is accepted as the philosophical and Islamic truth of being men and women. Specific attention is paid to the views of:

- gender thinking and its impact on hierarchical gender system
- the creation theories and the making of humanity
- the politics of reproduction and the impact on women's role in conception
- the masculine concepts and practices of feminine morality
- the performance of gender and self-process based on male superiority and supremacy
- the subordination of female self-determination and agency.

It argues that the diverse authoritative legitimacies of Islamic teaching—especially Muslims' interpretation of the expositions of certain practices in the Qur'ān and the *aḥādīth*—have formed a system that focuses on male humanity and supremacy, while at the same time disempowering the female self-becoming. This volume also examines the endeavors by feminists, womanists, and male advocates to disentangle the seamless relations of the existing gender system and foster the making of an egalitarian gender system and an inclusive humanity.

Gender and Self in Islam is a significant contribution to Islamic gender studies from an author who can provide a unique perspective as a Southeast Asian who is well versed in Islamic philosophy.

Etin Anwar is Assistant Professor of Religious Studies at Hobart and William Smith Colleges, Geneva, New York. She has published several articles on Ibn Sina, Meister Eckhart, Ibn Arabi, and women's movements in Indonesia in journals including *Islamic Studies, Islam and Christian-Muslim Relations*, and *Hawwa*.

Routledge Advances in Middle East and Islamic Studies

1 **Iraqi Kurdistan**
Political development and emergent democracy
Gareth R.V. Stansfield

2 **Egypt in the Twenty First Century**
Challenges for development
Edited by M. Riad El-Ghonemy

3 **The Christian–Muslim Frontier**
A zone of contact, conflict or cooperation
Mario Apostolov

4 **The Islamic World-System**
A study in polity-market interaction
Masudul Alam Choudhury

5 **Regional Security in the Middle East**
A critical perspective
Pinar Bilgin

6 **Political Thought in Islam**
A study in intellectual boundaries
Nelly Lahoud

7 **Turkey's Kurds**
A theoretical analysis of the PKK and Abdullah Ocalan
Ali Kemal Özcan

8 **Beyond the Arab Disease**
New perspectives in politics and culture
Riad Nourallah

9 **The Arab Diaspora**
Voices of an anguished scream
Zahia Smail Salhi and Ian Richard Netton

10 **Gender and Self in Islam**
Etin Anwar

Gender and Self in Islam

Etin Anwar

Routledge
Taylor & Francis Group
LONDON AND NEW YORK

First published 2006
by Routledge
2 Park Square, Milton Park, Abingdon, Oxon OX14 4RN

Simultaneously published in the USA and Canada
by Routledge
270 Madison Ave, New York, NY 10016

Routledge is an imprint of the Taylor & Francis Group, an informa business

Typeset in Garamond by
Newgen Imaging Systems (P) Ltd, Chennai, India
Printed and bound in Great Britain by
Biddles Ltd, King's Lynn

British Library Cataloguing in Publication Data
A catalogue record for this book is available from the British Library

Library of Congress Cataloging in Publication Data
A catalog record for this book has been requested

ISBN10: 0–415–70103–1 (hbk)
ISBN10: 0–203–79962–3 (ebk)

ISBN13: 978–0–415–70103–7 (hbk)
ISBN13: 978–0–203–79962–8 (ebk)

To
Siti Hasanah for the gift of life
and
Shalahudin Kafrawi for the gift of love

Contents

Acknowledgments ix
Note xi

Introduction 1

About the book 2
Philosophy as a method of inquiry into gender and self 5
The contents of the book 14

1 Gender thinking and the system it produces 16

The roots of the hierarchical and egalitarian gender systems 17
Gender and power difference in the family 32
Conclusion 44

2 The creation theories as the bases for ontological self and inclusive humanity 46

The creation of Adam and the making of humanity 48
Equality in human origin 61
Ontology and human equality 65
Conclusion 70

3 The transmission of generative self and women's contribution to conception 72

Female's roles in conception: an Islamic philosophical view and its Greek heritage 74
The politics of gender and reproduction in the post-Ibn Sīnān period 82
The stages of fetal development: a Qur'ānic view 86
Conclusion 92

4 **The embodiment of masculinity and femininity: the making of material self** 94

The narrative of the self and the making of material self 96
The formativity of material self 102
Conclusion 115

5 **The performance of the self: engendering dependency and pleasures** 117

The construction of the ethics and psychology of the self 118
Extensional and reciprocal dependency 123
The "Embodied Self," the truth of sex and pleasures 133
Conclusion 139

Conclusion 140

Glossary 147
Notes 149
Bibliography 177
Index 189

Acknowledgments

This book reflects my long quest on the subject of women in Islam, and my fascination with philosophy. It is rare to find these two topics spoken of in the same breath, particularly as regards the question of gender in Islamic philosophy. To fill this gap I have attempted in the following pages to create a new space for a philosophical discussion of gender and self in Islam. Philosophy, as a method of inquiry, can be an ideal method for understanding the current and historical construction of these topics. In so doing, I have tried to avoid overgeneralization and oversimplification of the diversity of issues affecting the lives of women in Muslim societies. Instead, I have attempted to describe the patterns of social realities in which Muslim women live, their oppression at the personal, familial, and societal levels, their resistance to the status quo and their empowerment.

My "innocent" worldview of women comes mostly from my deceased, illiterate grandmother, Ratna Komala, whose view of a woman's role and the world around her was simple, yet inspiring. Equally important has been the influence of my mother, Siti Hasanah, who has first and foremost taught me to act beyond the call of duty. She was generous in the first place by bringing me into the world, and even more so in doing everything she could to see that I would have a promising future.

My intellectual worldview of women has flourished under the influence of many inspiring teachers. I am indebted in the first place to Howard Federspiel, who introduced me to the academic study of Muslim women in Indonesia. I thank Bat Ami Bar-On, Ali A. Mazrui, and Anthony Preus for their insights at early stages of the book. I would also like to thank Stephen D. Ross, Marcia K. Hermansen, Nimat Hafez Barazangi, Mahmud Ayoub, Herman Landolt, Rebecca Alpert, Russel Blackwood, Jay William, Nelly Van Doorn-Harder, and Nanat Fatah Nasir for their generous support. I also thank Tim Elgren and Thomas Wilson for their assistance in finding me financial support during my stay at Hamilton College.

I want to express my infinite gratitude to Parviz Morewedge, Rosemarie Morewedge, and Pauline Mazrui who have been outstandingly supportive. My thanks also go to Elizabeth Bughaighis, Lisa Fischler, and Tracia Leacock for their contribution to this book. I would also like to extend my special thanks to Provost Teresa Amott and my collegues at Religious Studies Department at Hobart and William Smith Colleges: Lowell Bloss, Michael Dobkowski, Richard Salter, Susan Henking, and Hyo-Dong Lee.

Stephen Millier has read different versions of this book. I thank him for saving me from any embarrassments over *In*glish (Indonesian-English). Any mistake or imperfection, however, is entirely my own responsibility.

I also want to thank my entire family, especially, Hj. Siti Hasanah, the H. Bakri family, the H. Anwar family, the H. Kafrawi family, and their extended family who keep me in their daily prayers.

I am indebted forever to Sal, who appreciates my personal and intellectual life and has provided me with endless support, compassion, and love, especially when I need them most. Rizky, Fadly, and Jenna have given me the authority to speak first hand about what it takes to be a mother. While I am a daughter, sister, friend, colleague, stepdaughter, daughter, sister-in-law, neighbor, and citizen (not to mention other possible labels), my role as mother is special to me. To these three wonderful and fantastic children, my work is dedicated.

Bethlehem
August 4, 2006

Note

Reference

All references to the Qur'ān are indicated by Q.S., which stands for Qur'ān and Sūrah. The Qur'ānic translations are quoted from Muhammad Asad, *The Message of the Qur'ān* (Gibraltar: Dar Al-Andalus, 1980), otherwise they are noted. Other quotations of the Qur'ān and *aḥādith* are taken from the Islamic software, *Alim* (Multimedia CD edition). References are also made to the CD version of *Encyclopedia of Islam*.

Transliteration

The Arabic transliteration in this thesis will follow the system used by the Institute of Islamic Studies, McGill University with only slight modifications. It is as follows:

ب = b	ذ = dh	ط = ṭ	ل = l
ت = t	ر = r	ظ = ẓ	م = m
ث = th	ز = z	ع = ‘	ن = n
ج = j	س = s	غ = gh	ه = h
ح = ḥ	ش = sh	ف = f	و = w
خ = kh	ص = ṣ	ق = q	ي = y
د = d	ض = ḍ	ك = k	ء = ’
Short:	ـَ = a;	ـِ = i;	ـُ = u
Long:	ـَا = ā;	ـِيْ = ī;	ـُوْ = ū
Dipthong:	ـَيْ = ay;	ـَوْ = aw	

Ta Marbūṭah (ة) = h; in iḍāfah, it is written t.
Hamzah in the initial position is omitted.
Tashdīd is transliterated as double consonants.

Introduction

The contemporary construction of gender system in Muslim societies varies across cultures depending on the degree of the confluence between local beliefs, norms, laws and practices and global forces, such as post-colonization, globalization, feminism, human rights charters and Islamization. The seamless fusion of local and global forces combines with Muslims' quest to interpret and implement the Qur'ān and the *ḥadīth* within different Muslim localities and cultures, creating a cohesive production of knowledge that not only nourishes the intellectual pursuit, but also generates religious authoritative legitimacies. Within these different contexts—where hierarchical gender-minded Muslim men and women reiterate, strengthen and exercise the embodiment of religious legitimacies as appropriate for men and women at the theoretical and practical levels—many have embarked on an interpretation of Islamic teachings on gender issues and on questioning what Muslim societies perceive as "the truth." These attempts are not novel, since Muslims frequently revise their understanding of Islamic teaching in the face of new challenges, and have done throughout the history.

Muslims' different degrees of encounters with both local and global forces have produced, nurtured, and perpetuated the contradictory claims of gender system. Gender hierarchy claims that the natural difference between men and women entails ontological, moral, spiritual, financial, social, cultural, and political differences, whereas gender egalitarianism argues for intrinsic equality between men and women before God and their fellow humans, regardless of sexual and gender differences. While variations in hierarchical and egalitarian gender systems are part of the lived experiences of Muslims' daily lives, the existing gender hierarchy at the theoretical and practical levels continues to be dominant. The resilience of hierarchical gender system is mediated through the confluence of interpretation of Islamic teaching, hierarchical power relations in the family, masculine concepts of social order, and morality, Muslim images of body reflecting different places and cultures in the world and the reiteration of religious narratives and authoritative legitimacy that the public perceives as the truth.

Exposing the current established hierarchical gender system is a daunting task for many Muslim feminists,[1] womanists,[2] and male egalitarianists.[3] They have called attention to the variations of religious, social, and cultural construction of gender appropriation in Muslim communities. Their discussions focus on the analysis of the status of women, their roles, their identity, their participation in society, and their liberation from the shackles of unjust "religious," cultural, and social expressions and practices. Their works also address multilayered nuances of women's daily experiences in diverse cultures and communities.

The diversity of Muslim women's experiences and discourses reflects the variety in Muslim cultures and understandings of Islam from place to place, so that any attempt to generalize Muslim women or to define them as belonging to a homogenous group would entail "a specific version of Islam."[4] This reductionism often results in a partial Islam. The portrayal of partial Islam is definitely not an epitome of Islam since the multiplicity of religious expressions and practices in the Muslim's world represents ways in which the ideal Islam has been embodied and ingrained within different geo-political locality.

Muslims' diverse traditions and cultures capture the seamless assimilation of religious authoritative legitimacies with local beliefs and practices that is justified by reiteration of Qur'ānic discussions of the creation of Adam, the husband's superior position because of his financial responsibility in the family, inheritance, and testimony (Q.S. al-Baqarah, 2:30, al-Nisā', 4:34, al-Nisā', 4:176, and al-Baqarah, 2:282 respectively). The above-cited verses eventually provide the groundwork for such inconsistency in Islamic teaching. They appear to be in favor of hierarchical gender system. With this in mind, the present book elaborates on the religious, social, ethical and cultural roots of gender system, and their impact on the construction of the self. I argue that the dominant and hierarchical gender system operating in many parts of the Muslim world is supported by Muslims' justification of the conditional particularism of legal, social, and familial practices and expressions of Islam. Over the course of time, the religious legitimacies, expressions, and practices of conditional particularism tend to become universal.

While the hierarchical gender system is prevalent in the Muslim world, I am hopeful that gender egalitarianism as articulated in the Qur'ān and the Prophetic traditions (*aḥādīth*) will lead to equality of humans before God and their fellow humans. Any attempt to paint these sources as justifying un-Islamic thinking and behavior violates the universal ethical message of the Qur'ān. Muslim men and women have the responsibility to do their best to bring the Qur'ān and the Prophetic traditions (*aḥādīth*) into their daily lives since they are equally important moral agents for the internalization of the egalitarian gender system. To this end, my endeavor to deconstruct the web of gender thinking and system that determines the existing constitution of the self is extremely relevant and significant. This book attempts to contribute to nurturing a new epistemic production of egalitarian knowledge and system that works for the perpetuation of an inclusive humanity and the flourishing of a new constitution of self-becoming.

About the book

The resilience of the hierarchical gender system shapes what Ferguson calls "the self-process."[5] This self-process includes ways of doing, thinking, and feeling. Women's way of life, their customs, the laws pertaining to them, the institution of family, their dwellings, contours, facial expressions, bodily gestures, and ways of praying are visible and observable. As women's activities are visible at the surface, their activities and experiences reflect their cultural relativity. Thus, what is acceptable in one location may not be in other. For instance, guardianship, driving, and working in public are not important issues for Muslim women in Southeast Asia, but they are in Saudi Arabia. Regardless of the different mechanisms in which the self interacts and is constructed through those encounters with others, they are to a certain degree influenced by the way gender system operates in Muslim communities.

I interject the idea of the "self," which evolves within social, cultural, and historical constructs of gender. The question is: what does it mean to think about the "self"? How does the concept of the "self" relate to men and women? What is the manner in which the self is constructed? The answers to these inquiries vary, depending on how one defines the notion of the self. To begin with, the word "self" is one of the translations of '*nafs*,' which can denote soul, spirit, mind, life, animate being, living creature, person, individual, self, personal identity or nature.[6] In the Qur'ān, the word '*nafs*' stands for many of these meanings. Nevertheless, for our purposes, the word '*nafs*' will be interpreted in relation to the nature of humans.

The word '*nafs*' is used in conjunction with the creation of each human being. '*Nafs*,' as shown in the introduction to this book and its subsequent chapters, refers to the common origin of human beings in that male or female are created out of one living entity, self or soul (*nafs wāḥidah*).[7] Its consequent form is embodied in the ontological constituent of the self. What is called human denotes whatever has human form and the properties that grow along with their physical development and flourishing. The use of the word '*nafs*' to mean a human, self or person also occurs when it is used reflexively, such as in Āl 'Imrān, 3:61, "...ourselves and yourselves."[8]

The word *nafs* means the human soul, such as *al-nafs al-ammārah* (the blaming soul) (Q.S. Yūsuf, 12:53), *al-nafs al-muṭma'innah* (the tranquil soul) (Q.S. al-Fajr, 89: 27), *al-nafs al-lawwāmah* (the self-reproaching soul) (Q.S. al-Qiyāmah, 75:2), and *al-hawā* (base desire) (Q.S. al-Nāzi'āt, 79:40). These states of the soul also concur with Ibn Sīnā's philosophical discussion of psychological dimensions of the soul, even though he does not treat the soul or '*nafs*' the way the Qur'ān defines it. We will visit this issue in Chapter 5.

Nafs is also used interchangeably with *rūḥ* to denote spirit, angels, and djinn. *Rūḥ* is used to describe God's divine creative breath, as in the cases where God blew His spirit into Adam (Q.S. al-Ḥijr, 15:29), Mary received the Holy Spirit that resulted in the conception of Jesus (Q.S. al-Anbiyā', 1:91) and God sent *al-rūḥ al-amīn* (the divine inspiration) into Muḥammad's heart (Q.S. al-Shu'arā', 26:193). The Qur'ān does not explicitly indicate the similarity between *nafs* and *rūh*, but God does state that He blows His spirit (*rūḥ*) into human beings (Q.S. al-Sajdah, 32:9).[9] It follows, then, that the principle of life that philosophers designate as soul or self comes from God.

Even though the ontological self provides the basic foundation of the commonality of all humans insofar as they share a common origin and a similar human form (as discussed in Chapter 2), the way the material self is cited and the truth it produces are bound to the geo-political locality of the Muslim world. Since the embodied self grows up within a specific locality, the material self is subject to the coded gender system. The materiality of the self carries with it social, religious, and political constructs that have led to the establishment of hierarchical gender system and its various institutions at the personal, familial, and societal levels.

In this connection, the book examines the entangled systems and mechanisms that generate and nurture the theological, social, historical, and cultural roots of a dominant gender system and their impact on the construction of the self. I analyze the roots of gender hierarchy in the patriarchal system of Muslim cultures, especially Qur'ānic views of the creation theories and the making of gender, the politics of reproduction and its impact on women's role in conception, the masculine concept and practice of femininity, and the construction of gender based on male superiority and supremacy and female inferiority.

While the hierarchical gender construct is problematic, Muslims in general and Muslim women in particular do not usually see the constructed gender system as *their* problems. Most hierarchical gender-minded Muslims apparently do not perceive the problems underlying the gender system and its variations operating in Muslim societies since "a woman's role in Islamic society is clearly, at base, to rear children and create a wholesome and happy home."[10] Any deviation from this precept is actually "a problem." Muslims often hold anything Western—feminism, democracy and human rights—to be the source of the problems faced by Muslim men and women. Commenting on the calls for women's freedom, liberation and equal rights with men, Al-Sheha says that

> [I]t is stunning and surprising, however, to hear such calls in Islamic societies where women have been fairly treated and were given rights more than fourteen hundred years ago, and without any calls made by them, or rather by their advocates.[11]

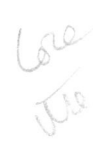

Muslims would not have any problems today if the liberation that started fourteen centuries ago had been carried on; if women were given all the rights they were entitled to; if they were not silenced in the realms of knowledge; if they were not alienated from politics; if they were not only confined to household tasks; if they were not economically deprived; if they received adequate protection from authoritarian fathers or abusive husbands; if children from previous marriages were guaranteed by law to receive child support; if divorced women received enough family and government support to be financially independent; if they were not despised for being single, widow, or unmarried; if they could pursue their personal goals and growth without mockery or opposition from their family and society. The list goes on depending on the problems and variations posed by women's conditions in different locations in the Muslim world. This reality is what Muslim women hope to change, although no such change can be introduced instantly. The only feasible option is to develop an attitude that gives Muslim women, along with Muslim men, the opportunity to introduce social, cultural, legal, political, and religious conditions that are more friendly to women. In this sense, Muslim women across the globe have the moral responsibility to reexamine actively what constitutes the "problems" and look for solutions that are workable and inclusive of women. Muslim women owe it to themselves to dismantle the patriarchal elements of Muslim culture that shape their thinking, life and knowledge.

Here, patriarchy refers to "a society in which older men are in positions of power and authority" and "a male-dominated society";[12] it also relates to a process and a system by which men and women give and participate in the construction of their sense of who they are.[13] Here, I borrow Johnson's definition of patriarchal culture as follows:

> Patriarchy's defining elements are male-dominated, male-identified, and male-centered character, but this is just the beginning... Patriarchal culture includes ideas about the nature of things, including men, women, and humanity, with manhood and masculinity most closely associated with being human and womanhood and femininity relegated to the marginal position of "other."[14]

Muslim women have for centuries lived within a social, cultural, and religious "system" that is not friendly to them. This structure systematically alienates women's worth as human beings. However, Muslim women do not recognize the alienation of their selves as a problem because the system in which they live their lives is so powerful and is sometimes alleged to be the system that women themselves unquestionably support. Following established sets of patriarchal beliefs, Muslim women contribute to and perpetuate that system as their own. This patriarchal culture depends on both men's and women's participation. And this participation beyond doubt shapes everyone's understanding of gender system, including gender thinking, construction, identity, equality, inequality, hierarchy, and relationship.

Given that woman's daily exposure to gender system is so intense, this book explores the elements contained within the gender system and its effect on the ontological, social, and cultural construction of the self. The following questions are some formulations of the problem of this book: What are the elements that constitute the prevalent hierarchical gender system? What mechanism perpetuates gender hierarchy? How does gender thinking work in light of the hierarchical gender system? What is the impact of the hierarchical gender system on self-becoming? Is the self recognized through extended or reciprocal dependency? What are the religious roots of the ontological, social, psychological, and ethical construct of the self? Indeed, these questions vary across Muslim societies as Muslims have different levels of theories and practices of gender. These variations lend themselves to various methodologies appropriate to the investigation of gender and self as follows.

Philosophy as a method of inquiry into gender and self

The methodologies employed in the study of gender in Islam vary, ranging from historical, social, and anthropological, to philosophical and mystical approaches. These modes of addressing the issue of women are not independent of each other, since women's lives and experiences are multifaceted and more complex than any methodology can capture. Despite the complexity of women's issues, however, most writers have preferred one methodology to others depending on the purpose of the research, the nature of the problem itself and how the subject-matter is analyzed and presented.

It should also be noted that an appropriate methodology does not necessarily warrant an objective conclusion, since researchers' worldviews will, in one way or another, inevitably affect their research.[15] Roald, a Muslim convert of Norwegian birth, points out that studies of Islam and Muslims in the West carried out by Westerners or Muslims who have adopted Western views and yet do not apply a "scientific methodology" often yield to other considerations, such as ideology or religion. Similarly, studies done by Muslims on Muslims can suffer from conflict of interest "between the various levels and directions of 'Muslimness.'"[16] At this juncture, it is not significant who the researchers are; what really matters is their commitment to the outcome of the research. Roald relates her own research commitment to her position as a person located "in between" Muslim and non-Muslim cultures.

I agree that being an *insider* to the subject of women or gender in Islam is a privilege, and yet having a methodological awareness of the subject matter in question is prerequisite to conducting an objective analysis of the problem. In my own case, I have the advantage of having learned the Indonesian version of Islam,[17] which is distinct in many respects from its Middle Eastern expression but not for that reason any less Islamic. One thing that Muslims, regardless of culture, have in common when perfecting their understanding of Islamic belief and practices is that they return to the *same* Qur'ān and Ḥadīth that Middle Eastern Muslims read and to which they refer. The main difference between the forms of Islam in the two regions is that Islam in Indonesia has absorbed the multifaceted cultures, practices, and perspectives that Islam has encountered in various parts of Indonesia. It is only to be expected that Indonesian Islam should vary, and that it should do so even within itself. The many varieties of Indonesian Islam expressed in the nation's history and culture have, to a certain degree, contributed to the multifaceted formulation of the hierarchical and egalitarian principles of gender.

I emphasize the position that I occupy as an insider, simply because the *insider's* views of the theory and practice of gender have multilayered nuances. The experiences of Muslim women contain their authentic encounters with the many kinds of oppression that arise from prescribed gender roles. Even if some Muslim women claim that they are not oppressed by their religion and culture, they must be given the opportunity to discuss their perspectives from the inside. Sometimes they will not interpret their experience in the same way that outsiders would. Outsiders often attempt as well to get into the insider's mind and experiences so as to interpret and develop certain theories of the insider's claims.[18]

My insider's claim also pertains to my experience as a *santri*, both as a class and as a religious identity that shapes my interpretation of gender and self in Islam. Clifford Geertz classifies Javanese Muslims into three classes: *santri*, *abangan*, and *priyayi*.[19] *Santri* refers to practicing Muslims who attempt to embody Islam in their everyday lives, best exemplified in the culture of the *madrasah* and *pesantren* (Islamic boarding schools). *Abangan* refers to nominal Muslims who declare their identities as Muslims, but whose religious practices are a mixture of Islam and pre-existing beliefs deriving from indigenous Javanese culture and Hindu and Buddhist remnants. Finally, *priyayi*—which Geertz mistakenly identifies as a religious category—refers to the traditional Javanese elite, most of whom are loyal to indigenous Javanese culture and its Hindu and Buddhist traditions. For my part, I attempt to incorporate my familiarity with the language, narratives, and logic used among the *santri* on the issue of gender in Islam. However, I use my cultural background as an Indonesian/Southeast Asian Muslim to show that this type of Islam is moderate and inclusive of women.

One may argue that the insider's view is disadvantageous because Muslim men and women may have been indoctrinated with certain teachings concerning women. Although a Muslim may start from the premise that Islam deprives women of their fundamental rights, his/her complex relations to Islam as a belief system can cause difficulties in reaching an objective conclusion. Here, objectivity becomes the heart of the question. Can an insider be objective in the production of knowledge relating to women's issues? Can Muslims generally research their own creed?[20] Can veiling Muslim women research veiling objectively? Can believing Muslim women do research on their own belief system?

To address these inquiries is not a simple task, since the way in which both insiders and outsiders interpret the phenomena of Muslim women will depend on the interpreter's mindset and experiences. For instance, Western scholarship on Muslim women often tends

> ... to accentuate certain specific practices in society, and to examine them using their own Western framework or value concepts. These studies often conclude that Muslim women are discriminated against, subordinated and ill-treated...
>
> These studies are so concerned with actual practices and specific matters in Muslim society that they often confuse Islam at practical level and Islam at "ideal" level. Thus they portray the image of women in Islam only from deduction, that is, they describe Muslim women based on Western viewpoint.[21]

This perspective shows how one's mindset and experience can quickly validate the insider's experience or, alternatively, develop an explanatory theory that totally dismisses the insider's perspective or his/her contentions.[22] Since validating and dismissing are common mistakes in studying human beliefs, actions, and experiences, neutrality is vital to any attempt to describe someone's claims about the truth. In this respect, both insider and outsider have the duty of understanding, explaining, and interpreting the phenomena of Muslim women fairly.

Beyond doubt, objectivity and fairness in the study of Islam raise the issue of the perennial relationship between faith and reason or science. For many Muslims, Islam in its ideological sense is a faith in which a person submits his/her whole life to God, Who continuously creates the cosmos (macrocosm) and human beings (the microcosm).[23] Because believing in God requires total submission, it is easy to suppose that Islam is not compatible with reason. Many often forget, however, that the Qur'ān is full of verses relating to zoology, astronomy, agronomy and human reproduction anticipated in modern research.[24] Indeed, Islam also teaches "the knowledge of the metaphysical subjects (*al-ghayb*, the unseen), such as the existence and the attributes of God, life after death, and purpose of man in the universe,"[25] which are not scientifically proven. Nevertheless, humans are inherently inclined to believing in any form of the unseen. The Qur'ān also invites humans to ponder God's massive creation, which often requires the use of the rational faculty in order to understand the magnitude of the world and its Creator.

Of course, methodology definitely shapes the outcome of research. Questions of gender, for instance, cannot be discussed within the boundaries of *Sharī'ah* (the legal dimension of Islam), according to Murata, because the *Sharī'ah* deals with something that is either accomplished or not. The *Sharī'ah* derives from the Qur'ān and "the *Sunnah* of the Prophet or of any subsequent authority under the *general* aegis of the Prophetic *Sunnah*."[26] It does not offer any deeper reason for questions such as why a woman receives less inheritance in comparison to her brothers. Even experienced jurists, when trying to answer such an inquiry, would have to conclude that God simply ordained it so. In a similar way, the ideology of gender cannot be addressed in the realm of theology (*kalām*), which is mainly concerned with the discussion of God and His attributes. Murata, therefore, points to mysticism (Ṣūfism) in the sapiential tradition as the ideal tool for studying the ideology of gender, because Ṣūfism addresses the structure of realities, that is, God, macrocosm and microcosm.[27]

Notwithstanding Murata's perspective on the relationship between the *Sharī'ah* and gender, I would maintain that the *Sharī'ah* remains an important element in the discussion of gender, since the notion of *Sharī'ah* refers to "the comprehensive principle of the total way of life."[28] In the *Sharī'ah*, there are principles known as *takhrīj al-manāt* and *'illah*—the method of derivation and a reason for legislation beyond preference for one ruling over another—which allow those "exercising legal reasoning (*mujtahids*) within a legal school" to produce laws that are just to women by virtue of taking into consideration the local legitimate interpretation.[29] While the *Sharī'ah* has been narrowly defined as dealing with obligation and prohibition, it can provide for the reform of legislation affecting women's well-being. The *Sharī'ah*, therefore, has the potential to function as an institution that addresses both men and women in a just manner. Given this fact, Muslims need to deal with the ways in which the interpreters of the *Sharī'ah* address the issue of women, so that they are able to pinpoint biased laws and perspectives on the issue of gender; otherwise, legal obligations and prohibitions will continue to be mainly imposed on women.

The interpretations of the *Sharī'ah* that "have been carried out via the process of *ijtihād*, attempt to reveal the conduct accepted by God."[30] *Ijtihād* functions as "the maximum effort expanded by the jurists to master and apply the principles and rules of *uṣūl al-fiqh* (legal theory) for the purpose of discovering God's law." Early scholars of Islam and the leaders of Muslim communities engaged in the renewal of tradition by exercising "a great deal of freedom and ingenuity in interpreting the Qur'ān, including the principles of *ijtihād* (personal reasoning) and *qiyās* (analogical reasoning from a certain text of the Qur'ān and arguing on its basis to solve a new case or problem that has certain essential resemblances to the former)."[31]

However, most Muslims no longer exercise the process of *ijtihād*, since the gate of *ijtihād* has long been believed to be closed.[32] Besides, *ijtihād* requires the ability to understand profoundly all the different branches of the Islamic sciences, like Ḥadīth literature, Qur'ānic exegesis, Islamic law, and other branches of Islamic knowledge, in order to finally reveal the truth in accordance with the Qur'ān and the prophetic tradition. Regardless of the long list of prerequisites involved in *ijtihād*, Hallaq argues that these requirements should be seen as attempts to facilitate the activity, rather than to hinder it. The *ijtihād* process itself carries on in both theory and practice.

Concurring with Hallaq's observation of the activity of *ijtihād*, Muslim modernists, Islamists, and reformists call for the implementation of *ijtihād* in every aspect of Muslim life. These efforts, more importantly, coincide with the stagnation of a contemporary Muslim society struggling with such problems as post-colonization, modernity, westernization, women's activism, feminism, human rights, and global capitalism.[33] Muslims' encounters with these current phenomena require new theories that can be channeled through *ijtihād* as "the effort to understand the meaning of a relevant text or precedent in the past, containing a rule, and to alter that rule by extending or restricting or otherwise modifying it in such a manner that a new situation can be subsumed under it by a new solution."[34] The practice of *ijtihād*, moreover—despite current rumors of its demise—is not a novel idea within Muslim communities: its practice can be traced back to the tradition of the Prophet and his companions in the seventh century.

In this respect, I see the *Sharī'ah* as potentially fruitful in terms of the discussion of gender. Islamic *Sharī'ah*, through the use of *ijtihād*, offers a possible means of generating the ethical teaching of an egalitarian concept of gender and the putting of this universal principle into practice. Gender equality is consonant with the *Sharī'ah*, which encourages (through its provisions) a way of life that is workable for both men and women. The *Sharī'ah* can produce a legal system that protects women's rights to life, education, property, voluntary divorce, and consented marriage as well as freedom from rape, abusive fathers or husbands, and violence. This endeavour is also certainly relevant to the cultivation of the moral teachings of Islam that all are equal before God and their fellow human beings and deserve the same protection and respect.

Even though the *Sharī'ah* promises instant solutions to the question of gender, this book is not a treatment of the legal aspects of gender and self. Rather, it attempts to analyze the complex web of ideas and practices that generate the dominant and hierarchical gender system. I argue that the diverse authoritative legitimacies of Islamic teaching—especially Muslims' interpretations of the expositions of certain practices in the Qur'ān and the *aḥādīth*—have formed a system that focuses on and empowers men, while at the same time marginalizing and disempowering women, including their construction of the self. I also argue that the existing condition of the majority of Muslim women in Muslim communities attests to a misunderstanding of the production of authoritative legitimacies, a process that was not originally meant to demean, exploit, or marginalize women's self-determination at the personal, familial, and societal levels.

Instead, I approach the question of gender from an Islamic philosophical standpoint. And yet, although I claim that philosophy can serve as a method of inquiry into the question of gender and self, the practice of philosophizing this kind of question is not a common one in the discipline. If we look at the contemporary philosophical literature in Islamic scholarship, we find that its content includes historical, epistemological, mystical, ethical, ontological, and political dimensions.[35] Contemporary writers therefore do not really pursue the question of gender as philosophical because the philosophical discourses in Islam still revolve around issues of medieval and modern philosophy. This trend is quite different from the Western philosophical tradition, where the question of gender is seen as an integral part of the contemporary philosophical discourse.

The question is: What does it mean to think of the question of gender as philosophical? How does the philosophical method work? In an attempt to respond to these inquiries, it is important to examine the problematic nature of applying philosophical methodology to the question of gender in Western feminist philosophy. Gould, for instance, argues that the question of woman or gender is a philosophical inquiry because philosophy can deal with the issues of "women's social role, their oppression, and liberation" as philosophical.[36] She bases her argument on the methodological distinction of an opposed criterion of universality, that is, "abstract" and "concrete" universality. The argument from the criterion of abstract universality or essentialism perceives the question of women or gender not as a philosophical issue, but as "an accidental and not essential or universal property of human beings, since one may be human and not female, or human and not male."[37] For essentialists, the question of women or gender cannot be part of philosophy because the proper subject-matter of philosophical investigation lies in whatever is common, universal, or *the same* to all members of a given class.[38] For them, the question of women or gender refers only to one segment of society: the one that shares the same biological and experiential characteristics as women; hence, it is excluded from philosophy. Based on the criterion of abstract universality, therefore, they refuse to recognize the relativity of essential properties. This view insists that the only category of phenomena deserving philosophical consideration is "what is essentially the same and excludes essential differences."[39]

In contrast to the criterion of abstract universality or essentialism, the criterion of concrete universality considers what is universal to be the totality of all features, encompassing both that which is in common and that which is not in common.[40] This criterion, therefore, regards human history and social differences as accidents that relate to each other in a systematic fashion. Those accidental differences contribute to the constitution of the universal.[41] As the criterion of concrete universality envisions society on the basis of social differences, it allows interpretation of what constitutes a society. For example, the way in which exploiters and the exploited in a class-based society interact,

> ...(a) is a social difference which constitutes the essence of that social form, (b) is a difference which is not present throughout time, but which developed historically, and (c) is a relationship which characterizes the individuals in terms of this difference and therefore in terms of their interactions with each other. Thus the universal form or essence of a class society involves an internal differentiation (between exploiter and exploited and a systematic relationship between the two).[42]

In such a society, the social interactions between men and women would determine the essence of what ought to be universal. Paradoxically, the "division" between the sexes entails—historically, socially, and culturally—"relations," including "such relations as domination, subordination, the division of labor, the various historical forms of love and dependence, and social forms of relation like family, slavery, and concubin[age]."[43] The complex relations of social structure, wherein women define their relations with other women, men, family, class, and society, are the contexts in which the question of women can be understood. And as the question of women is crucial to the essence of society, an attempt to analyze the past and present conditions of women can be made through a critique of the history of philosophy, contemporary philosophy, and the making of philosophy.

Given that the question of women or gender is philosophical, it remains to be shown that philosophy is an appropriate method for theorizing on gender issues. I refer to two senses of the meaning of philosophy as a methodological tool in women or gender studies. The first is to analyze previous philosophical works.[44] This approach will provide the philosophical foundation of the issue, illustrate the history of ideas, and situate one's own ideas or the meta-critique of philosophy within such a tradition. Clack argues for the development of a philosophical method that is closely linked to the way in which philosophical ideas developed within a certain philosophical tradition. For instance, the duality of matter/spirit, mind/body, reason/nature, and so forth can be traced to Plato and Aristotle and later on to modern philosophers such as Descartes and Kant. This philosophical heritage leads to a dualistic understanding of humanity in which male is associated with reason, spirit, and mind, while female is associated with nature, matter, and body.

In line with this argument, Islamic philosophy definitely contributes to the construction of hierarchical gender system, because Muslim philosophers have often revived the Greek philosophical ideas pertaining to the status of women, their role in procreation and their supposedly ideal virtues. In this respect, an analysis of historical and contemporary conditions, oppressions, and struggles borne by women can be made through a critique of philosophy in its historical and contemporary forms. The use of philosophical critique and analysis should focus on finding the root of oppression, a way to get around it and emancipation for women. In this way, Islamic philosophy can serve as a method of understanding women's oppression and their liberation as well.

The second use of philosophy as a methodological inquiry is to disentangle the patriarchal elements in which women live their lives. The cultural and social realities that have shaped these lives in Muslim societies have been recorded in the philosophical, theological, legal, and scriptural texts produced by male scholars and philosophers. For this reason, engaging in philosophy in the Islamic intellectual tradition should be a matter of transcending the boundaries of philosophical texts, since these texts often reflect the scholars' creative responses to the intellectual life and pre-existing patriarchal system in Muslim societies.

Since I am interested in producing what I call "a philosophical work," I use an inductive argument to form an abstraction of philosophical discussion on gender and self in Islam. I identify the common realities faced by women in many parts of the

Muslim world and the elements of hierarchical gender system that produce those realities without necessarily generalizing the lived experiences of women. Among these elements are the gendered interpretation of the Qur'ān and Ḥadīth, gender thinking that produces the construction of sexual and gender difference, the male superiority in both the private and public spheres, the mystification of the female status and role through the institution of the sexual division of labor, the use of religious narratives to construct femininity and morality, and a legal system discriminatory to women.

I examine not only the impact of these hierarchical gender systems on the construction of the self, but also the endeavors by feminists, womanists and male advocates to disentangle the seamless relations of the existing gender system and foster the making of an egalitarian gender system. While I address relevant gender questions in the contemporary discussion of gender and self, I extensively examine gender issues in Ibn Sīnā's writings, who was one of the greatest philosophers in the history of Islamic, and even world's civilization.[45] In this way, I can trace the historical and contemporary forms of women's lives, their oppressions and their resistance to what is accepted as the philosophical and Islamic truth of being men and women in Muslim societies.

Islamic philosophy is not only married to the norms and the practice of Islam, but it also reflects the way in which Muslim philosophers responded to the Greek philosophical heritage and the extent to which they incorporated this heritage into the Islamic intellectual tradition. As a consequence, Islamic philosophy came to be defined as a method to understand God and His attributes, the nature of human beings, and their relation to God and the world.[46] Later on, the philosophical tradition in the post-medieval period repeated and interpreted the philosophical understanding of God, humans, and the world. Even now, the task of Islamic philosophy basically consists of reinterpreting the living philosophical notions embedded in the historical and cultural contexts of the Islamic intellectual tradition as well as Muslims' encounters with contemporary issues, such as human rights, westernization, democracy, pluralism, and globalization.

Historically, Greek philosophy was introduced to the Muslim world through the translation of Greek works as early as the ninth century, when the Caliph al-Ma'mūn (813–833) established the Bayt al-Ḥikmah under the directorship of the famous translator Ḥunayn b. Isḥāq (d. 8730).[47] The establishment of this early Islamic philosophical school depended on the preserved traditions of two philosophical academies: the schools of Athens and Alexandria, which closed in the fifth and sixth centuries AD, respectively. The Nestorian Church adopted the teaching of the Athenian school, which was more Platonic in nature. This school advocated the translation of Greek literature into Syriac in Edessa and Nasibin, then moved to Jundashipur, and then found its way to Baghdad in the sixth century.[48] The Alexandrian school, originally based in Antioch, moved from place to place and finally reached Baghdad by the end of the ninth century. Both pagans and Nestorian Christian scholars of the Alexandrian school preserved Greek thought, which was eventually passed on to scholars in the Abbasid court in Baghdād.[49]

Culturally, Muslims integrate the notion of philosophy into their entire approach to life. Their philosophical thought embraces all aspects of living.[50] Philosophy not only centers on discussion of the metaphysical aspects of Islam, but it also includes different sets of knowledge in the natural sciences such as astronomy, mathematics, medicine, and physics, albeit in a more refined and abstract way. Islamic philosophy, therefore, develops as a "self-maintaining and self-developing system" in which Muslims employ Greek concepts and thought to rationalize Islamic faith.[51] Philosophy is, therefore, used as a method of inquiry to understand what Islam and its people have encountered.

While it is true that Islamic philosophy has its origin in Greek tradition, which is *foreign* to Islam, Muslim philosophers did not choose to adopt the language, humanistic values, or religion of the Greeks, but restricted their borrowings to the more technical and scientific aspects of Hellenism.[52] In fact, the character of Islamic philosophy relates to those aspects external to the Qur'ān or *Sharī'ah* and to the inner truth, or *Ḥaqīqah*, where the esoteric level of Islam is situated.[53] Therefore, Islamic philosophy not only records the encounter of Muslim philosophers with Islamic teachings, but also reflects the progress of their cultural encounters.

The close bond between philosophical activity and Islamic religious tenets sometimes leads to the assumption that Muslim philosophy is not a neutral method of analysis, but something that more or less resembles a religion. This assumption, however, fails to account for the fact that the philosophical teachings of Muslim philosophers do not always concur with the dogmatic aspects of Islamic teachings, especially with respect to such issues as the resurrection and punishment of the body, the theory of the eternity of the world, and God's knowledge of universals and particulars.[54] While Muslim philosophers were aware of such problems arising from the process of philosophizing, they were not always able to provide a philosophical proof that would be in accord with their personal belief.[55]

Before I conclude my discussion of the methodology of this book, I wish to distinguish between the notions of "universal Islam," "particular Islam," and "Muslim."[56] "Universal Islam" in its normative and ideal sense refers to the universal message of the Qur'ān and the tradition of the Prophet. In this sense, Islam has the potential to be universally valid, as indicated in the Qur'ān: "and we do not send you [O Muhammad] but for the grace of the entire universe" (Q.S. 21:107). The universality of Islamic teaching is not bound by any particular condition, but has the potential to be accepted into any locality in the Muslim world.

"Partial Islam" refers to the specific representation of Islam in any given location, time and culture. It entails Muslims' interpretation of Islam as embodied in the history of their exegeses, politics, and cultures that may not be valid universally. Since "partial Islam" is confined within its locality or to a particular time, it reflects the spirit of that particular culture. The attitudes toward women in Saudi Arabia thus exemplify the lived experience of "partial Islam" in that country. The Saudi image of women cannot be seen as a model for all Muslim women. In fact, the diversity of Islam in the Muslim world represents a cohesive mosaic of "partial Islams," since the universal Islam is inevitably diluted by local beliefs and practices.

"Muslims" refers to the followers of Islam and to their responses to the "universal Islam" as reflected in the fourteen centuries of their history. From an ideological perspective, some Muslims are cultural in that they perceive and embody Islam as their cultural heritage and as part of their life experience as Muslims, whereas others view Islam as political in that they see Islam as providing the solution to all kinds of problems, including that of political decadence in the majority of Muslim countries. On the level of practice, some are moderate in the sense that they, as Muslims, attempt to reconcile Islamic belief with the existing challenges at a given time whereas others are traditional in that they believe that Islam is fixed and requires no adjustment.

The contents of the book

In light of the preceding discussion, this book seeks to accomplish five purposes: (1) to elaborate on the roots of the existing discourse on the hierarchical gender system and its impact on the self-construct using a philosophical analysis; (2) to examine the notion of male superiority in the creation theories and reproduction; (3) to analyze the theological, cultural, and political apparatus of the masculine conception of femininity, which is projected onto women's bodies; (4) to examine the impact of gender system on the constitution of self-becoming; and (5) to provide an alternative reading of gender system that is egalitarian and friendly to women.

I have divided the book into five chapters. Chapter 1 discusses the way gender thinking shapes the variations of gender system in Muslim societies. I argue that while Muslims' quest to reveal and interpret Divine Will to produce a way of life (*Sharī'ah*) contributes to the definition of Islam, their endeavor is often tainted by gendered thought. This gender thinking can especially be seen in interpretations of particular concepts in the Qur'ān as universal through the reiteration of religious narrative, legitimacy, authority, and knowledge that is not friendly to women. Gender thinking gets in the way and molds the system in which men and women interact. I will in particular examine the way gender thinking and its effect produce the mechanism that perpetuates hierarchical gender system through the politics of difference in the way that sexual difference and the family are instituted in Muslim cultures.

Chapter 2 examines the public perception of human creation out of a male father, Adam. This chapter argues that Muslim authoritative legitimacies and perspectives on hierarchical and egalitarian gender systems depend on their interpretations of the original creation of human beings. Muslim interpretations often become the source material of the politics of gender differences, thereby reinforcing women's subordinate status and their exclusion from inclusive humanity. This status derives from the assumption that men are the primary creation and women the secondary, and that men play a more significant role in reproduction. This chapter also discusses the creation of humans out of the material substances necessary for human becoming and their creation out of a living entity (*nafs wāḥidah*).

Chapter 3 portrays the impact of authoritative legitimacies on the reproduction of human beings, and looks at the extent to which both men and women contribute to procreation. Even though the woman's role in conception is evidently very substantial, this role is often seen as secondary. The male contribution to conception tends to be seen as far greater than the contribution by women in the form of egg or menstrual blood. Even though this paradigm is of Greek origin, Muslim philosophers endorsed it as the truth. As a result, the inferior role of women in reproduction reinforces the overall notion of their subordinate status in society.

Chapter 4 observes how masculinity and femininity are embodied as repeated practices written onto the gendered material self. This chapter investigates the way the materiality of the self is constructed through religious narratives and pronouncements such as virginity, veiling, and circumcision. The citation and reiteration of normative "descriptions" of men as portrayed in the story of Joseph epitomizes "the prototype of rational, pious, and reserved man," whereas Zulaykhā is seen as "sexually dangerous", "intellectually deficient," and "religiously imperfect"—labels used to construct and reconstruct the material of the self in the current gender system. Along with the narrative of the self, religious expressions, and practices such as virginity, veiling, and circumcision are materialized onto women's bodies and have created the fixity of the feminine material self in the Muslim world.

Chapter 5 discusses the way the dominant and hierarchical gender system shapes self-becoming. In the first section, it elaborates the construction of the ethical and psychological self that shapes the lives of Muslims through the lenses of the Islamic and philosophical discourses. The second section examines women's self-becoming through an analysis of the self-extensional and reciprocal dependency in the family and communities. The last section looks at the constitution of the self cited in the embodied self and the truth it produces.

Overall, the book is organized around a common structure. It unfolds the theological, social, political, and cultural roots of the dominant hierarchical gender system and its impact on the self-construct, reveals the truth the body produces, and constructs a humanity inclusive of both men and women. The book also offers a new theory of the self that is gender sensitive, philosophically sound, and well grounded in the Islamic intellectual tradition. Hopefully, the book results not only in a more elaborate analysis of the existing discussion of gender system, but contributes as well to the body of philosophical discussion in general. With this in mind, the contents of the book move between reason and revelation, past and future, ideals and particulars, and, more importantly, theories and practices.

1 Gender thinking and the system it produces

This chapter seeks to examine how gender thinking shapes Muslims' deliberation on gender issues and its cohesive impact on the production of gender system and the constitution of the self. Gender thinking refers to the process of producing and reproducing public perception of the truth of how men and women's roles are appropriated in the Muslim world. This public perception evolves from the powerful influence of what Muslims consider valid and invalid, acceptable and unacceptable, lovable and hateful, and licit and illicit, as well as other norms as outlined in the Qur'ān, *ḥadīth*, and *Sharī'ah* and Muslims' diverse interpretations of them. While Muslims' expressions of Islam vary and are ingrained into local cultures, they perceive the correct interpretation of the Qur'ān as a thread that runs through all their lives.

The system that Muslim men and women are familiar with is gendered, since it is often defined based upon the politics of difference. Muslims use the politics of difference as a regime to produce a series of norms, values, rewards, prohibitions, disciplines, and punishments that shape male and female morality. This rhetoric perpetuates a public perception of the truth in which the natural differences of men and women entail different moral, social, cultural, and legal responsibilities in both private and public affairs. Muslims' emphasis on natural difference often in practice overrides the Islamic vision of human equality.

The gendered vision of the public perception of the truth is not an Islamic invention. It started long before the coming of Islam in seventh century Saudi Arabia. Marriage patterns, tribal relations, slavery, male seniority, female infanticide, and vendetta shaped women's lives and experiences during the pre-Islamic era. The pre-Islamic Arabs generally looked down upon women's moral qualities, "because the character of women is exactly the opposite to that which the Arabs considered as the model of the perfect men."[1] This misogynistic attitude infiltrated Muslim minds in such a way that women have persistently been defined in terms of the politics of difference between men and women in biology, the economy and politics. Of course, biological differences are innate, but this does not imply the economic or political supremacy of one over the other.

Not only did Islam improve the pre-Islamic practices respecting women's rights in the social and political spheres: its revolutionary vision of women as humans challenged the established view of the local culture whereby the female self was shaped through dependency on fathers, brothers, husbands, masters, and even tribes.

Within this context, women's honor and status were, on the one hand, closely related to the male members of their family and by extension their tribe, and on the other the chief factor determining the familial and tribal status. This gender thinking did not vanish with the progress of Islam. We see from the Prophet's life itself how his first marriage (to Khadījah) raised him in status into a respected circle. Later on, his marriages to a number of wives bestowed "honor and status" on them as *Ummu al-mu'minīn* (mother of the believers) and underpinned the honor and political alliances of the families and tribes from which his wives came. At the same times, his wives' actions affected the prophet's social, political, and divine status in the eyes of both his Muslim and non-Muslim neighbors.

What is at stake here is that the resilience of the pre-Islamic and local cultures with which Islam had been in contact perceived men and women as morally different. Women were categorized as the opposite of men (who were perfect), with the result that men had the power to define what was appropriate for women. This gender thinking has since been fixed in the Muslim mind, producing and reproducing relevant interpretations of the Qur'ān and selective recall of Prophetic tradition. Added to this gender thinking is a misogynistic attitude toward women that frequently addresses women as the other.

I argue in this chapter that gender thinking matters in interpreting the Qur'ān and in recalling the appropriate ḥadith to support one's authoritarian perspective on gender questions. Muslims' justification of their gendered views generates a politics of difference that in turn produces a wide divide between male and female worlds. Given that this mechanism appears to be consistent throughout Muslim history, I elaborate in the first section on the particular roots of the hierarchical and egalitarian gender system in Muslim communities. In the second section, I discuss sexual difference as a system that is well grounded in religious, social, philosophical, and socio-biological discourses. Finally, in the last section, I analyze the instituted concept of marriage that nurtures male superiority in both the private and public spheres, while portraying women as mothers and wives in the philosophical and Islamic discourses.

The roots of the hierarchical and egalitarian gender systems

Muslims' legitimate claims of hierarchical and egalitarian gender systems represent a valid attempt at interpretation of the Qur'ān and the *ḥadīth*, to which social and cultural values contribute greatly. Interpretation of this kind is obviously not scripture, since the application of this creative process to the normative, immutable, and divine Qur'ān involves human mind, experience, and gender thinking. What are now called the legal, scriptural, social, mystical, philosophical, ethical, religious, eschatological, and ontological dimensions of the Qur'ān in the history of the Muslim intellectual tradition all embody Muslims' quest for the meaning of the Divine. The Qur'ān is, indeed, a mine of ethics, law, eschatology, biology, philosophy, history, gender justice, and countless other categories of knowledge. Given this fact, Muslims' quest for gender justice often contains contradictory claims of gender hierarchy and egalitarianism, which in turn has an effect on gender system and self-becoming.

Gender hierarchy and its Qur'ānic foundation

The common source for the popular theories and practices of gender hierarchy in Muslim societies is said to be the social and legal provisions of the Qur'ān. Despite the fact that the number of legal and social verses (such as al-Nisā', 4:34, al-Nisā', 4:176, and al-Baqarah, 2:282) is quite small in comparison to the totality of the verses, their implication for non-egalitarian concepts and practices of gender system is enormous because they have traditionally been read in light of a hierarchical worldview. The impact of such readings generates authoritative legitimacies that govern an unequal and hierarchical gender system in Muslim communities at the personal, familial, and social levels.

The following verses are instances of the Qur'ānic verses that have been read according to such a hierarchical worldview:

> And Lo! Thy Sustainer said unto the angels: "Behold, I am about to establish upon earth [*khalīfah*—] one who shall inherit it." They said: "Wilt Thou place on it such as will spread corruption thereon and shed blood—whereas it is who extol Thy limitless glory, and praise Thee, and hallow Thy name?" [God] answered: "Verily, I know that which you do not know." And He imparted unto Adam the names of all things, then He brought them within the ken of the angels and said: "Declare unto Me the names of these [things], if what you say is true."
>
> (Q.S. al-Baqarah, 2:30–1)

> Men shall take full care of women with the bounties, which God has bestowed more abundantly on the former than on the latter, and with what they may spend out of their possessions. And the righteous women are the truly devout ones, who guard the intimacy, which God [ordained to be] guarded. And as for those women whose ill-will you have reason to fear, admonish them [first]; then leave them alone in bed; then beat them; and if thereupon they pay you heed, do not seek to harm them. Behold, God is indeed most high, great!
>
> (Q.S. al-Nisā', 4:34)

> ...and if there are brothers and sisters, the male shall have the equal of two females' share.
>
> (Q.S. al-Nisā', 4:176)

> And call upon two of your men to act as witnesses; and if two men are not available, then a man and two women from among [acceptable witnesses to you], so that if one of them should make a mistake, the other would remind her.
>
> (Q.S. al-Baqarah, 2:282)

Muslims' readings of the above Qur'ānic passages not only make the texts the center of a text-based legitimacy,[2] but they also generate public perception of the truth of how to treat women in Muslim societies. Such readings transform the specific historical contexts to which those verses responded and render them universal principles. In the process, Barazangi argues, "particular practices of certain expositions of Islam have replaced the underlying Quranic and prophetic principles. These practices have been transformed from temporal applications into principles themselves."[3]

As Muslims embrace particular truth as the only truth, women's daily experiences epitomize the truth of gender relationship and system in their communities.

Public perception of this truth is rooted in the following assumptions:

- Men's superiority arises from their biological origin as the primary creation, whereas that of females is secondary.
- Biological or sexual difference justifies male superiority in the perpetuation of the human race because men are seen as the moving principle of conception.
- Biological and sexual distinction justifies the division of labor in the family. Men are held to be superior because the Qur'ān gives men privileges over women in the following areas: economics, inheritance, power of divorce, the right to bestow a physical beating (on one's wife), and the right to act as witnesses.
- It is natural for husbands as the breadwinners to be in charge of the family's social standing and the morality of its members, whereas wives are the caretakers of the household and children.
- Sexual division of labor divides private from public, personal from political, appropriate from inappropriate, obedience from disobedience, virtuous from vicious, dignity from humility, and other categories that perpetuate the status quo of the hierarchical gender system.
- Men and women, therefore, are not equal in every respect.

Even though the abstraction of the hierarchical gender system is deduced from specific assumptions of human origin, the generative process and particular practices mentioned in the Qur'ān, gender-minded Muslims regard these particulars as universal. The acculturation of the particulars into what Muslims consider *Islamic* principles, along with prevailing local gender practices, has shaped Muslim women's life, experience, and knowledge.

While women regularly contribute to the status quo of this public perception of the truth, they have not actively been involved in the production of the knowledge that has shaped the epistemological status of women in Muslim societies. Muslim jurists, mystics, theologians, and scholars—who are mostly men—have been responsible for the interpretation of both the Qur'ān and the ḥadīth. Muslim women have not assertively produced their own interpretation; instead, they have become the object of male power, authority, and knowledge, whose effects are imprinted on their bodies. The confluence of perceived male superiority in sexuality, finance, marriage, politics, and leadership generates a hierarchical gender system, but also the constitution of the self. This existing gender system has benefited men, while condoning the subordination and alienation of Muslim women in most Muslim countries.

By contrast, the egalitarian principle in Islam has been uprooted from its religious, ethical, and social contexts. Muslim women have lived the whole of their lives within the existing hierarchical and patriarchal gender system, so that any challenge to the established system is hardly welcome. Equally important, women are used to receiving and implementing the power and knowledge produced by men. Women have, as a result, constantly been the object of religious interpretation and have continually been excluded from the quest for knowledge, genealogy, history, jurisprudence, and religious views based on their own interpretations. Women never make their own history: it is made for them.

For centuries, Muslim women have tended to reflect the image that men have of them. Women have abandoned thinking and talking about gender equality, especially with the male members of their families (father, husband, uncle, older sons, etc.) because such talk is very sensitive and intimidating and even perhaps *un-Islamic*. Women's opinions hardly count. They are discouraged from expressing their own voice in the public sphere for fear of inciting evil. Women are also dissuaded from speaking for themselves because fathers, brothers, and other male members of the family speak on their behalf—not because they are able to recognize the wishes of women, but because Muslim men are empowered to decide on what is best for them. Women are reluctant to disagree with or talk back to authoritative figures in the family and society, because disagreeing and talking back is seen as "ill-mannered." Women, therefore, are expected to be silent, obedient, and subservient to what are perceived to be culturally, socially, and religiously accepted behavior, conduct, and action.

This leads us to the question: To what extent does the Qur'ān advocate mistreatment of women? Barlas, for instance, argues that the Qur'ān is egalitarian in nature and that it advocates women's liberation.[4] She acknowledges that while its teachings do not promote inequality and discrimination, it does have the potential to be read in a patriarchal mode. Mostly, such readings are derived from "the secondary texts, the *tafsīr* (Qur'ānic exegesis) and the *aḥādīth* (s. *ḥādīth*) (narratives purportedly detailing the life and praxis of the Prophet Muhammad)."[5] Granting for the sake of argument that the Qur'ān does, in fact, promise equality and liberation for men and women, I will try to identify here the bases of gender egalitarianism in the Qur'ān.

The Qur'ānic view of gender egalitarianism

This section elaborates on gender equality as a component of universal Islam. I argue that the Qur'ān speaks of equality of men and women in their origin, in their responsibility as created beings in their life on this earth and in their preparation for eventual resurrection. One may argue that while the Qur'ān treats and recompenses men and women equally when dealing with ethico-religious responsibilities, it appears to discriminate against women when dealing with social and legal obligations.[6] The issue at stake is whether the variations of social, legal, and political discrimination against women in Muslim communities are to be perceived as universal principles as the result of excessive particularism.

Some examples of Qur'ānic verses that articulate equality in gender relationships are as follows:

> O mankind! Be conscious of your Sustainer, who has created you out of one living entity [*nafs wāḥida*], and out of it created its mate, and out of the two spread abroad a multitude of men and women. And conscious of God, in whose name you demand [your rights] from one another, and of these ties of kinship. Verily, God is ever watchful over you.
>
> (Q.S. al-Nisā', 4:1)

> Verily, for all men and women who have surrendered themselves unto God, and all believing men and believing women, and all truly devout men and truly devout women, and all men and women who are true to their word, and all men and women who are patient in their adversity, all men and women who humble themselves [before God], all men and women who give in charity, and all self-denying men and self-denying women, and all men and women who are mindful of their chastity, all men and women who remember God unceasingly: for (all of them) God has readied forgiveness of sins and a mighty reward.
>
> (Q.S. al-Aḥzāb, 33:35)

> ... And whatever [wrong] any human being [*nafs*] commits rests upon himself[/herself (*'alayhā*)]; and no bearer of burdens shall be made to bear another burden ...
>
> (Q.S. al-An'ām, 6:164)

> ... the rights of the wives [with regard to husbands are equal to the [husbands'] rights with regard to them ...
>
> (Q.S. al-Baqarah, 2:228)

These verses offer the following metaphysical, social, ethical, and eschatological grounds for an egalitarian gender system.

- Both men and women, by virtue of their being in the world, are God's creatures.
- Men and women as persons (selves), partners, members of society, and servants of God are obliged to respect each other.
- Men and women will receive rewards according to their actions and behavior.
- Men and women are jointly responsible for preventing evil and promoting good.
- Men and women as persons, partners, members of society, and God's creatures and servants are, therefore, equally expected to maintain each other's rights in order to be recompensed in the hereafter.

These formulations provide a basis for human beings to treat one another equally in such a way that none will offend others due to their sexuality, ethnicity, race, or religion. All persons, who form the building blocks of every social institution, are expected to fulfill the duty of maintaining their own rights and responsibilities proportionally. Each person is expected to preserve his/her rights and responsibilities toward others at the personal, familial, and social levels.

The egalitarian gender system is consonant with the ethical message of the Qur'ān. One example of this can be seen in Q.S. al-Aḥzāb, 33:35, in which God reveals the foundation for moral and spiritual equality. Feminists seeking to establish the principle of equality between men and women in Islam refer often to the following verse:[7]

> Verily, for all men and women who have surrendered themselves unto God, and all believing men and believing women, and all truly devout men and truly devout women, and all men and women who are true to their word, and all men and women who are patient in their adversity, all men and women who humble

themselves [before God], all men and women who give in charity, and all self-defying men and self-defying women, and all men and women who are mindful of their chastity, all men and women who remember God unceasingly: for (all of them) God has readied forgiveness of sins and mighty reward.

(Q.S. al-Aḥzāb, 33:35)

This verse offers a balanced view of virtuous behavior, which leads to rewards for all individuals, regardless of their sexual difference. By mentioning the same qualities for both sexes, it is clear that the verse identifies the foundations of morality as consisting in equal moral and spiritual obligations for human beings.[8] The implication of this verse is important in that ethical qualities such as piety, chastity, truthfulness, patience, charity, and kindness are not only appropriate for human beings as individuals, but are also relevant to their role as political and social beings. It also implies that women are vested with ethical, spiritual, rational, and social qualities that make them equally subject to blame, responsibility, reward, punishment, and discipline, just as men are.

A balanced egalitarian gender system in the Islamic intellectual tradition also relies on the depiction of the "sapiential tradition" regarding the nature of reality.[9] According to this framework, there are three basic realities: (1) God, (2) the cosmos or the macrocosm, and (3) the human being or the microcosm.[10] The relationship among these three could be portrayed in a triangular diagram in which God is at the apex and both macrocosm and microcosm are at the base as derivative realities. Other than God, everything, including human beings, perishes. In this sense, the created nature of human beings denies anyone the right to dominate others.

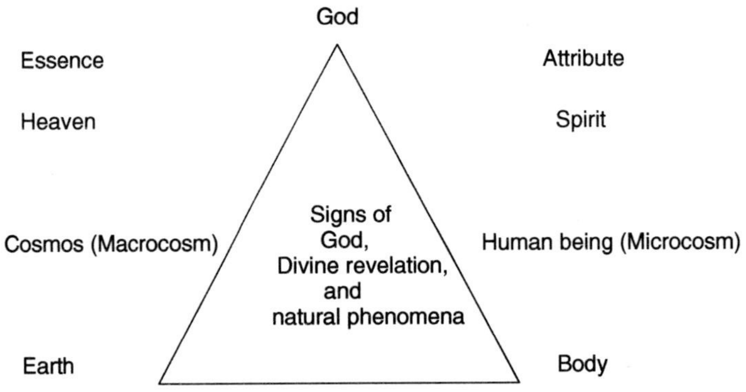

The above diagram shows that God manifests Himself in the Cosmos and human beings through His essence and attributes. God creates macrocosm and microcosm. He manifests Himself so that human beings see both macrocosm and microcosm as signs (*āyāt*) of God. By thinking about these signs, manifested in the phenomenal world and the revelation, human beings are supposed to understand God. The knowledge that is available to human beings through the macrocosm and the microcosm accords with the knowledge given to the prophets, from Adam to Muḥammad. For this reason, both natural phenomena and the divine revelation are signs of God that invite humans to contemplate God. As human beings are signs of God, their individual beings encapsulate all God's qualities. Both men and women have a unique role in the universe as God's representatives or vicegerents (*khulafā'*).[11]

Murata situates the issue of femininity within the framework of the three realities. She speaks of the duality of each reality, namely, God, macrocosm, and microcosm. Majesty and Beauty, for instance, are God's divine attributes, which are to be understood in terms of masculinity and femininity respectively.[12] Even though Majesty and Beauty are completely opposite, these attributes should be seen as a unity since they reflect God's Oneness (*Tawḥīd*). Similarly, the macrocosm also contains a binary opposition, in which the earth is usually identified as female and heaven as male. This polarity, however, is not to be interpreted as a total contrast, but a unity, in that male and female give rise to one of the relational pairs of the universe. The absence of either of the two would, in essence, make the creation of such a universe impossible.[13]

The materiality of the self too has the fluidity of masculinity and femininity. This fluidity generates an egalitarian relationality between men and women. Human equality is inherent within Islamic teaching, in the sense that individuals are responsible before God for their own selves (Q.S. al-An'ām, 6:164, Q.S. Ghāfir, 40:17, and Q.S. Ṭāhā, 20:15). Similarly, individuals, according to Islamic Sunnite doctrine, have equal access to God's Truth, regardless of sexuality, class, race, ethnicity, or gender,[14] in so far as they have the appropriate training, piety, and knowledge of Islam. In this sense, masculine and feminine tendencies are inherent in human disposition, although the construction of these tendencies is environmental. It happens that more individual men have been afforded the opportunity to interpret God's divine truth, leading not only to a lack of diversity in consciences, beliefs, and acts (despite the richness of Islamic doctrines), but also to perversity in the construction of masculinity and femininity, as will be seen in Chapter 4.[15]

Such an understanding of Islamic doctrines has shaped the way in which the fluidity of masculinity and femininity operates in Muslim societies. While universal Islam promotes gender egalitarianism as part of the harmony between God, macrocosm and especially microcosm, Muslims have adopted the concepts, expressions, and practices of gender that reflect their deliberative choices when dealing with women. In this sense, hierarchical and egalitarian theories and practices of gender system have always coexisted within Muslim cultures.

In a narrow sense, while Muslims have the crucial task of implementing the Qur'ān's teachings in daily life and of taking its universal ethical message into account, the Qur'ānic verses were themselves revealed over the course of almost twenty-three years on different occasions and addressing particular situations.[16] Yet, most interpreters (and I share their view) would contend that even though these revealed verses were inextricably linked to given sets of conditions, the ethics of the scriptural texts must be allowed to transcend those conditions in order to create a better and more just society. With this in mind, it is important to put Qur'ānic verses into their particular and universal contexts in order to find their meaningful divine messages.

Muslims generally view the authority of the Qur'ān as a unity, even though it was 'Umar ibn Khaṭṭāb (d. 644) who compiled the uncollected pieces (*ṣaḥifāt*) of the Qur'ān into its present form. While the Qur'ān is recognized as original in the sense that there is no revised edition of the Qur'ān, the literature interpreting it is extensive. The diverse interpretations of the Qur'ān often generate heterogeneous claims of what it means to be a Muslim man and a Muslim woman. These contradictions depend primarily on the way the interpreters read the Qur'ān and how its religious authority is carried over into everyday life. The Qur'ān itself never fails to inspire Muslims in their search for its divine meaning and truth.

Equally important in this connection are the Prophetic traditions (*aḥādīth*), which serve as further explanation of the Qur'ān and as a second authoritative source of Islamic teaching. History recorded Muḥammad's interactions with his wives, his speech with Muslim men and women and his wishes for the advancement of women's conditions. Yet while the Qur'an progressed along with the Prophet's life, the significance of the ḥadīth emerged after the Prophet's death. In the absence of direct consultations with and inspiration from the Prophet, Muslims looked for answers from his family and the first generations of Muḥammad's friends (*ṣaḥābah*), trusting that they would know what the Prophet had done and would have done. The recollection of the ḥadīth itself was juxtaposed to situations of chaotic political dissension leading to civil wars (656–60 and 680–92). Mernissi succinctly describes the appearance of the ḥadīth as follows:

> With the historical events as background, we can now appreciate in their true measure the two contradictory tendencies that were at odds with each other in elaboration of the Hadith: on the one hand, the desire of the male politicians to manipulate the sacred; and on the other hand, the fierce determination of the scholars to oppose the elaboration of the fiqh (a veritable science of religion) with its concepts and its methods of verification and counterverification.[17]

Compilation of the Prophet's actions, habits, thoughts, and wishes was clearly constructed with this historical specificity in mind. Muslims were interested in preserving the Prophetic tradition to validate and/or invalidate their behavior and political gains. Hence, the memory, intellectual rigor, personal integrity, and virtue of the Prophet's *ṣaḥabah* were of paramount importance to the validity of the ḥadīth.

Yet, despite this effort to produce and reproduce the interpretation of the Qur'ān and the collections of valid aḥadīth in order to reveal the divine message as expressed in the Qur'ān and embodied in the Prophet's life, the production of knowledge regarding women's issues has been gendered. Its discourses nurture the rival tasks of embodying Islam as a revolutionary religion that once liberated women from their traditions in their local culture and of instituting Islam as correct doctrines and practices—usually by those who are in power with (or without) Islamic knowledge and authority. Here, the message of liberating women becomes secondary to the implementation of the embodied institutions. Women are systematically barred from the political bodies that produce and reproduce authority, that regulate men and women by way of religious dogmas, and that treat women and men differently. This is partly because hierarchical gender-minded Muslims sometimes see the authority of *aḥādīth* as tantamount to that of the Qur'ān, when dealing with the issue of women. They hardly ever recount the extent to which the contents of the *aḥādīth* record the cultural, social, and political climate in which the Prophet and his companions lived. For this reason, it is important to recognize that there are *aḥādīth* whose contents and meanings cannot be taken for granted and/or separated from their actual contexts.

With the passage of time, the Qur'ān's verses have come to be interpreted independently from their historical contexts. The contexts are often unavailable to modern readers or are closed to them due to language or cultural differences.[18] The Qur'ānic text offers its meaning to readers, but those readers are prisoners of their personal experience and mindset; hence, individual verses do not always convey the same meanings for all readers. This explains why interpretations of the Qur'ān vary across Muslim cultures, even though these various interpretations should be understood as Muslims' valid attempts to understand God's Divine Will to the best of their capabilities.

While I share the passion for interpreting Qur'ānic texts as a means to embody the ethical teaching of Islam and to reveal the true meaning of the Divine Will, I strongly argue that Muslim interpretations of the Islamic teaching on gender issues shape not only the anti-egalitarian perspective that has persisted in Muslim cultures for the last fourteen centuries, but also that the female's self-becoming has left women with no choice but to give in to such a system.[19] The materiality of self-becoming consists of the resilient religious, cultural, philosophical, and socio-biological power and the production of women's experience and knowledge on the basis of their sexual difference and their extensional dependency to me in the family and society.

The politics of sexual difference and its impact on gender system

The existing hierarchical gender system highlights not only the male and female selves as manifestations of the sexual and material differences between men and women, but also as sites for social, cultural, and political construction. Even though sexual difference is naturally bestowed,[20] it establishes more than what material difference suggests; indeed, it carries with it certain regulatory norms that govern the progress of sexual development from childhood to adulthood. These biological differences are modified by social conventions; sex is "administered" by some sort of "policing mechanisms" that regulate the biological, religious, and economic domains through useful and public discourses.[21] In this sense, "sex" functions as an ideal construct that is materialized through time, while its materialization is accomplished through an enforced reiteration of certain norms and practices.[22] Given that gender thinking is among the most active and determinant principles for the appropriation of sex, I elaborate in this section on the religious, cultural, philosophical, and socio-biological constructs of sexual difference and on their comprehensive impact on gender system.

The religious category of sexual difference in Muslim societies serves to establish biological and material differences between men and women. The Qur'ān uses the word '*al-dhakar*' and '*al-unsā*' to designate a biological distinction between ma female respectively.[23] The word '*al-dhakar*' is the opposite of '*al-unsā*'.' Both the categorical identity of male and female bodies.[24] Such a biological distinction can be seen in the scriptural account of the birth of Mary (Āl 'Imrān 3:36), as follows:

> But when she had given birth to the child, she said: "O, my Sustainer! Behold, I have given birth to a female [*al-unsā'*]"—the while God had been fully aware of what she would give birth to, and [fully aware] that no male child [she might hope for] could ever have been like this female—"and I named her Mary. And verily I seek Thy protection for her and her offspring against Satan, the accursed."[25]

The phrase *laysa al-dhakar ka al-unsā'* is often translated as "the male child is not similar to the female."[26] In a similar vein, al-Ṭabarsī explains that being female is not the same as being male because the female is not as perfect as the male, in the sense that service to the Holy House (*Bayt al-Muqaddas*) is usually carried out by a male.[27] This service would not entail the same meaning if it were to be done by a female, especially when she menstruates or is in the midst of her postpartum period. Qatāda says that, culturallaysa, only men performed such devotions.[28]

When the phrase *laysa al-dhakar ka al-unsā'* is interpreted in gendered terms, it is generally understood to mean that "having a male child could not have been the same as having the granted female child."[29] This literal translation that "the male child is not and will never be like the female child" is embedded in Muslim unconsciousness. Such an interpretation reiterates and nurtures the common belief that male is generally superior to female and that the former is more perfect in every respect than the latter.[30] This reading of sexual difference as a normative criterion has been in play since Islam's early years. The gendered vision of sexual difference also nurtures the established view of the hierarchical principle of gender inequality to the extent that the materialization of male and female bodies revolves around biological difference. This distinction thus serves multiple functions, and is one of the many means used to impose order on society. It is also employed by such institutions as public perception of the truth and the economy, and is bolstered by the political regime. This cultural intelligibility engenders a multiplicity of signs and dominations empowering the body and mind.[31]

Public perception of sexual difference reiterates an exclusive and selective use of the Qur'ānic verses and the *ḥadīth*. Muslims restate certain *aḥādih* that contain exclusions based on women's biological functions.[32] Women are stereotyped as lacking in reason, apt to go wrong or defective in various ways so that they tend to act on the basis of irrational judgment. Their faults inevitably lead them to commit vice—rendering them incapable of existing as independent beings. No woman is exempt from this deficiency. Since all women are perceived to be faulty, imperfect, and blemished, their leadership would be terrible and damaging for the community.

Interestingly, despite this gendered thinking, several contemporary Muslim women have excelled in leadership as prime ministers or presidents of Muslim-dominated states such as Tansu Çiller (Turkey's prime minister, 1993–5), Benazir Bhutto (Pakistan's prime minister, 1988–90, 1993–6), Khaleda Zia (Bangladesh's prime minister, 1991–6), Megawati Sukarno Putri (Indonesia's president, 2001–4) and Sheikh Hasina Wajed (Bangladesh's prime minister, 1996–present).[33] Certainly, most of these women's political fortunes have benefited from their kinship relations to powerful male relatives. However, Muslims' humble acceptance of female leadership demonstrates that, with proper training, leadership is something that can be earned; it is not something that is associated with sexuality.

Muslim women are generally marginalized in the realm of political participation. Opponents of Muslim women's participation in politics regularly cite certain *aḥādīth* that are not friendly to women as the only truth, penetrating the Muslim subconscious in such a way that *ḥadīth* comes to seem independent of the Islamic vision of gender equality and justice. This process bolsters public perception of the truth of sexual difference as a system. Muslims embrace this truth to the extent that any deviation from it must be tantamount to deviation from the scripture. Daring to challenge the *ḥadīth* means defying Islam or risking the charge of denying the tradition (*inkār al-sunnah*) or even of being a *kāfir* (a non-believer). For this reason, Muslims rarely question the validity of *ḥadīth*, knowing the kind of religious and communal punishment he/she may face.

Muslims take *ḥadīth* at its face value. For example, when Abū Bakr, the narrator of the *ḥadīth*, commented on the defeat of 'Ā'ishah b. Abī Bakr at the Battle of the Camel (d. 656), he cited what the Prophet Muḥammad said regarding female leadership. The *ḥadīth* reads as follows:

> During the days (of the battle) of al-Jamal, Allah benefited me with a word I had heard from Allah's Apostle after I had been about to join the Companions of al-Jamal (i.e. the Camel) and fight along with them. When Allah's Apostle was informed that the Persians had crowned the daughter of Khosrau as their ruler, he said, "Such people who are ruled by a lady will never be successful."[34]

While this *ḥadīth* is often quoted and reiterated to exclude women's political participation, it remains questionable whether it was appropriate for the *ḥadīth* narrator to cite any *ḥadīth* that had historical specificity and was echoed in a different context.

Mernissi draws attention to the historical context in which the ḥadīth was first pronounced. Abū Bakr was a former slave who had led a humiliating life and had thereafter became a very well-known figure in Iraq after embracing Islam.[35] 'Ā'ishah contacted him and asked him to participate in her army by taking up arms against 'Alī (the chosen fourth caliph). 'Ā'ishah perceived 'Alī as an unjust leader because he did not persecute the killer of 'Uthmān (the third caliph). By that time (656 AD), public opinion was divided into supporters of 'Ā'ishah, supporters of 'Alī, and a neutral group. Abū Bakr neither responded to 'Ā'ishah's letter nor participated in the battle; instead, he quoted the above *ḥadīth* to justify the fact that the defeated party was led by a woman. Abū Bakr recalled and reiterated this ḥadīth one-quarter century after the death of the Prophet. The context of the ḥadīth itself was female leadership in the midst of political unrest (629–632) in Persia where two women had been appointed after their King had been assassinated. As for Abū Bakr's reliability, it may be pointed out that he was once flogged because of his false testimony against a companion, al-Mughīrah Ibn Shu'bah, who was accused of the crime of *zinā*.[36]

Just as Abū Bakr's integrity and honesty as the narrator of the ḥadīth are questionable, the content of the ḥadīth, if it is applicable to all Muslim women, does not seem to be an accurate reflection of the fundamental teachings of the Prophet Muḥammad. He taught equality between men and women as humans by abolishing the tradition of killing female infants, a custom practiced prior to the coming of Islam. He gradually introduced women's rights as a means toward empowering women's agency. He also summoned his followers to protect women by commanding his fellow Muslim not to kill women or children in wartime and to treat them well in everyday life.

Yet even though the context of the above mentioned *ḥadīth* has nothing to do with a Muslim woman's leadership, it became the most prominent example of the construction of sexual and gender difference, one in which the multiplicity of culture, religion, and politics may be seen to be interwoven.[37] Surprisingly enough, the focal point of the image is not 'Ā'ishah's involvement in the political arena, her religious authority or her piety rendering her an excellent model for Muslim women to imitate (for she reportedly regretted what she had done),[38] but the portrayal of her transgression and rebellious attitude. 'As Ā'ishah's political participation in the Battle of the Camel was portrayed by the tradition as leading to the greatest *fitnah* (social chaos) and was denounced for having caused much bloodshed in the early history of the Muslim community,[39] Muslim women have been generally barred from politics and particularly from the public space by virtue of their sexuality.

This account has two implications. On a personal level, women are relegated to an inferior status and are identified as sinful, sexually dangerous, irrational, defective, and easily susceptible to going astray. Women cannot be trusted to manage and lead their own lives because they tend to obey their illogical premises and impulses. As a result, women have hardly any authority in any field. Women generally comply with what male judges, shaykhs, scholars, and theologians have told them with regard to their bodies. To this extent, Butler is right in saying that "the judge does not originate the law or its authority; rather, he 'cites' the law, consults and reinvokes the law and in that reinvocation, reconstitutes the law."[40]

On a social level, the implication of the usual sexist reading of 'Ā'ishah's leadership in the Battle of the Camel—which has been interpreted, reinterpreted, and reinforced from time to time as an innovation (*bid'ah*)[41]—is that women are unfit for political and social roles. Some argue that women are not endowed with the skills to participate in public life and manage public affairs, so that women have no political significance in history.[42] Others refer to the Qur'ān, *ḥadīth*, practical experience, and the Islamic legal principles of the consensus (*ijmā'*), *maṣlaḥah* (*welfare*), and cutting pretext (*shadhdh al-dharā'i'*).[43] Such beliefs and interpretations have been materialized for ages.

Even though the retreat of women from public participation has caused a major setback for Muslim women in comparison to the way women participated in the public arena during early Islam, it has shaped the public perception of the truth that women's political participation is inappropriate and out of place. There are indeed exceptions where women have been admitted into public office, but these women have usually been connected to the male members of the family and benefited politically from kinship associations. The overwhelming practice, by contrast, is to confine women within the biological and social regime that gives them no option but to make peace with family life.

The politics of sexual difference for some Muslims is not only religiously endorsed, it is also rooted in Muslims' social-cultural construct. The socialization of maleness and femaleness starts when children are born. This enduring identification is manifested in how gender identity and the learning of gender roles take shape.[44] Gender identity refers to the consciousness that one is either a boy or a girl with a corresponding role to play in the society where one is born and/or brought up. A child develops within the role that is socially and culturally assigned to each sex through the internalization of what it means to be a girl or a boy. Therefore, gender identity is formulated even as both males and females develop, internalize, and embody their expected roles in society.

Gender identity also carries value judgment, as certain cultures prefer one sex to the other. Even though the extent of male preference in Muslim culture is not as extreme as it is in other religious traditions where filial piety and ancestor worship can only be done by male descendents (in the case of Confucianism),[45] Muslims generally look at the male with a greater favor. Indeed, there are cases where having a female body in many Middle Eastern countries makes a human being "incomplete" or causes her to be seen as having "something missing."[46] In fact, it is a great embarrassment in some cultures for a family to consist mainly of baby girls.[47] Some families keep trying to have a baby boy after having several girls. This is especially true for many Muslim parents, who would freely admit that they prefer to have baby boys because it saves parents from such complications as financial liability, guardianship, wedding celebrations, and threat to family honor. Muslim parents perceive sons as a form of insurance that will assist them as they are aging. This extreme preference for boys reflects the enduring influence of pre-Islamic culture in which female offspring were perceived as a "potential source of the familial dishonor."[48]

Still, some Muslim parents welcome daughters, as may be seen in Southeast Asian Muslim cultures, such as Indonesia, Malaysia, and Singapore.[49] In the societies where bilateral kinship relations and uxorilocal residents are common, such as in the greater part of Java, Sunda, Minagkabau, and South Sulawesi, female babies are sometimes more desirable, because when the parents get older, they can move in with their daughter's family. In other societies, where kinship hierarchy and partilocality are more dominant such as Bali, the Anganen of the Southern Highlands Province of Papua New Guinea,[50] and North Sumatra, the parents' preference for male descendants will be stronger since this inclination goes along with the societal assumption of men's position in that particular society.

Whatever the parents' rationalization for preferring a boy or a girl, the fact remains that male and female sexuality marks anatomical distinctions of a biological nature. This sexual difference is only the beginning, since the sexual category to which the sex of person is assigned by social categories is in the making.[51] Gender is an active process of the "enactment of social categories" within historical and cultural contexts.[52] With this in mind, the appropriation of sexual difference perpetuates the status quo of the existing gender system, since it is enacted through the interplay of religious, cultural, and social norms that are profoundly ingrained in the everyday lives of Muslim men and women.

Given the social, cultural, and historical construct of sexual and gender difference, feminist theorists ask, "[if] gender is a cultural interpretation of sex or [if] gender is culturally constructed, what is the manner or mechanism of this construction?"[53] This question has traditionally been at the core of philosophical discussion. Simone de Beauvoir in *The Second Sex* points out that the construction of gender is developed in conjunction with the view of the opposite: "man represents both the positive and the neutral, as is indicated by the common use of *man* to designate human beings in general, whereas woman represents only the negative, defined by limiting criteria, without reciprocity...."[54] De Beauvoir depicts women's alienation, inessentialness, and inferiority as being the *other*. This *other* has always been an opposite, which arises out of the one. The *other* is the opposing significant, which is socially and culturally constructed and inscribed in every culture. As a result, men's and women's relations to humanity are defined in such a way that humanity embraces only the male, while women are identified relative to and dependent on men.

In contrast to de Beauvoir, who refuses to recognize women as "the other," Irigaray proposes to identify them as "another."[55] She argues that the negation of women as others implies the refusal of "another" as the equal of the masculine subject. It demands the stability of the fundamental form of human being as "one, singular, solitary, and historically masculine...with the many always subordinate to the one."[56] This ideal mode of humanity results in obedience to the singular model of subjectivity, which belongs to traditional philosophy and is historically masculine. Irigaray maintains that women should view themselves as *another* subject, which is irreducible to a masculine subject. Thinking of women as *another* also implies that women enjoy a position equal to that of men. In order that men and women become coexistent subjects, what constitutes humanity should be predicated on "the two." Here, the salient feature of the "two" is to be found in "sexual difference" which implies[57] that two subjects should not be situated in either a hierarchical or a genealogical relationship, and that these two subjects have the duty of preserving the human species and of developing their culture, while respecting their differences.

Even though de Beauvoir and Irigaray appear to discuss the idea of woman from opposite poles, both of them are concerned with the historical oppression of women. The core of their discussion is the way in which women have been constructed as reducible to masculine subjects. Both de Beauvoir and Irigaray attempt to escape from the epistemological structure of knowledge, which posits women as secondary to men in the history of philosophy. Such a position should not come as a surprise since the fundamental paradigm of philosophy is built on masculine reasoning. If de Beauvoir demands that women be recognized as components of a single humanity, like their male counterparts, Irigaray proposes that the idea of humanity be acknowledged to consist of two sexes and two genders. Both of them, therefore, seek a concept of humanity that is friendly to, and inclusive of, women.

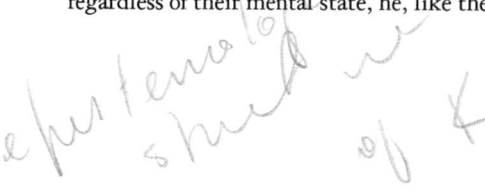

The philosophical construct of female self-existence in Islam is also conceptualized on the basis of sexual difference. Even though Ibn Sīnā believed that the self (the soul) marks humanity which is equal for all humans in that they have self-knowledge, regardless of their mental state, he, like the majority of Muslims in his day and in the contemporary world, viewed women as sexual, disloyal, and less rational. In his own words,

> Since woman by right must be protected inasmuch she can share her sexual desire with many, is much inclined to draw attention to herself, and in addition to that is easily deceived and is less inclined to obey reason; and since sexual relations on her part [with many men] cause great disdain and shame, which are well-known harms, whereas [sexual relations] on the part of man [with other women] only arouse jealousy, which one should ignore as it is nothing but obedience to the devil; . . .[58]

The Islamic prohibition against women having multiple sexual relations with several male partners carries with it the assumption that women are sexual beings. When it happens that women have sexual relations outside marriage, they can easily be condemned to corporal or even capital punishment, whereas the men with whom these women have sexual relations can go unpunished.

The idea that the female sexual drive subdues their rational capability has resulted in their being classified as irrational and emotional. Ibn Sīnā's view of the strength of female sexual desire is in line with the theory of form and matter. Form represents the male, whereas matter represents the female. The female always desires the male, just as matter yearns for form. This view is Aristotelian origin in that "The truth is that what desires the form is matter, as the female desires the male and the ugly the beautiful—only the ugly or the female not in itself but accidentally."[59] It should not come as a surprise that women are seducers who allure men to forbidden pleasure.

Aristotle's view on the inequality between men and women is grounded in the theory of the female's inability to exercise authority (*akyron*). Indeed, all parts of the soul—vegetative, animal, and human rational—are to different degrees present in women. However, women, like children, are unable to exercise their deliberative faculty, so they cannot have any authority. Children, especially male children, have the potential to be authoritative once they mature.[60] It follows that women's deficiency in authority obliges them to obey men's rules, while men are never subjected to the female demand for obedience, if there is any.

Central to the constructed role of Muslim women at the personal, familial and communal levels is the lack of authority. At the familial level, the hierarchical gender-minded fathers (and later husbands) have the authority to decide what is best for women. In this kind of environment, women are denied the opportunity to exercise fully their personal authority in knowledge, public affairs, and power relations. This systematic cycle has remained unchallenged for as long as the history of Islamic civilization.

Perceiving women as lacking in character and authority was not only regarded as philosophically sound, but it has also been "proven" by the socio-biologists who maintain that gender role is genetic in nature.[61] Embedded in biological difference is the inherent expectation that males are "to be aggressive, hasty, fickle, and undiscriminating," whereas females tend to be "coy, to hold back until they can identify males with the best genes."[62] This distinction in human behavior is based on three assumptions: "there are widespread genetic differences; genetically controlled behaviours that have an effect on biological fitness; and genetic differences lead to behavioral differences."[63] The saying, "like father, like son," extends not only to shared physical characteristics, but also inherited character traits.

However, while it is true that generative self is genetically inherited from the parents, self-becoming is constructed within the locality of the self. Each self receives his or her genetic code that marks a human as human at the moment of conception.[64] The 46 chromosomes of each individual have a set of genes, consisting of 50,000–100,000 genes, known as the human *genome*.[65] This genome, which is stored in the nucleus of every cell, is the blueprint of a human being. And this genetic information contains certain characteristics, "the biological carrier of the possibility of human wisdom" and "a self-evolving being."[66]

Since genetic codes are something inherent within humans and tend to confer certain characteristics that are unique to the parents or their ancestors, socio-biologists claim that gender is biological. In this sense, humans exhibit the characteristics that are rooted in the genetic code. Yet while such a perspective could be true to the extent that some human characteristics are passed down through genes, the construction of these behavioral traits does evidently occur within the bounds of social relations and first and foremost in the family and its immediate environment.

The resilience of the religious, socio-cultural, philosophical, and socio-biological construct of sexual difference that nurtures and generates the existing gender system in the Muslim world is the concurrent effect of gendered thought with the emphasis on the social ordering of female sexuality. Mernissi argues that the construction of Muslim social order in Muslim communities is based on the assumption that women are sexual beings who pose a threat to society in general.[67] This assumption suggests further that, in order to establish and perpetuate social order, women's sexuality should be controlled, because it is the source of social chaos (*fitnah*), "a living representative of the dangers of sexuality and its rampant disruptive potential."[68] For this reason, women should be kept at home and confined to the household world; otherwise, they would invite disorder in society.

To say that women are a constant threat to the Muslim social order is, in de Beauvoir's eyes, to perceive women as "the other," in that men represent the positive, while women represent the negative. Men are considered to embody the positive because they are the main constituents of social order. Conversely, women are considered to be the negative, for they are seen, with their sexual distractions, to work against the orderliness of the society. Indeed, there are cases in which women are included within the Muslim social order. Yet, their inclusion is not seen as the primary agent, as men are, in dignifying humanity, but as agents destructive to the "social order."[69] Given that women's sexuality is seen as the active cause of the misery of society, women need discipline first and foremost in the family where sexual difference becomes the axis of a religious, social, cultural, and political regime of power.

Gender and power difference in the family

Gender thinking marks the appropriation of sexual and gender difference for any regime or system that is to be established at the personal, familial or communal levels. I will, however, argue that the politics of gender difference operates forcefully at the level of the family, where gender expectations and appropriations become materialized. In normal circumstances, the politics of sexual difference is first instilled in the family, where women receive their extensional status as wives, mothers, and/or daughters in the family. They learn how to control their voice, behavior, contours, and dress; otherwise they can be subjected to punishment, discipline, blame, and responsibility. They also learn to accept public perception of what is socially, culturally, and religiously up to standard in terms of ethical and unethical, shame and dignity, honor and dishonor, responsibility and irresponsibility, and other embodied concepts.

Interestingly, gender thinking not only penetrates the theoretical and practical Islamic understanding of gender difference, but also extends to philosophical discourse on the truth the system of gender difference can produce. Muslim philosophers do not consider gender difference as an isolated issue, for they are interested in the multifaceted relations between Islam and philosophy. The difference between philosophy and religion lies in linguistic terminology.[70] Religion conveys philosophical truth in popular language, whereas philosophy seeks truth by way of reasoning. Adopting this line of thought, philosophers call for the rationalization of Islamic revelation.

The effort to philosophize Islam is more well-defined in Ibn Sīnā's metaphysics in that he integrates the necessity of the Prophet as a legislator, with special reference to the revealed nature of this legislation. He elaborates the idea that the *Sharī'ah* was beneficial for the masses and even for the elite. However, the philosopher sage should be able to deal with the details of the *Sharī'ah*, wherever revelation overrides reason.[71] Despite the different tones in the Islamic and philosophical expressions of the role of women in family and society, self-professed Muslims and philosophers, especially Ibn Sīnā, share something in common. In this section, I elaborate on the intertwined commonalities of the role of marriage in the Muslim family, male superiority in marriage, and the appropriate and ideal role of women as mothers and wives, all of which serve as "policing mechanisms" to perpetuate the existing gender system in the Muslim world.

Ibn Sīnā schematizes the marital institution based on the metaphysics of prophecy.[72] He asserts that the presence of the legislator as ruler over society is of absolute importance. The task of the ruler is to enact legislation, build the city, and divide the leadership between three groups: administrators, artisans, and guardians.[73] Each group would have a multiplicity of leadership until they could create a common ground for the establishment of a democratic and just vision for the city. To maintain the city, there should exist a common public fund, punishment for crime, and fair distribution of welfare. One of the tasks of the legislator is also to establish laws, including those on marriage, and to encourage people to obey these laws. According to him, marriage is the institution that perpetuates the species, through which the proof of the existence of God is manifested.[74]

Ibn Sīnā's view of marriage is very much in line with the majority of Muslims in that marriage serves as a means to produce progeny and to perpetuate humanity. The significance of marriage also embodies the doctrine of *Tawḥīd* (the Oneness of God) and humans' responsibility toward Him at the Day of Judgment[75] in that different individuals with different sexualities, backgrounds, and worldviews are brought together by their human need for each other, embodying the Qur'ānic view of mutual affection and mercy—defined as the foundation of marriage (Q.S. al-Rūm, 30:21).

Ibn Sīnā also shares a common view of marriage with the Greek philosophers. It is, in fact, quite plausible that his writing on the management of the household responds to the philosophical discourse on women expressed by Aristotle and Plato. Aristotle, for instance, frequently discusses the relationship between men and women within the boundary of marriage. Husband and wife are the main components of the household. The bond between them is based on the marital relationship. The rule that governs this relationship is constitutional, just like the rule of the intellect over the appetite.[76] In practice, this kind of rule manifests itself in a discussion of the virtues of commanding and obeying, according to which men are expected to command and women to obey.[77] The relationship between female and male is traditionally unequal. In one of the passages, Aristotle confirms that "[a]gain, the male is by nature superior, and the female inferior; the one rules, and the other is ruled; this principle, of necessity, extends to all mankind."[78]

Ibn Sīnā also responds to Socrates' proposal of the community of women in the new constitution of the state. Socrates believes that women have the potential to become successful if they receive the right training or education. Socrates is said to have used the following analogy to make his point:

> Do we expect the females of watchdogs to join in guarding what the males guard and to hunt with them and share all the pursuits or do we expect the females to stay indoors as being incapacitated by the bearing and the breeding of the whelps while the males toil and have all the care of the flock?[79]

By this analogy, Socrates intends to show that both males and females share all things in common. The difference is that we tend to treat "the females as weaker and the males as stronger."[80] If women, Socrates argues, receive education, like gymnastics, music, and the office of war in the same manner as men do, the former will surely be able to hold official jobs, just like men.

Indeed, Socrates recognizes the reality that men and women have different natures and that these differences may lead to different pursuits.[81] However, this difference in nature does not interfere with women's endeavor to pursue the same goals. This is to say that the difference is not found in the fact that the female bears and the male begets. This distinction has not yet been proven to be in conflict with equal pursuits.[82] Both men and women, to different degrees, have the ability to be guardians or administrators of a state, except that women have been inhibited by the biased stereotype that "the woman is weaker and the man is stronger."[83] At this point, we may notice that Socrates could not fully free himself from the notion that women are naturally weaker than men.

Socrates was aware of the different degrees to which men and women can pursue their pursuits. He did not however let this stop him in his goal to include women in the new constitution. To achieve this goal, he believed that women should be part of a community of wives through the commonality of marriage and childbearing. Marriage would be arranged, and the lawgiver would match couples based on their similarities of temperament. The couple would then proceed to procreate. After the birth, the child would be surrendered to officials, either men or women, who would take care of the baby. All men would be able to claim the children born after the seventh and/or tenth month of marriage as their sons or daughters. The commonality of wives, marriage, childbearing, kinship, and property would reduce the tension of heredity, paternity, and other such disputable matters. The state would then be able to function in a just manner.

Ibn Sīnā would definitely have disagreed with such an arrangement, as would many Muslims. Marriage is indispensable in order to perpetuate the human species, but more importantly, it also provides an assurance of heredity and paternal origin for the child, and assures one clear-cut line of paternity. Marriage should also be a permanent union so that there will be less social dislocation. In fact, the most powerful mechanism for general good in his view is love: "love is achieved through friendship; friendship through habit; and habit is only produced through long association."[84]

Ibn Sīnā's strong support for marriage is coincidently analogous to Aristotle's refutation of Socrates' proposal for having women, children, and property in common. Aristotle bases his objection on three reasons. First of all, Socrates does not provide a valid argument by which the institution could operate.[85] As a means to an end, such instruments are impractical, because the nature of the state requires plurality. Socrates' premise "that the greater the unity the better the state" does not make sense, as state comprises different types of men and groupings.[86] These groups of citizens share something, if not everything, in common, as they inhabit one place.[87]

Second, the greatest unity also results in ambiguity in the familial relationship. Socrates' notion of the state demands that each person should refer to the same boys as their sons and call the same women their wives.[88] This kind of extended family creates a scenario in which the guardians would perceive all sons and daughters as their own,[89] according to Socrates, since each citizen would share an equivalent sense of belonging. Aristotle argues that the ability to claim parenthood is only possible within a particular relationship. It would be impossible for the first generation of citizens of the state to really feel that they belong to an extended family.[90] The familial bonds become less significant due to the fact that: "Whereas in a state having women and children in common, love will be diluted; and the father will certainly not say 'my son', or the son 'my father.' "[91]

The familial relationship would lose all meaning because there is no motivation for the father to take care of his sons or daughters.[92] In a similar manner, the children would also feel neglected and abandoned because they would experience maternal and paternal deprivation. Such a psychological condition does not provide a firm foundation for a good state.

Finally, Aristotle refutes the proposal of communal property, because it is much better for property to be privately owned than for it to be used in common.[93] Having private property, to a certain degree, celebrates personal achievement and symbolizes love of the self. Ownership is an innate need of every being, since it is a means to have pleasure, to live well, and to be generous to family, relatives, and friends. Lack of property, according to Aristotle, will diminish temperance toward women and hinder the liberality of using property.[94] Here, Aristotle makes the strong point that it is important for men to have property so that they can modestly support women. But women are obviously not expected to have their own property, because, as Aristotle argues, if women were given the same liberty as men to engage in society and to have property, who would therefore look after the home? And even if Socrates were to retain private property while still making women common property, the men will attend the fields, but who will see to the house? And who will do so if the agricultural class have both their property and their wives in common? Once more: it is absurd to argue, from an analogy on animals, that men and women should follow the same pursuits, for animals have never managed a household.[95]

Aristotle obviously thinks that the most fitting role for women is to engage in activities in the household, rather than in public life. This role accords with his understanding of the nature of women and his earlier premise regarding women's lack of authority. A woman does not possess the ability to engage in public affairs because her role in the household, especially that of domestic laborer, requires different training from that necessary for intellectual pursuits. Aristotle does not seem to have admitted the possibility that women could also receive training similar to that of men so that both could pursue the same pursuits. He believed that what is universally proper for women is to be in the house. Hence, it would have been impossible, for him, to foresee the possibility that men and women could share household activities.

Ibn Sīnā shares many facets of thought with Aristotle. Both of them believed that a marital relationship is important for the establishment of the city. The familial bond gives a better chance for the family to maintain a marital relationship. Ibn Sīnā even mentions that it is important for the couple to maintain their marriage so that both of them can provide the best education for their children.[96] Both Ibn Sīnā and Aristotle also believed that women's primary task is to maintain the household, and that men's responsibility is to provide the means of subsistence. As men are responsible for financial security and commanding the family, women are expected to obey their husbands completely.

Ibn Sīnā and the majority of Muslims share the view of the truth of marriage as an institution that favors men's superiority rather than equality.[97] There are ample mechanisms that evidently support male superiority in marriage, such as financial responsibilities, inheritance, and divorce. The ability to be *qawwāmūn* (caretakers) has granted men higher status "*because* God has made the ones excel [*faḍḍala*] the others and because they support them from their means" (Q.S. al-Baqarah, 2:34).[98] According to Mawdūdi, the word *faḍḍala* means

> God has endowed one of the sexes (i.e. the male sex) with certain qualities which He has endowed the other sex with, at least not to an equal extent. Thus it is the male who is qualified to function as the head of the family. The female has been so constituted that she should live under his care and protection.[99]

A husband's economic responsibility for his female relatives is thought to warrant him biological and social superiority over women in general. With this in mind, every aspect of a man's life is appropriated in relation to his economic power and access to the public. The husband's financial support, in Ibn Sīnā's account, entails ownership of the female genitalia. This is certainly the logic behind the control of women's sexuality. If genitalia, which are the most powerful asset of women, can be bought by their husbands' maintenance and support, then women can expect no control over sexuality, body, liberty, and individual growth and even life itself.

Similarly, God's command that men receive a double share of inheritance has lent them superiority (Q.S. al-Nisā', 4:11). Yet, while men receive a greater share, they are expected to spend their share or what they earn on their family. In contrast, women need neither provide sustenance nor spend any inheritance on their families, unless they do so by choice. Thus, despite the practical reason for men's double share of inheritance, it is used to demonstrate male superiority and female inferiority, based on the assumption that God's favor toward men demonstrates their superior status. This assumption is flawed, however, for the law of inheritance is framed within a socioeconomic context in which women are not accustomed to economic independence. In fact, the inclusion of women as recipients of inheritance was intended to improve women's social condition at that particular time, when women in general were seen as chattels.

Equally important to mention is that the Qur'ān grants men the right to divorce women, even though it is often abused for male personal interests (Q.S. al-Baqarah, 2:228). Certainly, women can propose the marriage's dissolution (*al-khul'*) for a genuine reason by returning the dowry (*mahr*) that was given to them on the wedding eve.[100] But, divorce, which is a useful option for unresolved marital problems is effectively a male prerogative. Because husbands are in a position to divorce women, men often use this privilege to divorce women for any possible reason. Yet, what is easily forgotten is that the notion of divorce must be seen in light of the protection afforded by the Qur'ānic injunction: "the right of the wives [with regard to their husbands] are equal to the [husbands'] rights with regards to them" (Q.S. al-Baqara, 2:228). Even if a man has "precedence" (*darajah*) over the woman, this is only viable if a woman wants to maintain the marital relationship; otherwise, the divorce continues to proceed. However, as *darajah* is sometimes translated as "superior," men yet again abuse the institution of divorce in order to regulate women's lives and, in doing so, cause them emotional and psychological trauma.

But why should men be entitled to sever the marriage bond, whereas women may not? Women, according to Ibn Sīnā, cannot be trusted in the matter of divorce, because women are irrational, less inclined to follow reason, and get angry easily.[101] Ibn Sīnā is well-aware that women are not in charge of the divorce process, but acknowledges that the institution of divorce can easily be misused against women. For this reason, he argues that while divorce "must not be placed in the hands of the less rational of the two, the one more prone to disagreement, confusion, and change," judges are a necessary part of divorce proceedings, especially in cases of women's mistreatment by their partners.[102] The judges' involvement in the divorce process is to ensure that women's rights are not jeopardized when separation occurs. In cases where the separation has already occurred, the opportunity to renew the marriage should be available, except for those couples who have divorced three times. In that case, the woman has to marry somebody else in a genuine marriage before being able to return to her previous husband.

Above all, God's ordinances granting the rights to financial sustenance, double inheritance and divorce to men oblige the latter to do what is right and to ensure women's well-being and their rights in the marriage. If, in reality, a man fails to serve God's ordinance and maintain justice in his reciprocal dependence with his family, the account will be between him and God. Clearly, God does not ordain the subjection and oppression of women as parts of His agenda, but encourages co-existent dependency and partnership between husband and wife at every level of interaction. In this respect, the Qur'ānic verses 3:34 and 2:228 are, as noted by al-Faruqi, meant to depict husband and wife as

> ... indeed complementary partners with equal rights. The difference between males and females is rooted in the socioeconomic distribution of communal responsibility rather than gender.... The ultimate aim of the socioeconomic construct of the Qur'ān is to create a system of interdependence in which the extended family unit is the norm and in which, therefore, the community is set to take full care of its members on both legal and moral grounds so whatever happens on the wider social and political scale, the individual is still protected. It adjusts the imbalance of biological tasks by countering them with socioeconomic responsibilities.[103]

Therefore, men's responsibility for financial sustenance, double inheritance, and divorce are not legalized in order to oppress women's biological nature and their roles, but to protect their rights so that women as daughters, wives, and mothers can advance their self-fulfillment in both the private and public spheres.

Despite the Qur'ān's exposition of the importance of mutual love and respect within marriage, there are avenues that can be used and abused to perpetuate the subordination of women. The repeated theory and practice of male superiority in leadership, guardianship, financial maintenance, inheritance, and divorce show male dominance over women. To rule is natural for men, because women, according to Ibn Sīnā, are easily deceived and less inclined to follow reason.[104] With their weak deliberative skill and irrational disposition, women are considered to be unable to manage their own lives. Because women cannot control their own bodies, or even their sexuality, they cannot be trusted as independent agents. Thus, immediate relatives become the extension of women's eyes, ears, and minds.

Ibn Sīnā's view concerning who rules whom is not alien to Mediterranean culture and philosophy. Aristotle too argues that it is more fitting for men to be rulers and for women to be ruled. The types of rule range from the despotic and constitutional to the royal.[105] The first type of rule is used to manage slaves, who are usually possessed by their masters. The second type, as mentioned earlier, is a "government of freemen and equals."[106] And the last is the rule of fathers over their children. While men enjoy the privilege of ruling over women and slaves, Aristotle makes a clear-cut distinction, saying that by nature the female and the slave are different.[107] The females are free and equal to men in that they have the deliberative faculty. Slaves who are singled out for subjection[108] are considered to have no deliberative faculty at all.[109]

Even though men and women both possess the deliberative faculty, they do not share an equal degree of authority. Women's tendency toward irrationality prevents them from attaining authority. As virtue is the standard that decides who rules, men are automatically judged to be more deserving of this authority. It is thus justifiable to administer women's bodies, life, morality, and financial support by placing them in seclusion. When a woman is secluded from public life and confined to the household, she has no need to look for money or other means of subsistence. It remains a man's responsibility to provide for and to fulfill a woman's needs. But where men are responsible for the expenses of women, they are clearly superior to women. Because women, according to Ibn Sīnā's account, are no more than property to men:

> ... unlike man, she should not be a bread-earner. For this reason, it must be legislated that her needs be satisfied by the man upon whom must be imposed her sustenance. For this the man must be compensated. He must own her, but not she him. Thus she cannot be married to another at the same time. But in the case of man this avenue is not closed to him though he is forbidden from taking a number of wives whom he cannot support. Hence the compensation consists in the ownership of the woman's "genitalia." By the ownership of the genitalia I do not mean sexual intercourse. For the [pleasure] of sexual intercourse is common to both. The woman's share is even greater, as is her delight with the pleasure in children. By this I mean that no other man can make use of them.[110]

Ibn Sīnā's concept of women seems more radical than those of any other Muslim's scholars. His hostility towards women extends beyond marking women's bodies as sexual, dangerous, disloyal, and irrational. He bluntly states that a woman's genitalia are the property of a man, and yet to say such a thing is to imply that she, as a whole, is a piece of property or an object. Indeed, Ibn Sīnā states that a husband must "own" his wife's genitalia so that she will not make them available for other men. Yet, even if Ibn Sīnā expresses his concern for a couple's fidelity, why did he rest the argument upon the ownership of genitalia? On what basis should a husband own a wife's genitalia, a part that belongs to the female body and is external to the male body? Of course, we can all own something external to us and incorporate it into our bodies. However, a human bodily part cannot be subject to ownership unless we have it transplanted into our bodies, as in the case of organ or tissue transplants. The genitalia of a woman belong to her, however, and as a human being, she exists as an individual and as a separate entity from a man. Indeed, the bonds of marriage, in a sense, join two different bodies into one union. However, marriage in Islam does not dwell on the ownership of a woman's body and her organs, but on mutual and shared love and compassion.

The male superiority in marriage is reaffirmed by the appropriate (in the eyes of Muslim philosophers, at least) construction of women in terms of men's needs and interests in society. Like Muslims in general, Muslim philosophers generally view the most fitting roles for women—suiting their natural disposition and serving male interests at the familial and societal levels—as those of wives and mothers. Muslims' pride in motherhood and wifehood finds its profoundest support in the Qur'ān and the prophetic tradition. While the Qur'ān mentions motherhood in terms of women's reproductive ability (Q.S. al-Nisā', 4:1 and Q.S. Luqmān, 31:14), the cultural social construct demands that every woman become a mother.

The Prophet equates motherhood with the hardship a woman has to go through. Other *aḥādīth* state that the woman who is pregnant and breastfeeds the baby for as long as necessary and dies in the process will receive a reward equivalent to that of a martyr.[111] Martyrdom in the time of the Prophet—whose life was dedicated to building and defending the newly founded religion, often at a great price—was yearned after by all Muslims, both women and men.[112] Muslim women, for their part, had asked the Prophet for the right to fight alongside men on the battlefield, but the Prophet's answer was to encourage them to reproduce instead, equating this with military service. At the same time, he did not rule out the possibility of women partaking actively in wars.[113] He even on many occasions brought his wives along on campaign. In this sense, he acknowledged the military skills of both men and women.

In the course of time, his wife, 'Ā'ishah, left her quarters to lead an army at the battle of the Camel. Her leadership required her to be on the front lines of the battle. One may wonder why 'Ā'ishah decided to get involved in a military expedition against 'Alī, who was also the Prophet's most beloved cousin and his son-in-law. What would the Prophet have said if he had been asked for his advice? Would he have forbidden 'Ā'ishah to participate in the war, for the reason she was a woman? 'Ā'ishah was the Prophet's favorite wife: her courage and intelligence stood out and, in fact, her religious authority remained strong even after the death of the Prophet. However, 'Ā'ishah's personal, political, and religious authority never generates a model of autonomy as a significant feminine trait, because the society in which she lived was in the midst of a transition into more segregated private and public spheres.

What the jurists construe from the prophetic saying is that the most appropriate role for a woman is to be a mother, while they care less about other prophetic examples that are friendly to women. The jurists' legal opinions are interwoven with other received notions, as follows:

- a wife's proper place is in the house[114]
- the potential harm a woman causes from going out and its prohibition[115]
- a good woman does not lay eyes on other men[116]
- a wife's obedience to her husband and its reward[117]
- the parents' obligation to marry off their daughters[118]
- the prohibition to spend a husband's earning without his permission[119]
- a wife's devotion to her husband in the house and its reward[120]
- a wife's obligation to educate children, especially after the death of her husband and its reward.[121]

While Muslim jurists nurture, reiterate, and perpetuate these prophetic teachings, Muslim men impose these values upon *their women*. Muslim women for their part do not feel that they are the object of the male imposition of prophetic teachings: they materialize them as the expressions of their unconditional devotion to God and the Prophet. With this in mind, Muslim women are never in the position to question the validity of the prophetic practical guidance. This reality is quite the contrary to what early Muslim women were accustomed to do, since they had direct access to the founder of Islamic authority.

The centrality of the Prophet Muḥammad in his newly founded community made him a religious and community leader whose thoughts and sayings constituted a "political body" that carried authority. Muslims came with all sorts of questions, including the issues of Muslim women and their rights. Not only was Muḥammad eager to answer them, he also frequently answered in a way that showed high regard for women. He was known for calling upon Muslims to be affectionate to their mothers, sisters, and wives. He also extended his compassion to Muslim women by treating them as humans and encouraging them to participate in education, public affairs, military, and the economy.

Showing kindness to close female and male relatives is a good habit and instills the virtue of kindness in others. It conveys the ethical message that if all Muslims learn to show respect to their female and male relatives out of duty, they will pay a similar respect to others. It is often said that husbands in the Muslim world do not respect their wives as much as western husbands do, but that at the same time, sons in the Muslim world respect their mothers more than sons in the West.[122] This statement begs for further explanation. If sons are trained to respect their mothers, it follows that they would pay a similar respect to women in general. Given the context of respecting and caring to one's mother in the middle of the war, the Prophetic saying of respecting and caring for mothers three times[123] conveys the ethical message of respecting women as class. In this sense, if sons are taught to hold their mother in high esteem, they would treat their wives, female friends, and daughters in good manner.

Even though the prophetic practical guidance shows that respectful of the mothers are due to their biological sacrifice for their children, it does not rule out the possibility to respect women as a whole. By this, it does not mean that all women should become mothers since many women could not bear children, just like many barren husbands could not beget offspring. Regrettably, wifehood and motherhood are withheld high as if women's worth as humans are determined by these two ideal roles. Philosophers look at these ideal roles of women on the ground of their disposition and characteristics, which eventually lead them to posit a universal concept of what is appropriate for women. In this regard, the concept of gender is constructed based on what women do rather than who they are. Even if women are seen as who they are, these women are described as the opposites of men, because the female nature is more fitted for childbearing, nurturing, and care taking. Their self-existence is also defined as the extension of the family whose dependency lends them financial support, control, discipline, and guardianship.

The conflated concept of a woman as a wife and/or a mother remains the locus of gender construction in Muslim societies. The importance of these roles as "the most sacred and essential one" that shapes the future of the nation is a common view.[124] In the Middle East, the view of women "as wives and mothers, and gender segregation is customary, if not legally required."[125] Youssef shares a similar view with Moghadam's observation that[126]

> Tight control through an early and parentally supervised/controlled marriage, as well as strict seclusion before that event, instill the idea that only one life exists for the woman. Motivation is channeled in the direction of marriage by creating desire for familial roles, by extolling the reward accruing from the wife-mother status, by severe community censure of spinsterhood.

Muslim women in the predominantly Muslim countries, such as Malaysia and Indonesia, experience the same faith, just like their sisters in the Middle East in that they are succumbed to the conflated view of women as reproduces and mothers.[127] The same is true for Muslim women as minorities in China and Australia in which their lives are confined to the role of motherhood.[128] At any rate, motherhood appears to be woman's priority in every culture regardless of their religious affiliation. Eisentein argues that[129]

> ... the sexual division of labor that assigns childbearing/rearing and domestic labor to women applies cross-culturally and produces significant similarities in women's lives. Motherhood remains the domain of women.

Wifehood and motherhood are, therefore, not simply associated with women's reproductive organs, but mark their existence and identity in the world. Accordingly, not only are girls encouraged, and sometimes forced to get married, they are systematically domesticated to the household world. I am not arguing that being a homemaker as a wife and/or a mother is not rewarding. My concern is that the systematic "housewifization" and the mystification of a caring wife and nurturing mother negate women's self-determination, choice, and autonomy. Mothers and wives could definitely choose to be full-time mothers or wives as they wish depending on the priorities they are committed too.

The cultural and religious mystification of wifehood and motherhood restrict women's world to the household of her parents or, later, husband. Indeed, many women have access to public life to work, study, or perform other duties, but they do not enjoy the same liberty and opportunities as their male counterparts would enjoy. Women continue to be subjected to a multiplicity of restrictions and limitations because they are constantly seen as a potential threat for social disorder.[130] In Saudi Arabia, for instance, women are not allow to drive because

> [w]omen driving leads to many evils and negative consequences. Included among these is her mixing with men without her being on her guard. It also leads to the evil sins due to which such an action is forbidden. The Pure Law forbids those acts that lead to forbidden acts and considers those means to be forbidden also.[131]

Women are not allowed to work, but to remain in their houses because interaction with men at workplaces would be a "very dangerous matter that has dangerous consequences and negative results."[132] Similarly, if women were absent from the house, no one would take care of the family, especially the men. Since taking care of the family and being in the house suit the nature of women, they are destined to be morally responsible for it. If the family prospers, society will be more prosperous and there would be no promiscuity.

It is quite understandable that some women should want to stay home for religious and personal reasons, but to generalize that all women should do so is to ignore the need of some women to provide sustenance for their families. It is true that the patriarchal agnatic family system requires fathers and later husbands to provide finance, shelter, food, and clothing for those in their care. However, there are horrendous and irresponsible hierarchical and gender-minded Muslim fathers and husbands who get away from responsibility to care for their families. They leave women with nothing but the responsibility to care for the children's well-being and education. Women also often stay with their abusive fathers and/or husbands for the reason they do not have any capital to exit an abusive relationship. Muslim governments usually lack infrastructure and legal system that protect women from abusive families. Instead, violence against women is often justified with religious beliefs. Women cannot return to their parents' houses since such an act is the threat to the family's honor and good social standing.

Women's lack of ability to decide for their lives and of access to education and opportunities that upgrade their life's condition impinge on the self-realization of their potential. One may argue that this kind of life is not universal to all women. Certainly, exceptions exist. There are women who excel in religion, politics, wealth, and career. But, this is not what the majority of Muslim women have. If women were to work, they have to compete with other male prospective workers within the workplaces that are specifically designed for male workers. Many women have their jobs as the extension of their household responsibility, like cooking, taking care the family, and cleaning. While privileged Muslim women stay home, they also at the same time have imported their Muslim sisters from the less fortunate Muslim countries in wealth to do dirty jobs. While privileged Muslim women are forbidden to work outside the houses for religious reason and for preventing any unforeseeable dangerous consequences, some foreign Muslim sisters work, eat, and sleep in these houses. While privileged Muslim women travel for vacation or study abroad, these households' workers extend their services to cater their needs in the foreign countries. These foreign Muslim sisters embark to work in the unknown world to fulfill their religious obligation to care for the family left behind in their home countries.

However different the lived experiences women have illustrates the multitude of sexual, gender, and familial constructs in Muslim societies. Philosophical texts capture the intertwined pronouncement of what is appropriate and inappropriate for women in Muslims' context, as an expression of what the public perceives as the truth. In this sense, the confluence of Islamic doctrine, gender difference, and power relations perpetuates the status quo of gender thinking, expectation, and appropriation.

In this multiplicity of religious, cultural, and social expressions, women continue to be subjected to the production hierarchical theory and practice of gender at the private and public spheres.

Conclusion

I have argued in this chapter that gender thinking shapes the ways Muslims interpret the expositions of particularism in the Islamic teaching and apply particular interpretation into the religious, social, and philosophical constructs of sexual and gender difference and the system it produces. In particular, I have elaborated how the religious legitimacy in the different locality in Muslim countries has an effect on the construction of sexual and gender difference that is materialized at the personal and familial levels.

As the appropriation of sexual difference entails gender difference, women's roles are conceptualized relative to men's roles and needs. Women as wives are frequently expected to be sexually available, economically beneficial, and efficient manager in household works, fertile child-bearers, as well as nurturing, caring, and loving mothers. Remarkably, many women embrace the constructed roles as rewarding. They internalize the care for household responsibilities, children and even elderly as fitting their natural disposition. They never in a wink think that the strict sexual division of labor tyrannizes them.

Many women tirelessly maintain the inherited status quo of the dominant hierarchy of gender as their own constitution of their self-becoming. Their participatory engagement in constituting male demands, needs, and interests drives women to becoming others without any reciprocal and mutual relationship. What is considered a "reciprocal and mutual" relationship at this point is the satisfaction and appropriation women get for meeting the male need. Even if women desire for "reciprocal and mutual" relationship in the sense that they could speak their mind to their parents, husbands, or male counterparts, they would hesitate to embody authority, rationality, and independence. Not because all these characters belong to men, but socially and culturally, women with these traits will find life more complicated. Hence, it is more convenient for women to comply with the ruling ideology and norms.

The existing status quo of sexual and gender difference as the system is not only exercised by men on their immediate family members, but also are among women who instill their ideal portrayal of women in their in-laws. Mothers share the kind of gender thinking in that they make every attempt to ensure that their sons continue the legacy of masculine depiction of ideal Muslim men who are in charge of their wives. The fathers and sons set a model in which mothers are the ideal women to which the gendered construction of being an ideal woman succumbs. For this reason, the whole construct of dominant and patriarchal gender system is so profoundly rooted in each individual so that to uproot it sounds impossible.

In this context, the conformity and acceptance to the cultural elevation of women in their capacity as wives and mothers as necessary for the perpetuation of the human race[133] find its justification in the gendered interpretation of the creation theories.

The appropriation of gender difference as a system reiterates the intentional creation of women and their origin depicted in the Adam story, as will be seen in Chapter 2. Embedded in this story is the partnership of men and women in reproduction, in which a woman's womb is intended to as the "place" multiply. It follows that the female's role in reproduction and its extended responsibility is not only natural, but is also religiously divine, socio-culturally rewarding, and politically fulfilling the female's interest in the household and the male's need to take care the public affairs.

2 The creation theories as the bases for ontological self and inclusive humanity

This chapter discusses the contradictory claims of the creation theories and their subsequent impact on the ontological self, gender, and humanity in Muslim scholarship and societies. The hierarchical view of the standard creation theory generates the premise that human beings originated out of the male father, Adam. Drawing on the story of Adam and Eve (or Ḥawwā'), both Islamic scholars and lay Muslims believe that Adam was created in a manner superior to Eve. This interpretation has become the public perception of the truth governing how the status of men and women as humans is materialized. In its subsequent interpretation, the concept of gender relationships is often founded on gender inequality and difference. Such inequalities are further accentuated within the patriarchal system, whose power operates throughout different legal, economic, social, political, and cultural apparatus.

Even though the "Adam's rib" story has been interpreted in such a way as to support the moral inequality of the sexes, it is not the only Qur'ānic account of the origin of human beings. The Qur'ān, like the Bible, tells several stories about human origin. It introduces different creation theories: that of the creation of humans as narrated in Adam's account; that of the creation of man and woman out of one entity (self/*nafs wāḥidah*); and that of the creation of humans out of material substances. While these creation theories point to the common origin of human beings—created out of one entity and the material substances that constitute humans—the first creation theory describing Adam's status as the primary being and that of his partner, Ḥawwā', as secondary, has shaped the public perception of what dictates the self, gender, and humanity. This interpretation is extremely popular in Muslim cultures: even the verses suggesting that creation occurred from one entity (*nafs wāḥidah*) (Q.S. al-Nisā', 4:1) are interpreted to fit the traditional theory of Adam's creation.

The theories of human creation have long fascinated exegetes, philosophers, Ṣūfīs, and feminists. Exegetes deal with human creation as they interpret the Qur'ānic verses either thematically or holistically.[1] Philosophers address the question of how human beings are created in relation to the way in which the reproductive organs work within human bodies, and how organic and inorganic materials grow in a woman's womb.[2] The Ṣūfīs[3] symbolically relate the creation of human beings to God's power.[4] Scholars examine the theories of human creation within the framework of the Qur'ān and Islamic sciences.[5] Feminists construe the public discourse on the creation of human beings as the source of gender inequality[6] and call for a reinterpretation of the

Qur'ānic verses dealing with the creation of human beings to promulgate a new understanding of gender equality in Islam.

Muslim feminists have taken the issue of the creation of humans and its implication for the making of gender inequality seriously.[7] Hassan, who has pioneered the reinterpretation of the creation theory in Islam, considers the issue of equality in creation as "more basic and important, philosophically and theologically, . . . because if men and women have been created equal by Allah who is the ultimate arbiter of value, then they cannot be unequal, essentially, at a subsequent time."[8] Wadud-Muhsin also argues that the different treatments in the Qur'ān of the creation of humankind does not attribute any essential difference in the importance of men and women.[9] Men and women are two co-existing creatures that constitute humanity. Likewise, Barlas echoes the Qur'ānic vision of the ontological equality and similarity between men and women in that "the two sexes were meant to co-exist within the framework of mutual love and recognition."[10]

In line with feminists, I argue that the hierarchical view of the creation theories and its subsequent impact on the construction of gender has eliminated the female self from its potential to constitute humanity. Humanity is reduced into what fits male standards, values, philosophy, culture, and other attributes. Women are in the process marginalized through the embodiment of norms and virtues that are male derived. They internalize such knowledge as theirs to the extent that they are not inquisitive in producing their own knowledge, philosophy, culture, and civilization.

Despite the denial of women's "full worth as human beings,"[11] hence excluding them from humanity, I argue in this chapter that the nature of humanity is inclusive of all attributes possible for human flourishing, regardless of sexuality, social status, religious affiliation, racial and ethnic backgrounds, moral values, and other contextual attributions. Men and women are joint components of humanity since both are responsible for creating a just and democratic relationship between humans. Such a relationship would be impossible if it assumed an unequal relationship between men and women.

In an attempt to establish a new vision of humanity, I first recapitulate the theory of the creation of Adam and its role in constructing humanity. My purpose in doing so is to open up discussion on whether the creation of Adam implies the superiority of men over women and an exclusive claim to humanity as well. It also shows the extent to which the interpretation of the creation of Adam has been internalized into the lives of women. To facilitate this discussion, I probe the religious discussion of Adam's creation theory and trace its roots in the Judeo-Christian tradition.

In the subsequent section, I analyze the commonalities between the creation of Adam in particular and the creation of human beings in general. I argue that the creation of human beings points to a common origin. Its commonality lies in the fact that human beings are composed of substances, such as fluid/water (*mā'*), clay (*ṣalṣal* or *ṭīn*), and dust (*turāb*). This common origin was also applied to Adam, for the Qur'ān (Q.S. Āl 'Imrān, 3:59) mentions that he was created out of clay (*ṭīn*). While the material substances constitute the bodily origin of human beings, the self or living entity (*nafs*) animates human bodies.

I finally present an alternative interpretation of the fundamental religious structure of how human beings are created as described in Q.S. al-Nisā', 4:1 and its impact on the ontological view of humanity. This interpretation reflects the Qur'ānic view of equality in human creation, which to a certain degree invalidates the accepted misogynistic perspective on creation theory according primacy to Adam over Eve. I also highlight Ibn Sīnā's metaphysical discussion of the self and its effect on the making of humanity.

The creation of Adam and the making of humanity

I argue that the Qur'ān never intended the story of the creation of Adam to serve as the basis for a theory of "male" humanity founded on a male father. The Qur'an appears to introduce the archetype of human creation in general and Adam in particular. When the Qur'ān speaks of the archetype of human creation, it generally refers to the created nature of humans and their purposive mission in the world. Likewise, the Qur'ān illustrates the creation of Adam to show his commonalities by and large with other humans. To elucidate these commonalities, in what follows, I discuss the creation of Adam *vis-à-vis* humans (*khalīfah*, *bashar*, and *al-insān*), the creation of Eve, and their impact on humanity.

The creation of Adam vis-à-vis *humans (khalīfah, bashar, and al-insān)*

The Qur'ān introduces the creation of Adam and human beings in several places without always distinguishing between them, such as Q.S. al-Baqarah, 2:30–4, Q.S. al-Ḥijr, 15:26–34, and Q.S. Ṣād, 71–77. In these instances, the Qur'ān begins by introducing generic language, such as *khalīfah* (vicegerent), *bashar* (human being), and *al-insān* (human being) to describe the universal human origin, trait, and disposition. Adam's narrative later on appears in related verses to show the process and progress of what constitutes human origin and their nature and how these dispositions fly in the face of God's other creatures, namely angels (*malā'ikah*) and Satan (*Iblīs*), the two competing powers that continue to interfere in the human search for right and wrong. In this connection, I present three contexts in which the Qur'ān mentions the creation of Adam *vis-à-vis khalīfah* (vicegerent), *bashar* (human being), and *al-insān* (human being).

In Q.S. al-Baqarah, 2:30–4, the Qur'ān introduces Adam's name within the context of the creation of a *khalīfah* (vicegerent):

> And Lo! Thy Sustainer said unto the angels: "Behold, I am about to establish upon earth [*khalīfah*—] one who shall inherit it." They said: "Wilt Thou place on it such as will spread corruption thereon and shed blood—whereas it is who extol Thy limitless glory, and praise Thee, and hallow Thy name?" [God] answered: "Verily, I know that which you do not know."
>
> And He imparted unto Adam the names of all things, then He brought them within the ken of the angels and said: "Declare unto Me the names of these [things], if what you say is true."

They replied: "Limitless art Thou in Thy Glory! No knowledge have we save that which Thou hast imparted unto us. Verily, Thou alone art all-knowing, truly wise."

Said He: "O Adam, convey unto them the names of these [things]." As soon as [Adam] had conveyed into them their names, [God] said: "Did I not say unto you, 'Verily, I alone know the hidden reality of the heavens of the earth, and know all that you bring into the open and all that you would conceal'?"

And when We told the angels, "Prostrate yourself before Adam!"—they all prostrated, save Iblīs, who refused and gloried in his arrogance: and thus he became one of those who deny the truth.[12]

In other verses, the Qur'ān describes Adam within the context of the creation of human (*bashar*) as in Q.S. Sād, 38:71–77 as follows:

(71) Behold thy Lord said to the angels: "I am about to create [hu]man [*bashar*] from clay:"
(72) "When I have fashioned him (in due proportion) and breathed into him of My spirit fall ye down in obeisance unto him."
(73) So the angels prostrated themselves all of them together;
(74) Not so Iblis: he was haughty and became one of those who reject Faith.
(75) (Allah) said: "O Iblis! What prevents thee from prostrating thyself to one whom I have created with My hands? Art thou haughty? Or art thou one of the high (and mighty) ones?"
(76) (Iblis) said: "I am better than he: Thou createdst me from fire and him Thou createdst from clay."
(77) (Allah) said: "Then get thee out from here: for thou art rejected accursed."[13]

In Q.S. al-Ḥijr, 15: 26–34, the Qur'ān describes Adam within the context of the creation of human (*al-insān*) from sounding clay (*ṣalṣāl*) as follows:

(26) We created [hu]man [*al-insān*] from sounding clay, from mud moulded into shape;
(27) And the Jinn race, We had created before, from the fire of a scorching wind
(28) Behold! Thy Lord said to the angels "I am about to create [hu]man [*bashar*] from mud moulded into shape;
(29) "When I have fashioned him (in proportion) and breathed into him of My spirit, fall ye down in obeisance unto him."
(30) So the angels prostrated themselves, all of them together:
(31) Not so Iblis: he refused to be among those who prostrated themselves.
(32) (God) said: "O Iblīs! What is your reason for not being among those who prostrated themselves?"
(33) (Iblīs) said: "I am not one to prostrate myself to man, whom Thou didst create from sounding clay, from mud moulded into shape."[14]

While the exegetes read these verses in relation to the particular creation of Adam, the universal context that the Qur'ān addresses is the creation of *khalīfah* (vicegerent), *bashar* (human being), and *al-insān* (human being). The medieval exegete al-Rāzī points to Q.S. al-Baqarah, 2:30 in particular as referring to the manner in which Adam was created and the way God elevated him above other creatures, just as God continues to honor the children of Adam.[15] Like al-Rāzī, the contemporary exegete Bint al-Shāṭī' remarks that Q.S. al-Baqarah, 2:30 refers to the creation of Adam, the first human being, from which the chain of humanity (*al-bashariyyah*) begins.[16]

The verses further elucidate the dialectics of the creation of Adam, *vis-à-vis* God and his existing creatures, such as angels (*malā'ikah*)[17] and Iblīs (Satan). Made of the *created* light, the angels foresee the problem posed by humans as the ones who "will spread corruption thereon and shed blood" (Q.S. al-Baqarah, 2:30). They also measure their superior nature, roles, and characteristics *vis-à-vis* humans. Al-Rāzī depicts the nature and characteristics of angels as follows:[18]

- The angels are God's messengers entrusted with conveying His message (Q.S. Fāṭir, 35:1 and Q.S. al-Ḥajj, 22:40).
- They are close to God in their high rank (*sharīf*), but not in physical proximity (Q.S. al-Anbiyā', 21:19 and Q.S. al-Ṣāffāt, 37:42).
- They are obedient to God in three senses: (a) they constantly praise and glorify God with full devotion (Q.S. al-Baqarah, 2:30 and Q.S. al-Ṣāffāt, 37:166); (b) they are prompt in executing God's command (Q.S. al-Baqarah, 2:30); and (c) they do not do something except what God orders them to do (Q.S. al-Anbiyā', 21:27).
- They have powerful abilities in four senses: (a) they carry the Throne of God (Q.S. Ghāfir, 40:7); (b) the loftiness of the Throne to which the angels and inspiration (rūḥ) ascend daily (Q.S. al-Ma'ārij, 70:4) is beyond imagination; (c) they are in control of the trumpet of the Day of Judgment (Q.S. al-Zumar, 39:68); and (d) Gabriel was sent to destroy the people of Lot (Q.S. al-Ḥijr, 15:72–3).
- They are in reverent awe (*khawf*) of God in three senses: (a) while the angels fully devote their lives to the service of God, they fear God (Q.S. al-Naḥl, 16:50 and Q.S. al-Anbiyā', 21:28); (b) they are in awe of God's intercession in the Day of Judgment (Q.S. Saba', 34:23); and (c) they execute their mission with God's permission.

Notwithstanding the angels' superiority in origin, rank (*sharīf*), speech (*kalām*), and skill, they obey God's command to bow down to Adam (Q.S. al-Baqarah, 2:30). This attitude reflects the angels' constant devotion, obedience, and reverent awe shown to God. This is not the case with Iblīs and his devil companions, whose superiority and seniority drive them to defy God's command to bow to Adam. Devils feel more superior in their origin since they were created from fire in comparison to Adam, fashioned from clay (Q.S. Ṣād, 38:71 and Q.S. al-Ḥijr, 15:27). They also deem themselves to be senior since they were created prior to Adam. The nature and attitude of Iblīs are more revealing when they deceive Adam and Eve into betrayal to God's command.

But who was Adam? And what made this creature so special in the eye of God? The Qur'ān refers to Adam as an individual and as the archetype of humankind.

It mentions Adam as an individual with respect to his role as a prophet (Q.S. Āl 'Imrān 3:33 and Q.S. Maryam, 19:58) and to the manner in which he was created: "Verily in the sight of God, the nature of Jesus is as the nature of Adam, whom He created out of dust and then said unto him, 'Be'—and he is" (Q.S. Āl 'Imrān, 3:59).[19] Asad notes that while this verse mentions both Jesus and Adam by name, it does not necessarily exclude them from the common origin of human beings, as they were created out of dust like anyone else.[20]

The term "Ādam" may also denote the human race, because the last word of the above sentence '*kun fayakūn*' ("Be"—and he is) employs the present tense.[21] It stands for the archetypal human as "a self-conscious, knowledgeable, and morally autonomous humanity."[22] Bint al-Shāṭī' argues that *al-Ādamiyyah* is neither angelic nor satanic (*Iblīsiyyah*).[23] It is neither angelic in the sense of total submission and obedience nor satanic in the sense of mere evil, passionate disobedience, and a persistent will to go astray; instead, it is the realization of the faculty of distinction, consciousness, and will. "Adamness" also refers to humans' ability to stand the trial when wickedness prevails, when their consciences feel uncomfortable, moving them to repent and ask for forgiveness. They will constantly experience the cycles of good and evil along with moral responsibility for their deed and choices.

The use of the term "Ādam" as the archetype of humanity has a bigger implication, because it mingles with the universal context of the creation of the human race. The Qur'ān always reiterates the origin and portrayal of Adam in relation to broader generic terms, such as *khalīfah* (vicegerent), *bashar* (human being), and *al-insān* (human being). The term *khalīfah* (vicegerent), according to al-Rāzī, refers to Adam as one who inherited the earth from the *jinn* who preceded him and who was entrusted by God with leadership (*ḥukm*).[24] It also refers to the children of Adam in that they succeed one generation after the other (Q.S. al-An'ām, 6:165, Q.S. al-Naml, 27:62, and Q.S. Fāṭir, 35:39). Asad, however, construes the word *khalīfah* as signifying human supremacy on earth and humanity's endowed capacity to discern right and wrong as God's vicegerent.[25]

If the term *khalīfah* denotes to the human's superior role and his/her qualification to carry out the mission of successors on the earth, the word *bashar* (human being) stands for the physical function of human being in the world. The Qur'ān often employs the term *bashar* (human) to demonstrate the humanity (*al-bashariyyah*) of the prophets in that they were just human beings who ate food (Q.S. al-Anbiyā', 21:8), were mortal (Q.S. Ibrāhīm, 14:11, Q.S. al-Mu'minūn, 23:24, Q.S. al-Kahf, 18:110, and Q.S. Hūd, 11:27), and went to the market (Q.S. al-Furqān, 25:7). Just like mortal humans in general, the prophets shared physical needs, lived in their communities, and acquired what was essential to their needs.[26] The physical need for food as a means of life sustenance is also present in the account of Mary's life, even though she was granted with an immaculate pregnancy and gave birth to Jesus, who was created in the manner of Adam (Q.S. Āl 'Imrān, 3:37 and 59).

The use of the term '*bashar*' with regard to the creation of Adam suggests that Adam shared a common origin with other human beings. He was created out of clay (*ṭīn*) like other mortal humans originating "from mud moulded into shape" (Q.S. al-Ḥijr, 15:28). This implies that whoever is created in the manner in which humans are moulded and shaped into human form, they share the same physical form as humans and the same bodily need and fill their lives with human activities, such as eating, walking, sleeping, and going to the bathroom, just like all mortal beings do. Humans are required to fulfill their physical needs by making the right choices (*ikhtiyār*), since they are morally responsible for the choices they make and for what they do. This role coincides with the potential of humans to be God's vicegerent (*khalīfah*), as long as they are able to work out the inevitable tensions and moral struggles that arise in daily life. Otherwise, humans would be more inclined to do evil, like the one who "will spread corruption thereon and shed blood" (Q.S. al-Baqarah, 2:30).[27]

The use of such terms as 'Adam,' '*bashar*,' and '*ṭīn*' has suggested to some that several words in the Qur'ān have Syrian Christian origin.[28] O'Shaughnessy, for example, suggests that many phrases of Syriac origin have found their way into the Qur'ān, as follows:

> *Bashar* and *ṭin* have close cognates in Syriac; Aphraates, a Syrian monastic writer of the fourth century, speaks of God creating man alone of all creatures "with His own hand." Iblīs, too, the name used for Satan, a corruption of the Greek *diabolos*, probably entered the Qur'ān through the Syriac, and the epithet *rajīm* (stoned, deserving of death by stoning, accursed) in [38/Ṣād: 77–78] is a transliterated Syriac adjective also applied to him in the works of St. Ephrem. Finally the phrase "breathed into him of My spirit (*nafakhtu fīhī min rūḥī*) used here and elsewhere in the Qur'ān to describe God's creative breathing into Adam, is found in Syriac cognates arranged in the same partitive construction both in Aphraates and the *Liber graduum*, an anonymous collection of moral and ascetical sermons dating from the early fifth century.[29]

Obviously, there are similarities between Islamic and other Judeo-Christian accounts of the creation of humans. The creation of Adam "out of dust"[30] implies a common origin of human beings in general. God teaches Adam the names of all things;[31] settles both Adam and his companion in paradise;[32] forbids both to eat the fruit of the tree;[33] and expels Adam and Eve from the Garden.[34]

In this connection, the question of whether or not these similarities justify the charge of Islamic borrowing from the Judeo-Christian tradition has given rise to a heated debate. Haas argues that Muḥammad had no direct contact with the Genesis accounts.[35] He points out that the Qur'ān consistently employs the word '*khalaqa*' to indicate the creation of human beings, whereas Genesis uses the word *bāra'* exclusively to denote the creative activity of God, which Muḥammad would have known either from the Jews of Medina or probably from the Christians of the north.[36] In fact, the word *bara'* itself is not alien to the Qur'ān, as it employs the word in many different forms, like *nabra'ahā* ((to bring into being), Q.S. al-Ḥadīd, 57:22), *al-Bāri'* ((the Shaper), Q.S. al-Ḥashr, 59:24), and *bāri'ikum* ((your Maker), Q.S. al-Baqarah 2:54). These passages were revealed in Medina in connection with the events in which the Prophet encountered the Jews.

In addition, the common similarities between Islam and Judeo-Christian tradition should not come as a surprise, since Muslims perceive Islam as the last link in the chain of the Abrahamic religions, which, from the Islamic perspective, emphasize the Oneness of God (*tawḥīd*). Muḥammad did not usher in a new religion; he merely renewed the religion of Abraham, Jacob, Isaac, and Ishmael (Q.S. al-Baqarah, 2:131 and 133). In fact, the verses dealing with creation generally accord with the prophetic mission of proving the Oneness of God (*tawḥīd*), which is the core teaching of Islam. This proof derives in part from the conviction that God has power over humankind with respect to creation and punishment. Since God is able to create humans from either a drop of water or dust, He is also able to resurrect human bone and dust in the hereafter.[37] This implies that human life is finite, whereas God as Life-giver (*muḥyī*) is infinite.

In the case of the creation theory, Islam shares with Judaism the use of the term "Adam." In Judeo-Christian tradition, the term Adam is not only used in reference to the biblical name of the first "human" (Genesis 1–5), but also alludes to humankind in general (Genesis 1:27).[38] In Hebrew, however, the term itself never occurs in the plural, but instead appears in a phrase indicating plurality, that is, *benei Adam* (the sons of Adam, Ps. 36:8). The term is, moreover, sometimes employed to designate men and women (Leviticus, 24:17). In light of these different usages of the word "Adam," Genesis 1:27 can be read as saying that "Adam" was "created male and female."[39]

While the terms '*khalīfah*' and '*bashar*' seemingly connote a universal humanity that is male derived and that is construed in relation to male prophets, the term *al-insān* appears to advocate a humanity that is inclusive of men and women. The Qur'ān consistently employs the word *al-insān* in relation to the commonalities of humans' origin and their common properties. The very first revelation that Prophet Muḥammad received talks about the creation of the human (*insān*):

> Read in the name of thy Sustainer, who has created—
> Created hu[man] out of a germ-cell
> Read—for thy Sustainer is the Most Bountiful One
> Who has taught [hu[man]] the use of the pen—
> taught [hu]man what he did not know.[40]

These verses parallel the creation of *khalīfah* and *bashar* in that humans were created out of material and immaterial substances, such as germ-cells, dust, clay, and mud. They share physical human form and need to live their life on earth. They are also endowed with knowledge to fulfill their mission as God's vicegerents and to exert themselves in moral perfection so that they are able to manage the inevitable tension of good and evil and exercise intelligent ability to choose morally responsible actions and avoid wrongdoing.

The notion of humanity, therefore, signifies humans' role to become God's vicegerents on earth, with the capacity to follow up their trust responsibly.[41] They are endowed with the knowledge, explanation, intelligence, and conscience to discern the trial of good and evil, to inquire into deception, and to feel proud of their high status as humans. These properties are not only male constructed, but are also appropriate for women as well. For this reason, the universal message of the creation of *khalīfah*, *bashar*, and *al-insān* shows that humanity in Islam is inclusive of men and women. This assertion is in line with the fact that the Qur'ān never directly addresses the question how Eve was created.

The creation of Eve or Ḥawwā'

It should be noted that, as the Qur'ānic verses (Q.S. al-Baqarah, 2:30–4, Q.S. al-Ḥijr, 15:26–34, and Q.S. Ṣād, 71–77) dealing with the creation of humans (*khalīfah*, *bashar*, and *al-insān*) have been interpreted in relation to the creation of Adam, Muslims have formed a notion of humanity that is male derived. This perception to a varying degree concurs with the Qur'ānic view of the creation and intellectual progress of Adam, since it does not refer at all to how his female partner was created.[42] I argue, however, that despite the Qur'ān's silence as to the manner in which Eve was created, it does not reduce the importance of Eve's creation along with Adam's, God's first vicegerent. The universal message of the creation of Eve also reiterates God's intention that creation was irreducible to one or the other since both Adam and Eve mirror the micro-model of humanity as consisting of the two.

The ambiguity of how Eve was created has led to a vast array of interpretations. The most common, as previously noted, is that woman was created from one of Adam's ribs.[43] Al-Ṭabarī,[44] for one, reports the circumstances of Eve's creation as follows:[45]

First opinion:

Ibn 'Abbās, Ibn Mas'ūd, and a group of companions:

> Then Iblīs was exiled from the Garden when he was cursed, and Adam was put to dwell in the Garden. He went around alone with no wife in whom he could repose. Then he fell asleep and woke up to find a woman sitting beside his head whom God has created from his rib. So he asked her: "Who are you?" And she said: "A woman." He said, "Why were you created?" She said: "So that you could find repose in me." Then the angels asked him, to see how much he knew: "What is her name, Adam?" He said: 'Ḥawwā' (= Eve)." They said: "Why is she called 'Ḥawwā'?" He said: "Because she was created from something living (*ḥayy*)'. Then God said to him: 'Adam, dwell, you and your wife, in the Garden, and eat thereof easefully where you desire.

Second opinion: Others said that she was created before Adam dwelt in the Garden. Ibn Isḥāq:

> When God had finished reprimanding Iblīs, He turned to Adam and taught him all names. Then He said <<"Adam, tell them their names">> up to (*sic*)—<<"Surely You are the All-knowing, the All-wise.">> (...) Then He cast slumber upon Adam—according to what has reached us from the people of the Torah among the scripture, and from other people of knowledge, through 'Abd Allāh b. 'Abbās and others—and then He took one of his ribs from his left side, and joined together and place where it had been with flesh. [Meanwhile] Adam slept, and he did not stir from his sleep until God had created his wife,

> Eve, from this rib of his. And He arranged her as a woman in whom [Adam] could find repose. When his slumber was lifted from him, and he stirred from his sleep, he saw her beside him, and he said—according to what they claim, and God knows best—: "My flesh, my blood, and my wife." And he found repose in her. When God had duplicated him, and made a means of repose for him from himself, He spoke to him face to face: <<Adam, dwell, you and your wife, in the Garden and eat thereof easefully where you desire; but do not draw near this tree, lest you become evil-doers>>.

The above accounts illustrate the manner in which Eve was created, the naming process, her self-knowledge, and her relation to a man. Ḥawwā' was created out of Adam's rib. This interpretation implies that Adam was intended as the primary creation, and that Ḥawwā' was subsequent and therefore subordinate to him. While Ḥawwā' had the self-knowledge of being "a woman," Adam did the naming and appropriated the name on the basis of her origin from something living, referring to his being. Ḥawwā's role is also extensional in that her existence is not independent of Adam. Adam might find repose in her, but Ḥawwā' had no place to turn for her repose.

The story also emphasizes Adam's intellectual properties. It was Adam, not Ḥawwā', who was taught all the names necessary for surviving and for carrying out the prophetic mission. In line with this, the majority of prophets, jurists, leaders, teachers, ṣūfī masters, exegetes, and Ḥadīth narrators have been male. Men, not women, have been the ones to engender knowledge, history, religion, civilization, and other institutions necessary for the survival of the society. Women are constantly depicted as lacking the reason needed to generate their own knowledge, culture, religious interpretation, and institution.

The story likewise illustrates God's acceptance of Adam's repentance, as the Qur'ān states in Q.S. al-Baqarah, 2:37: "Thereupon Adam received [of guidance] from the Sustainer, and He accepted his repentance: for, verily, He alone is the Acceptor of Repentance, the Dispenser of Grace."

However, Ḥawwā''s repentance is not mentioned individually because she was dependent on Adam—a fact repeated in most interpretations of the Qur'ānic verses and prophetic traditions dealing with the issue of women.[46] Again, a woman's voice is dissolved into a man's, even though the story shows that Adam and Ḥawwā' sinned and betrayed God's command to not touch the tree.

Al-Ṭabarī's interpretation of the verse (Q.S. al-Baqarah, 2:35), reflects the common understanding of the Prophet's Companions. Four centuries after al-Ṭabarī we find Muḥammad Ibn 'Abd Allāh al-Kisā'ī reiterating, repeating, and retelling, in his *The Tales of the Prophet*, the story that God created Eve out of Adam's left rib.[47] Such an interpretation clearly highlights the continuing theme of male superiority from the outset of Islam. This interpretation continues to shape the resilience of gender thinking as a mechanism that runs for generations and centuries to come.

It needs to be stressed that the concept of Eve being created out of Adam's rib has a common origin in one of the two creation stories in the Judeo-Christian tradition.[48] I am not saying that all three religions are misogynistic in their account of women, since the authoritative texts also provide the basis for gender egalitarianism. What I am trying to demonstrate here (and in this book generally) is that the gender thinking ingrained in the politics of the interpretation of religious texts amplifies the misogynistic attitude toward women. The resulting interpretation has become the pillar of the patriarchal system of Muslim culture.

A hierarchical reading of the religious texts is not exclusive to Islam. The same reading is unfortunately found in Genesis 2:18–24, which narrates the manner in which Eve was created out of Adam's rib.[49] The creation story in Genesis 2 is often read as signifying that a woman is subordinate to a man, and that, therefore, he is dominant over her by virtue of a "creation ordinance," as reflected in the following arguments:[50]

(a) Woman was created after man and is therefore secondary to him.
(b) Woman is "taken from man" and is therefore secondary to him.
(c) Woman is named by man and is therefore subordinate to him.
(d) Woman is created to be a helper for man and as such is subordinate to him.

While these and other similar arguments are associated with the creation story in Genesis 2, such statements are not essential to the text.[51] The creation of man and woman, in other words, can be seen as parallel and its order as belittling neither gender.[52] The equal importance of men and women in human creation invalidates the argument of male superiority over female. Similarly, the argument that woman is derived from man does not imply that woman is inferior, but that she is his equal, without whom he would be incomplete.[53] It also shows that, like man, she possesses an essential and equal identity as human.[54] The fact that the name of her gender is derived from that of man is not a strong argument for women's inferiority, for "woman" is not a proper name; moreover, the word "name" does not occur in the verse Genesis 2:23.[55] Even the fourth argument, which rests on the assumption that woman was created as "a help meet for him"[56] need not denote the inferiority of woman, but the recognition of woman as fitting to be "his counterpart, his complement, his partner, his companionship and his associate, bone of his bone, and flesh of his flesh."[57] In addition, the word "helper" in other translations of Genesis 2:18 is sometimes given as "a sustainer beside him."[58] Overall, the ethical message of Genesis 2–3, according to Yahwistic narrative, is that God intends to complete His primary creation by making a woman, for whom the man has waited and longed.[59] The woman is, thus, to be recognized as "the other that completes him."[60]

A non-hierarchical reading of another verse, Genesis 1:27, provides the most explicit biblical account of how man and woman were created equally. The passage reads as follows:[61]

> And God created the human ['ādām][62] in his image
> in the image of God He created him
> male and female He created him

The aforementioned passage contains two noteworthy statements. The first one asserts that the human animal is distinct from any other creation in that it was made in the image of God.[63] Being created in the image of God, according to Westermann, means[64]

1. Having certain spiritual qualities or capacities (soul, intellect, will)
2. Having a certain external (corporeal) form (i.e., upright carriage)
3. Having both spiritual and corporeal features characteristic of humankind
4. Being God's counterpart on earth; able to enter into partnership with God
5. Being God's representative on earth (based on royal theology, humankind as God's viceroy/administrator).

The second statement indicates that the essential nature of the genus, 'adam, consists of being male and female.[65] The passage suggests that humankind is made in the image of God. Unlike God, humankind is constituted of male and female, which becomes the condition for their multiplicity.[66] Humanity, therefore, consists of the two.

The notion of "image" (*ṣūrah*) in Islam refers to what is perceivable through appearance.[67] The image of humans, for instance, differs from that horses due to their respective appearances. Humans are also distinguished from animals because they are endowed with such properties as reason, will, and emotion. The Qur'ān frequently uses the term '*ṣawwara*' ("to shape" or "to form") in describing human development from the embryonic stage to maturity and to their role as humans (Q.S. al-A'rāf, 7:11 and Q.S. Āl 'Imrān, 4:6). The human image, therefore, denotes self-evolving individuals as well as their relationship to God, the macrocosm and other human beings.

Regarding the creation of Adam in particular and of human beings in general, the concept of "image" in Islam refers to the perfect physical form of human beings, to intellectual properties and moral qualities, to their excellence as God's creation in comparison to other creatures, and to their authority (as God's vicegerents).[68] Even though humans are created in the image of God, it is inferred that neither did God become part of the human race nor are humans God's equals. When the notion of the image of God is mentioned, it means that God bestows honor on humans for their superior being in comparison to the macrocosm. This "image" is common to all humans, regardless of any physical, mental, and moral qualities they have. Humans are inviolable and irreducible to any object. Humanity in Islam is, therefore, inclusive of all humans regardless of their specific biological anatomy, mental properties or moral perfection.

The making of humanity

The Qur'ān contains ample verses on the creation of human beings that can be read in the light of inclusive humanity. Muslims have taken the issue of human creation for granted, as if there were no theological and philosophical implications to being men and women in this world. However, Muslims are confined to the established argument that the existence of gender difference points to the premise of Adam's superiority over Eve. Subsequently, these differences in their creation have led the descendants of Adam and Eve to different legal, moral, and ethical responsibilities in society. In view of this, I argue that the account of Adam and Eve's downfall has shaped the gendered view of humanity.

Despite the fact that the creation theories in both the Islamic and Judeo-Christian traditions provide the basis for inclusive humanity, in which men and women are both the primary and intentional creation, and are made for each other,[69] Muslims often restate the misogynist understanding of the creation theory in Genesis 2:18–24, to support the creation of Ḥawwā' and its subsequent construction of humanity. The introduction of the message of Genesis 2 into Muslim scholarship, according to Hassan, was not direct since few Muslims would have encountered and read the Bible.[70] Instead, the manner in which Ḥawwā' was created from Adam's rib sounds very familiar to Muslim ears because several *aḥadīth* record the creation of women in this fashion, such as the following:

> Allah's Apostle said, "Treat women nicely, for a woman is created from a rib, and the most curved portion of the rib is its upper portion, so, if you should try to straighten it, it will break, but if you leave it as it is, it will remain crooked. So treat women nicely."[71]

The Prophet also said,

> Whoever believes in Allah and the Last Day should not hurt (trouble) his neighbor. And I advise you to take care of the women, for they are created from a rib and the most crooked portion of the rib is its upper part; if you try to straighten it, it will break, and if you leave it, it will remain crooked, so I urge you to take care of the women.[72]

These *aḥādīth*, according to Hassan, are weak with respect to their lists of transmitters (*isnād*) and even their contents (*matn*).[73] To say that women were created out of a rib contradicts the Qur'ānic message about the creation of human beings. Muslim scholars agree that all the *aḥadīth* whose contents are in opposition to the Qur'ān ought to be rejected. However, this does not diminish the significance of the *aḥādīth* recorded by such compilers as al-Bukhārī (810–870) and others, since these reports have been accepted as authentic by the majority of Muslims. For in the end what concerns women most is the increasing popularity of such *aḥādīth* that discredit their status and force them to remain in a subordinate position.

The male's superiority over the female, in Hassan's eyes, is furthermore rooted in three theological assumptions:

> ...(1) that God's primary creation is man, not woman, since woman is believed to have been created from man's rib, and is, therefore, derivative and secondary ontologically; (2) that woman, not a man, was the primary agent of what is customarily described as "Man's Fall" or expulsion from the Garden of Eden, hence "all daughters of Eve" are to be regarded with hatred, suspicion, and contempt; and (3) that woman was created not only from man but also for man, which makes her assistance merely instrumental and not fundamental importance.[74]

Hassan maintains that the misogynistic assumption that Eve was created out of Adam's rib has become the normative basis of the construction of the status of woman. Tragically, both scholars and ordinary Muslims have in essence endorsed this creation theory. It has also contributed to the entrenchment of the notion of male supremacy and to the subordination of women. Subordinate and inferior are among the attributes (if not virtues) assigned most commonly to Muslim women. These attributes are cited, coded, reiterated, and interpreted as representing the normative. Scholars likewise perpetuate this belief in the legal dimension of the faith (*Sharīʿah*), so that women are obliged to conform to this mistaken understanding of their roles.

A gendered view of humanity is also found in the different portrayal of the dispositions of men and women. Women are, for instance, associated with vicious characteristics more often than men. A woman is often seen as naturally seductive, crooked, and deceitful. This characterization stems from the creation story where Eve tempted Adam to eat the forbidden fruit at the urging of Iblīs. Seeking to cause the downfall of Adam and Eve, Iblīs took on the form of a snake, and entered Paradise. Picking some of the forbidden fruit of the tree and presenting it to Eve, he persuaded her to eat. With some of the fruit in her hand, Eve went to Adam and said: "Look at this fruit! How sweet does it smell! How good does it taste! How beautiful is its color! Thus, Adam ate of it."[75] According to al-Ṭabarī's account, God accused Eve of deceiving Adam,[76] whereas in other accounts, Adam admitted that Eve made him eat of it.[77]

Certainly, the Qur'ān does not attribute Adam's fall to the temptation of his spouse. Instead, Iblīs tempts both of them and causes them to be exiled from Paradise (Q.S. al-Baqarah, 2:36). But Iblīs had already experienced such a fall

> ... from God's grace because he refused to bow to Adam, in direct contravention of divine order. Satan's disobedience resulted from his arrogance, which was justified by a self-serving world-view. Satan believed that he was better than Adam because God created him from fire and Adam from clay.[78]

Satan's fall from paradise resulted from his self-serving belief in the loftiness of his origin, whereas the fall of Adam and his spouse reveals the nature of human beings as vulnerable to making mistakes. In the case of Adam's and Eve's downfall, both were morally responsible for their wrongdoing. However, their fault did not cause them to remain in the state of "a lasting defect of human primordial nature," nor did it make them the bearers of "original sin."[79] Both men and women are free and equal agents in battling Satan and they are both entitled to serve as God's vicegerents on earth, as well as to receive knowledge, inspiration, reward, and forgiveness as long as they seek God's guidance in their life. For this reason it should be stressed that the Qur'ān maintains its egalitarian perspective in portraying the subjectivity of Adam and Ḥawwā' and human beings in general.

Despite this, however, Eve in Islamic literature was repeatedly portrayed as responsible for Adam's expulsion from paradise. Eve was blamed for being so easily persuaded by the serpent to disobey God and enlist Adam in this defiance of the Divine Will.[80] Eve symbolizes women's seductive nature, their potential to invite temptation, and their tendency to be disobedient to men and God. This misogynistic portrayal often fails to convey the truth that both Eve and Adam suffered the consequences of what they had done. Evans argues that while Genesis 3:1–6 assigns the immediate responsibility to Eve, Genesis 3:7 makes it clear that the consequence of eating from the tree became apparent to both of them: "the eyes of the two were opened and they knew they were naked."[81] Therefore, both Adam and Eve not only sinned and fell as individuals, but also as a pair.[82]

What then does this story in its manifold forms mean for the gendered construction of humanity? Both men and women have different traits. Adam becomes the figure of how masculinity, superiority, independence, rationality, and spirituality are constructed. Men are superior because they are the primary creation on this earth. They are also independent creation because they exist primordially without necessitating any other condition. By contrast, Eve's existence is contingent upon that of Adam. Men are also rational because they are more able to make their choice on the basis of deliberation, just as Adam could have resisted Satan's temptation but for Eve's efforts at seduction. Men also have more potential to be spiritually endowed because Adam was a prophet and all of the prophets were male, whereas a woman cannot possibly be a prophet.

In stark contrast to traditionally masculine traits, women's femininity is usually portrayed as inferior, dependent, emotional, docile, rebellious, and less spiritual. Women are generally regarded as subordinate to men because they are not the primary creation. Such assumptions have impacted on women's lives to the extent that they are regarded as less entitled to rights and opportunities than their male counterparts. Women will never be religiously equal to men because men are superior in their origin. Women are also unable to exist as independent agents because they were originally dependent upon men. Women will never be consistent because, as is shown in the story of their origin, they are too vulnerable to change. They are also emotional because they base their choices on emotion and desire, just as Eve relied on these traits in deciding whether or not to follow Satan's instruction. Women are less spiritual because they are not capable of observing all religious obligations due to the constraints placed on them by menstruating, delivering a baby, and experiencing the postpartum period.

This image of women deriving from the particular interpretation of Islamic teaching dictates how Muslim women are treated in Muslim communities. Muslim women across the globe are frequently portrayed as submissive, inferior, oppressed, and backward. Regrettably, such a portrayal is often understood as synonymous with Islam. Hence, Islam is analogous to oppression, backwardness, subordination, and hostile human rights, and other labels that do not represent Islam in an ideal sense. Hekmat, for instance, contends that Islam has degraded the social status of women to a point where they have been "humiliated, abased, mistreated, and ignored."[83] In fact, "millions of Muslim females, under rigid and inexorable Islamic laws, have been deprived of their fundamental inalienable rights and driven into seclusion for many centuries."[84] Caner and Caner echo the same account saying, "Islam has deserved its reputation around the world for stifling and even enslaving women."[85]

While such candid accounts are accurate to the extent that this situation results from the gendered view of humanity and the mistreatment of women in the Muslim societies, those portrayals, nonetheless, fail to recognize the ethics of the egalitarian principle of gender, which is inherent in the Qur'ānic message. Said argues that "we should isolate the basic teaching of the Muslim religion as contained in the Koran, which is considered to be the word of God... This is the bedrock identity of Islamic faith..."[86] The Qur'ān, over the course of time, has become the point of departure for various interpretations, often at odds and conflicting with one another, which nowadays "make up the numerous Islamic sects, jurisprudential schools, hermeneutic styles [and] linguistic theories,"[87] not to mention the hierarchical and egalitarian theories of gender. For this reason, Said describes Muslim societies as "the communities of interpretation" whose creative interpretive energy augments what we call Islamic culture.[88]

The mistreatment of women in different Muslim localities does not, therefore, derive from the ideal teaching of the Qur'ān. It more or less reflects the particular interpretation of Islam and the embodiment of unjust practices that have culturally and socially existed in or have been assimilated to Muslim societies. As the hierarchical gender-minded Muslims are responsible for sowing the seed of a non-egalitarian view of gender, it is absolutely important to reinterpret the creation theories that are in line with the basic message of universal Islam and that favor the flourishing of gender egalitarianism.

Equality in human origin

I will argue in this section that the equality of humans is inherent in the creation of Adam, who was constituted of form and matter. The form refers to Adam's human form, whereas matter denotes to the constituents of material causes, such as clay (*ṣalṣāl*[89] or *ṭīn*)[90] and dust (*turāb*).[91] This argument may seem to contradict the assumption that Adam was created "out of nothing." It is often said that he existed "out of nothing" because there was no other human being prior to him. Accordingly, any discussion of the creation of human beings is linked to the assumption that Adam was created "out of nothing" and Ḥawwā' "out of something." Since the archetype of human beings does not share a common origin, they are consequently not equal. The assumption goes further in that this inequality is relevant to all human beings.

Quite contrary to the common assumption, the Qur'ān introduces the common origin of human beings. It suggests that human beings share one single origin of human form and are composed of organic and inorganic materials.[92] Humans, thus, have affinities with other earthly substances. When the Qur'ān speaks of Adam's creation (Q.S. Āl 'Imrān, 3:59), it mentions clay (*al-ṭīn*) as the substance of Adam's origin. In light of this argument, I will explore the religious views of "what human beings come from" as well as the philosophical insights when it is relevant.

The Qur'ān introduces the origin of human beings either as coming "out of something" or as coming "out of nothing." In explicating its argument, the Qur'ān introduces different terms that denote the act of creating.[93] These terms[94] are '*khalaqa*' (to create/to mold),[95] '*ja'ala*' (to create/to make),[96] '*banā*' (to create/to form),[97] '*rafa'a*' (to raise/to build),[98] '*madda*' (to furnish),[99] '*ṭaḥā*' (to expand),[100] and '*ṣawwara*' (to shape/to form).[101] The proper noun of the efficient agent who creates is usually *al-Khāliq*, which refers only to God and is one of His Divine Names.[102] The Divine Name of *al-Khāliq* also concurs with the names *al-Bāri'* (the Maker) and *al-Muṣawwir* (the Shaper), as indicated in the verse al-Wāqi'ah, 56:4: "He is God, the Creator, the Maker [and the Shaper] who shapes all forms and appearances!"[103] God is also sometimes called *al-Badī'* ("the Originator of the heavens and the earth," Q. S. al-An'ām, 6:14). Such names as *al-Khāliq*, *al-Bāri'*, *al-Muṣawwir*, and *al-Badī'* refer to God's Infinite Power over His creation.

Among these terms, *'khalq'* (a noun of the verb *'khalaqa'*) is the most commonly used verb root to indicate the creation of both the entire universe and human beings.[104] Most philologists understand the meaning of the term *'khalaqa'* in one of two opposite senses. Al-Iṣfahānī, for instance, interprets *'khalaqa'* as "innovating something without having a model or imitating something," as in the creation of the heaven and earth. It also means "to bring something into being out of something else," like the creation of human beings.[105] Ibn Manẓūr also notes that *'khalaqa'* denotes the act of "innovating something without a previous model," as well as "to create something according to its model," and "to measure."[106] Al-Zabīdī in *Tāj al-'Arūs* adds that *'khalaqa'* sometimes means to determine how much leather is needed to make a bag or water bottle before it is cut.[107] All of these indicate that creation (*'khalq'*) has two distinct connotations, namely, creation out of "nothing" and creation out of "something."

The equivocal meaning of the word *'khalaqa'* makes the idea of creation in general one of the main controversies in Islamic philosophy.[108] This debate centers on the question of how the world came into being. The theologian-philosopher al-Ghazālī maintains that the credit for the creation of the world belongs entirely to God. God has power over His creation. He can create, change, and intervene in what He creates; as the Qur'ān states: "His Being alone is such that when He wills a thing to be, He says unto it, 'Be'—and it is" (Q.S. Yāsīn, 36:82).[109] Therefore, it is possible for God to exist and the world not to exist. Al-Ghazālī puts this argument as follows:

> ... God is prior to the world and time, that He was and there was no world and that then He was and with Him was the world. The meaning of our statement, "He was and with Him was the world," is only [the affirmation of] the existence of the Creator's essence and the non-existence of the world's essence. And the meaning of our statement, "He was and with Him was the world," is only [the affirmation of] the existence of two essences.[110]

Al-Ghazālī's emphasis on God's divine omnipotence reinstated the problem of theodicy in Islam, which was emphasized by the Ash'arite school of theology in the fourth/tenth century.[111] The formulation of theodicy in Islam was a reaction in particular to the Mu'tazilite school of theology, which asserted God's limited omnipotence with a rationalistic view of divine justice.[112] According to the Ash'arite concept of divine omnipotence, which leads to an occasionalistic view: "God is the only agent; He alone creates actions (*af'āl*)"[113] and "the author of good and evil."[114] Consequently, everything in the world results from the direct and inevitable effect of God's omnipotence and decree.

While al-Ghazālī restates the Ash'arite doctrine of God's omnipotence to prove God's power to create and not to create, his conception of creation was primarily intended to refute Ibn Sīnā's theory of emanation. The latter argues that the whole universe emanated from the Necessary Existent and that it is through this that His essence radiates the Universal Intellect, Soul, Nature, Body, and the multiplicity of the world.[115] Al-Ghazālī for his part opines that Ibn Sīnā's theory of emanation deviated from Islamic belief because the latter's teaching, in his view, does not accord with the Qur'ānic verse, which clearly indicates that "I did not make them witnesses of the creation of the heavens and the earth; and neither do I [have any need to] take as my helpers those [beings] that lead [men] astray (Q.S. al-Kahf, 18:51)."[116]

While the existence and multiplicity of the world have been explained through creation and emanation theories, the creation of human beings is usually said to have originated either "out of something" or "out of nothing." In one instance, the Qur'ān states that human beings are created "out of something." The Qur'ān uses different terms to show the material causes of the creation of human beings. The materials out of which human beings are constituted include cloth (*'alaq*),[117] fluid/water (*mā'*),[118] a drop of sperm (*manī*),[119] a germ-cell (*nuṭfah*),[120] clay (*ṣalṣāl*[121]/*ṭīn*),[122] and dust (*turāb*).[123] In other instances the Qur'ān says that God created human beings out of nothing (*lam taku shay'ā*).[124] There are two other verses, moreover, which are usually cited in support of the notion that human beings were created "out of nothing": "But does man bear in mind that We have created him aforetime out of nothing?" (Q.S. Maryam, 19:67).

(8) [Zachariah] exclaimed: "O my Sustainer! How can I have a son when my wife has always been barren and I have become utterly infirm through old age?"
(9) Answered [the Angel]: "Thus it is; [but] thy Sustainer says , 'This is easy for Me—even as I have created *thee* aforetime out of nothing.' "

(Q.S. Maryam, 19:8–9)

These verses allude to God's power in bringing life into being and in resurrecting human life after death, with the first in particular to allegedly establish the idea that human beings were created "out of nothing" (*lam taku shay'ā*).

Nevertheless, the term "out of nothing" (*lam taku shay'ā*) is debatable. Al-Bayḍāwī interprets the term *lam taku shay'ā* in both verses as "absolute non-existent" (*ma'dūm ṣarfā*)—whereas nonexistent is to be understood as "nothing."[125] Such an interpretation is not surprising, since it accords with the school of thought that holds the theory that creation is from "non-existence" (*ex nihilo*). Another Qur'ānic verse that upholds this theory is: "His being alone is such that when He wills a thing to be, He but says unto it. 'Be'—and it is" (Q.S. Yāsīn, 36:82).

Taking a different view from al-Bayḍāwī, al-Zamakhsharī argues that the phrases "I have created *thee* aforetime out of nothing" and "We have created him aforetime out of nothing?" are to be understood as referring to a condition in which the state of human existence is not even counted.[126] Such an understanding is in line with the ethical message of the following verse in the chapter of Q.S. al-Insān, 91:1, which states:

> Has there not been over Man a long period of Time when he was nothing—
> (not even) mentioned?
> Verily We created Man from a drop of mingled sperm in order to try him: so
> We gave him (the gifts) of Hearing and Sight.[127]

In a similar vein, Asad interprets the statement "as I have created *thee* aforetime out of nothing" as placing an emphasis on God's unlimited power to bring "into being a new chain of causes and effects."[128] The verse "We have created him aforetime out of nothing" is also to be interpreted as "when [or "although"] he was nothing."[129] The meaning of the term '*khalaqa*' in both verses indicates that God created human beings "out of something"—either out of congealed blood, dust, or other related materials. And yet the state of being a parcel of blood, sperm, ova, and dust is not the state of being human. It takes certain actions and an organizing principle to make these potential materials into a human being. Along the same line, al-Alousī argues that these verses (Q.S. al-Insān, 19:8–9 and 67) have nothing to do with the creation of human beings *ex nihilo*.[130]

Chronologically, both the aforementioned verses belong to the Meccan period when the Prophet attempted to elucidate revelation by pointing at numerous instances from nature and history. They treat in particular the signs of God's power in nature and discuss as well the earlier prophets.[131] However, as shown in the previous discussion, philologists and exegetes have arrived at a twofold understanding of the verb '*khalaqa*'—to bring something out of nonexistence and to create something out of something. Even though linguistically the term '*khalaqa*' for the Arabs means "to make or to create" something out of something already existing, such as when the cobbler makes shoes from leather, it was left to the exegetes to transform the meaning of the word '*khalaqa*' into something that supports the theory of creation *ex nihilo*.[132]

To render the term '*khalaqa*' as meaning to create something out of an absolute nonexistence is problematic since it does not give an answer to the question "from what human comes." The Qur'ān proffers its answer by situating the creation of human within its constituents, such as fluid/water (*mā'*), clay (*ṣalṣāl* or *ṭīn*), and dust (*turāb*). For instances, while Q.S. Ṣād, 38:71 mentions that the human beings was created "out of clay" (*khāliqun basharan min ṭīn*), Q.S. al-Ḥijr, 15:26 states that humans are created "out of sounding clay [*ṣalṣāl*] or out of dark slime transmuted [*ḥama'in masnūn*]."[133]

The material cause, such as fluid/water (*mā'*), clay (*ṣalṣāl* or *ṭīn*), and dust (*turāb*) are, indeed, absolute nonexistence with regard to human. The philosophers call the act of giving existence to these absolute nonexistent entities "creation" (*ibdā'*).[134] The existence of human from absolute nonexistence or after nonexistence represents the highest mode of creation because it gives actuality to nonexistence. And actuality is better than nonexistence. It is also called creation because it satisfies the description of giving existence to nonexistence without intermediary. Others, however, may not call it creation since humans come into existence from the First Cause by means of emanation.[135] Transforming fluid/water (*mā'*), clay (*ṣalṣāl* or *ṭīn*), and dust (*turāb*) into humans requires intermediary process by absorbing these material causes into human body to finally function as the efficient cause of generation as will be seen in the Chapter 3.

However, it suffices us to say that the material causes such as fluid/water, clay, and dust are the constituents of human body, which are common to both men and women. Added to this bodily anatomy with its need for subsistence is the moral perfection, knowledge, and leadership, which to a varying degree represent human's disposition to become God's responsible moral agents on the face of the earth. This natural disposition is inherent within men and women, so that they function responsibly as moral agents in their daily life. This view is in line with the universal context of the creation of *khalīfah*, *bashar*, and *al-insān* in that humans share the common origin of humanity, namely self, as follows.

Ontology and human equality

The Qur'ān generally refers to the creation theory out of "one entity" in relation to the equality of all human beings regardless of their gender, race, kinship, tribe, and nation. However, this creation theory is not always offered as an alternative account of human creation since the creation of a woman out of Adam's rib has been repeatedly retold, reiterated, and restated as the only human creation theory in Islamic teaching. This tendency demonstrates that there is a systematic attempt to generate, nurture, and perpetuate the hierarchical principle of women's status, so that women never fully enjoy equality in their social, cultural, and political flourishing. In this section, I propose to examine the ontological equality between men and women from both Qur'ānic and philosophical perspectives.

The creation of humans out of one self (nafs wāḥidah)

The creation of male and female out of one self (*nafs wāḥidah*) is not a novel idea, for it is as old as the Qur'ān itself. What is new, however, is the attempt to reinterpret this creation theory in light of an egalitarian worldview. The basic premise of this theory is that each human being is created out of one single entity and that out of this entity is also created its mate.[136] Wadud-Muhsin, a contemporary American womanist, puts forward the idea that man and woman are created as a pair. Like that first pair, men and women share a "single point of origin" and are endowed with individual moral responsibility to God and to society.[137] Accordingly, the equal status of men and women in society is common to all members of society.

While the Qur'ān represents the continuous theological message of the prophetic tradition in that it was revealed by God to fulfill the true mission of all revealed religions, its depiction of the creation of women departs from the Judeo-Christian tradition. The Qur'ān explicitly mentions that both men and women originated from one soul:

> O mankind! Be conscious of your Sustainer, who has created you out of one living entity, and out of it created its mate, and out of the two spread abroad a multitude of men and women. And conscious of God, whose name you demand [your rights] from one another, and of these ties of kinship. Verily, God is ever watchful over you.
>
> (Q.S. al-Nisā', 4:1)

> It is He who has created you [all] out of one living entity, and out of it brought into beings its mate, so that men might incline with love towards woman. And so, when he has embraced her, she conceives [at first] a light burden, and continues to bear it. Then, when she grows heavy [with child], they both call unto God, their Sustainer, "If Thou indeed grant us a sound [child], we shall most certainly be among the grateful!"
>
> (Q.S. al-A'rāf, 7:189)

The above verses attest to the origin of humankind from one self, one living entity. Asad assigns to the word *nafs* the connotation of "soul, spirit, mind, animate being, living entity, human being, person, self (in the sense of personal identity), humankind, life essence, and so forth . . ." [138]

Interestingly enough, even though these verses profess a sense of human equality in that both male and female originate from the same self (*nafs*), exegetes are divided over how to interpret it. Al-Bayḍāwī[139] and al-Zamakhsharī,[140] for instance, offer two different understandings of the phrase '*min nafs wāḥidah*.'[141] The first relates to the creation of human beings out of one entity, that is, Adam, who was created from dust, and Ḥawwā', who was created out of his rib. The second refers to Adam who was created out of one self or soul, from which Ḥawwā' was made. Such an interpretation is not surprising because the understanding of '*min nafs*' as "the extraction of self from another soul" may be understood to mean that "the first created being (taken to be a male person) was complete, perfect, and superior. The second created being (a woman) was not his equal, because she was taken out of the whole and, therefore, derivative and less than it."[142]

Abduh, however, disagrees with the biblical-minded interpretation of the above verses.[143] He interprets the '*min nafs wāḥidah*' as referring to humankind as much as the common origin of human beings and the equality of all races.[144] This interpretation, although it is in line with the word *nafs* as self, soul, or living entity, is never actually reflected in the Qur'ān, except on one occasion where there is a discussion of the creation of human beings.[145] Like Abduh, Wadud-Muhsin interprets the word '*nafs*' as referring to all human beings. This single entity was the origin of Eve and Adam, whose offspring developed into different tribes, ethnicities, and nationalities with different languages, cultures, and civilizations.

The other idea that supports the interpretation of the common origin of all human beings is the word '*zawj*,' commonly understood as "mate," "spouse," or "pair" as the essential nature of creation. The word "pair" in respect to human beings refers to their origin as "two co-existing forms" of a single living entity.[146] This pair constitutes male and female. Maleness and femaleness are contingent upon one another. Being a male is comprehensible only in relation to the female and vice versa, just as the existence of night is relevant to day, since the Creator has had created all things in pairs (Q.S. 36:36; 51:49). Men and women, therefore, are equal components of humanity.

As men and women share equality in origin and humanity, what constitutes humanity, to a varying degree, demands human plurality, respect for each other and tolerance for differences. While the application of these demands is relative to the operative standard within societies, the universal value of humanity is inherent in any culture. Human is inviolable subject whose existence calls for recognition and protection. The call for recognizing other humans requires all citizens of the world to consider that each human is unique in himself/herself since no human is an exact copy of the other; otherwise, there will be uniformity in what we call humans.

Certainly, the dominant entity quite often defines the subordinate. The dominant religious group actively engages in "othering" religious minority. The dominant race and ethnicity perpetuate their superiority. By the same token, men as a dominant class by social, biological, and cultural construct, have drawn a pattern of humanity that imposes "male humanity" into the female. This pattern, however, fails to recognize what the notion of humanity entails for both men and women. In truth, what has been going on in many parts of the Muslim world is the resilient of othering process directed to women through political, social, and legal policies and practices that keep men as the dominant and women as the subordinate.

In the Muslim world where power and authority are held by the male politicians, policy makers, and religious scholars, they are bound with the duty to call for the recognition of human's plurality, diversity as something intrinsic to humans. The fact that we are born to different parents, races, cultures, languages, religions, nations, and civilization speaks for the condition of plurality, something the Qur'ān has predicted in al-Ḥujurāt, 49:11:

> O men! Behold, We have created you all out of a male and a female, and have made you into nations and tribes, so that you might come to know another. Verily, the noblest of you in the sight of God is the one who is most deeply conscious of Him, Behold, God is all-knowing, all aware.

Diversity, multiplicity, and pluralism in a Muslim's view are part of God's creation, or His intended purpose, designed to ensure so that human beings develop mutual understanding and that they respect differences.

Plurality calls for respect for each other in that one must equally recognize the shared vision that we are all humans. Of course, recognizing humanity that is constituted of differences is easier to say than actually acknowledging it in practice. Humans in one way or an other have engaged in dehumanizing the others, by reducing these others into non-humans along with the flourishing of the derivative institutions that maintain the binary opposition of master/slave, the self/the other, modern/backward, and first world/third world.[147] This view in a larger level of human relation leads to the suppression, control, colonization, occupation, and invasion of the others; in the micro gender relationship, it causes the oppression of women. To avoid a systematic injustice treatment of other human beings, we call upon the recognition of humanity that is inclusive of both men and women because both of them share equal metaphysical self as follows.

The ontological view of the self

The question is whether or not the concept of '*nafs*' (self) lends itself to a discussion of humanity in general. Brison argues that the self at a metaphysical level is "bodily continuity that accounts for personal identity; another, . . . it is continuity of memory, character traits, or other psychological characteristics that makes someone the same person all the time."[148] Like Brison, I argue that the self marks the humanity of human beings. Human beings belong to the same genus as other animals. What marks the difference between human and animal is the self. The presence of the self or soul is equal for both women and men, inasmuch as it consistently marks humanity.

As humans equally share the self, they contain the "same" human identity, for each human being is aware of who he or she is and continues to be himself/herself. Similarly, being male or female does not make any difference, because sexual differentiation is not unique to humans. Animals of the same species display different sexuality as well. In this respect, personal identity continues to persist regardless of one's physical appearance or the change in the skin, hair color, or bodily organs. Of course, such physical changes may change the way one perceives himself or herself, but overall, they do not alter the ontological constitution of the self.

While humans equally share the self (*nafs*) in the sense of humanity, the *nafs* marks the differentia of human from other species. Ibn Sīnā proposes the metaphysical dimension of the self on the basis of his theory of being.[149] His metaphysical proof of the existence of the self can be found in the hypothetical example known as the "Flying Man." According to Marmura, there are different versions of the "Flying Man" in Ibn Sīnā's writings.[150] Nonetheless, what is of interest here is Ibn Sīnā's third version, found in his *al-Ishārāt wa al-Tanbīhāt* (*Remarks and Admonitions*)—one of the late works that probably represents the culmination of his philosophical system. Ibn Sīnā presents this version in a short paragraph under the heading "*tanbīh* (awakening)." This account, which falls under the subtitle "On the Terrestrial and Celestial Soul," reads as follows:

> Return to your self and reflect whether, being whole, or even in another state, where, however, you discern a thing correctly, you would be oblivious to the existence of your self (*dhātaka*) and would not affirm your self *(nafsaka)*? To my mind, this does not happen to the perspicacious—so much so that the sleeper in his sleep and the person drunk in the state of his drunkenness will not miss knowledge of his self, even if his presentation of his self to himself does not remain in his memory.
>
> And if you imagine your self *(dhātaka)* to have been at its first creation mature and whole in mind and body and it is supposed to be in a generity of position and physical circumstance where it does not perceive its parts, where its limbs do not touch each other but are rather spread apart, and that this self is momentarily suspended in temperate air, you will find that it will be unaware of everything except the "fixedness" *(thubūt)* of its individual existence (*ananiyyatihā*).[151]

The purpose of this illustration, according to Marmura, is to prove that self-knowledge is the very core of human cognition.[152] The first *tanbīh*, Marmura explains, implies that the self is immaterial. Another implication is that self-knowledge is "direct, not mediated, on the basis that the example excludes awareness of anything other than the self." The second *tanbīh* signifies that "the self cannot be body since the body is apprehended by the external sense."

Ibn Sīnā acknowledges a twofold dimension of the metaphysics of the soul. At the outset, he establishes the equality of all humans based on their innate recognition of themselves, despite the fact that their embodied self falls apart. The self is also inherent within each human being and makes humans human. The individuality of the self is conjoined with the life of the individual. Brison argues that "a dead body cannot be said to be anyone's self, nor can a living but permanently comatose one."[153] For this reason, Ibn Sīnā remarks that human beings have self-knowledge about who they are regardless of their physical, mental, and psychological states. What marks a person to be a person is therefore "self-consciousness."

Ibn Sīnā's human recognition of oneself is analogous to Adam's and Ḥawwā's self-knowledge. They recognize each other, at least in al-Ṭabarī's account, by acknowledging differences. Ḥawwā' recognized her self-knowledge by acknowledging to Adam that "she is a woman." While she has the full potential to actualize her self-knowledge, the narrative was constructed in such away that Adam was responsible for naming her with Ḥawwā', just like the male members of the family, such as fathers or grandfathers, are assumed to naming babies when they are born.

As the process of naming is constructed within the Muslim culture, women's very existence is conditioned upon the naming culture and its derivative institution. Although women are born as individuals with full potential for self-becoming, men and women experience different socialization of self-knowledge so that they are never equal with respect to their self-becoming in both the private and public spheres. Women's opportunity to the actualization of self-knowledge is hijacked with the multifarious powers that operate at individual, familial, and societal levels.

Had Muslims construed Adam's and Ḥawwā's self-knowledge in terms of their commonalities as humans, they might have generated different discourse of self-knowledge. Certainly, this is the bedrock of the story. Like other humans, Adam's and Ḥawwā' were created in the human forms constituted of material substances. They are endowed with the intellectual, moral, spiritual, and social capabilities to rule the earth as God's vicegerents (*khalīfah*). They ought to make good and responsible choices in order to receive reward. When they did make bad choices and were counted for personal responsibility and accountability. As humans, Adam's and Ḥawwā' were required to reconcile with each other, and at the same times ask for God's repentance. This cycle is also true for Muslim men and women in general.

In addressing the second dimension, Ibn Sīnā demonstrates that men and women have self-knowledge of their own being. This knowledge does not depend on any prior knowledge gained through sensory experiences or activities; rather, they possess self-consciousness, which, in turn, signifies their existence.[154] Human's self-knowledge is not mediated through the sensory medium due to the immateriality of the self in that it does not take form in the human bodily anatomy. However, humans' exposures to the sensory medium can shape what constitute their perception of personal identities.

The immateriality of the self also bestows humans with their intellectual and spiritual heights. With proper training, human's immaterial self is potential to have a direct ascent to the Active Intellect, which is understood by the Ṣūfī to be a direct link to God. It is on this point that Ibn Sīnā's theory of the soul has a mystical connection with the soul's origin, in that the soul knows that her very essence is her existence. This state of personhood reflects humans' ability to be fully conscious of who and what humans are, while having a direct union with God that will allow them to manifest God's attributes. This kind of state does not require any prior experience, but is immediate, direct, and spontaneous. With this in mind, Ibn Sīnā's discussion of the metaphysical dimension of the soul prepares the *'ārif* (the Gnostic mystic) to meet and unite with God as will be discussed in Chapter 5.

Ibn Sīnā's metaphysical discussion of the self sheds a new light on the inherent equality amongst humans. It also complements the concept of equality in human origin, whereby a human being—regardless of sexuality—consists of material substance and immaterial self (*nafs*). This implies that what constitute the common origin is the material substances and the living entity in the human form (*nafs*). These constituents are equal to both men and women, inasmuch as they are of the same kind (genus) and share the same humanity. Humans too have the self-knowledge of their existence regardless of their physical changes in their body and appearance. Even if any part of the body is corrected, transplanted, removed, or undergone any medical procedure, he/she remains who he/she is.

Conclusion

In light of the creation of humans out of one self (*nafs*), I have argued for an inclusive humanity in which all accidental differences, such as race, ethnicity, religion, sexuality, and nationality are acknowledged as components of this humanity. This inclusion accords with the Qur'ānic texts that teach the principle of equality, according to which men and women share the same origin, namely, one self (*nafs wāḥidah*), and are created in pairs. Each member of the pair completes each other, without which humanity would be incomplete. The pairs also constitute humanity as whole. Equality, then, is the main force for establishing equal moral responsibility, since men and women are equally endowed with rights and responsibilities as God's vicegerents on earth.

The equality of human creation—which is the very foundation of an egalitarian gender system—is, unfortunately, little respected as a notion due to the popularity of the theory of humanity's creation out of a male, highlighted in the creation of Adam. Certainly, the Adam story entails the equality of humans in that all humans are, just like Adam, created out of material substance such as dust (Q.S. Āl 'Imrān, 3:59), fluid/water (*mā'*), clay (*ṣalṣāl* or *ṭīn*), and dust (*turāb*). In fact, the Qur'ānic account of the creation of Adam is narrated in relation to the commonalities of humans as expressed in different terminologies such as *khalīfah* (vicegerent), *bashar* (human), and *al-insān* (human), which denote human form and perfect faculties.

Despite the Qur'ānic account of the universality of the creation theories, they are schematized within conditional universalism. This is to say that, while the Qur'ān speaks of a particular archetype of human creation in the form of Adam, Muslims use this model to generate a universal claim, as if all humans are created out of a male father. This premise is at odds with the Qur'ānic version of human origin from material substances such as fluid/water (*mā'*), clay (*ṣalṣāl* or *ṭīn*), and dust (*turāb*) and self (*nafs wāḥidah*). The Qur'ān also speaks of how humans beget humans (through which the generative self is inherited from parents), whose sexual difference is necessary for the perpetuation of humanity.

Regrettably, the Adam and Eve story generates a genre of knowledge, a gender system and a constitution of the self that is male derived. The biological difference even entails the hallmark of what it means to be human, from which it follows that men's and women's roles are constructed on the basis of natural-biological disposition. This sexual difference not only shapes the making of the hierarchical gender system, but also dictates what constitutes the self and humanity. The perpetuation of such a system is buried deep within patriarchal Muslim cultures, where maintaining a division of labor based on sex is the rule in both the private and public spheres.

An assumed unequal humanity has become the underlying principle of hierarchical gender system in the Muslim world. This existing practice hinders women from having access to religious interpretation, knowledge, education, public life, and even the most private aspects of life, namely, sexual relationships. Women often have no say in deciding whether or not to have sex. This situation is condoned by the assumption that, while men and women are complementary in procreation, they do not contribute equally to the production of a new human being—a view that we will discuss in Chapter 3.

3 The transmission of generative self and women's contribution to conception

This chapter examines the conflicting claims of parental role in conception and their impact on the self and gender construct. I argue that neither the Qur'ān nor the ḥadīth establishes male superiority in reproduction. There is no specific verse that categorically declares male superiority in reproduction; likewise, no verse signifies the inferiority of women in conception. The Qur'ān depicts the parental roles in reproduction in a complementary manner in that men and women produce the generative self in the form of sperm and egg (the material causes necessary for generation) and explains how those materials develop in the womb of the mother. The Qur'ān also views the roles of male and female in conception as equal: unless they both contribute to procreation, reproduction would be impossible.

Almost ignoring the actual Qur'ānic account of the conception of human beings, the interpretative tradition on the Qur'ān declares male superiority in conception. There are three primary assumptions that perpetuate the inequality of men and women in reproduction: (1) the male superiority in human reproduction; (2) women's intended purpose as reproducers; and (3) the wives as husbands' tilth. These three assumptions along with other religious, social, cultural, and political apparatus are imposed on women's bodies to the extent that women are valued only as reproducers. It follows that women's roles are constructed according to their reproductive organs.

Let's address the three assumptions one by one. First, the notion of male superiority in human reproduction is often the result of interpretation of some verses of the Qur'ān independently of other related verses. For example, the verses that states that male and female are created out of a mere drop of sperm (Q.S. al-Najm, 53:45–46) are repeatedly held up as the foundation of male superiority in reproduction.[1] Based on these verses, Albar, a contemporary Saudi scholar, draws two conclusions: (1) that the male's semen determines the sex of the fetus because male and female are formed out of "semen ejected from men"; and (2) that only a small portion of seminal fluid is necessary for generation.[2] While both assertions are scientifically proven, the male's sperm (*manī al-rijāl*) is regarded as central to the whole reproduction process as if the female contribution does not count at all.

The male's sperm (*manī al-rijāl*) is considered to be the life-giving element in shaping a new individual, whereas the female's egg is merely the material upon which the sperm works. The effect of the interpretation that the male's semen is the prime determinant in forming a new being has been transformed into the public perception that the male's role in conception is far superior to and greater than the female's. Given the hierarchical manner in which the role of women is conceptualized, it is therefore predictable that the female role in the reproduction of a human being should be seen as inferior. This assertion circulates not only within religious circles, but also finds support in philosophical discussion of the parental contribution to conception.

Second, while it takes both a man and a woman to produce a new individual, the compatibility between male and female occurs "only" in reproduction, with the emphasis on the role of women as reproducers. This role stems from the assumption that women's primary *raison d'être*, that is, the purpose for which they are created, is to serve as the "place" for men to repose and multiply. The most fitting role for women, therefore, in many cultures and religious traditions, and not just Muslim culture, is not far removed from her biological state as either a mother or a wife. The cultural and social perception of mothering and wifehood in turn becomes one of the essential elements in the perpetuation of the patriarchal system in Muslim communities.

This view brings us to the third assumption: that male–female compatibility does not suggest equality in conception, for a wife in Muslim societies supposedly functions "as a tilth" for a husband (Q.S. al-Baqarah, 2:223). This verse is often interpreted to mean that husbands can demand sexual favors from their wives anytime they want to. They do not need to be considerate about their wives' feelings, desires, and satisfactions. The existing assumption and practice not only regard women as sexual objects, but also give men the power to assert their sexual drive at their convenience. Because women are treated as the objects of sexual pleasure, they have no say in their reproductive rights. Certainly, this practice does not reflect the ethics of the Qur'ān, which postulates a spiritual relationship between men and women as the essential basis for sexual relations, as the verse al-Baqarah, 2:223 requires men to purify their "selves" before actually engaging in intimacy with their wives.

> Your wives are your tilth; go, then, unto your tilth as you may desire, but first provide something for your souls, and remain conscious of God, and know that you are destined to meet Him. And give glad tidings unto those who believe.

Quite contrary to the above assumptions, I will argue that women's contribution to conception is as essential as men's and that the view of the male as the originator and motivator of human generation is not theologically, philosophically, or even scientifically sound. Both men and women are the principles of generation in that they produce and pass down the generative self in the form of sperm and egg necessary for the formation of a new individual. The fact that the male's sperm determines the sex of a new being does not imply the superiority of one over the other. With this in mind, I will discuss the Qur'ānic and philosophical views of the female's contribution in conception and the way in which the fetus develops in the womb. I will also discuss the resilience of the politics of reproduction that produce and reproduce the view of women as reproducers.

Female's roles in conception: an Islamic philosophical view and its Greek heritage

The question of how both male and female come into being has preoccupied the minds of Muslim thinkers ever since the advent of Islam. The Qur'ān straightforwardly asserts that God is the source of all human being.[3] God is the Creator and humans are His creatures, as is made clear in Q.S. al-An'ām, 6:2, "He is who has created you out of clay and then has decreed a term [for you]—a term known only to him."[4] The Qur'ānic emphasis on the common origin of human beings therefore depends to a large extent on their created nature. While God retains His role as the active agent in the creation process, men and women are, however, fully responsible for making it happen.

I argue that even though the Qur'ān envisions an equal role in reproduction, in that parents pass down the generative self, Muslim exegetes and philosophers have utilized the Qur'ān to justify their belief in the male superiority in conception. While both camps have an interest in common with regards to male dominance in reproduction, they normally use different criteria in articulating most matters of doctrine, including the issue of reproduction. The exegetes produce their arguments based on their interpretation of the Qur'ān, whereas the Muslim philosophers and biologists embark on reconciling the scriptural and philosophical traditions by giving them both rational justifications. In so doing, they develop a theory of reproduction primarily using Greek science and philosophy, hoping to demonstrate that human knowledge does not conflict with God's revelation. Only when they encounter irreconcilable differences on reaching their final conclusions, would philosophers have to choose between philosophical reasoning and religious justification.

Like early scholars, contemporary Muslim thinkers continue to argue whether Islam and science are dichotomous or compatible.[5] This debate goes along with the rapid development of Western scientific discoveries and Muslims' attempts to regain their identity in the post-colonial period. Hoodhboy, for instance, argues that the Qur'ānic verses are not compatible with modern science because science "begins with the assumption that there exist facts."[6] The Qur'ān's perennial Truth cannot, therefore, be explained in terms of scientific truth, which is abstracted from experiment and conditioned by the expected assumption. By contrast, Sadar argues that, although the primary theme of the Qur'ān is God and His Creation, it teaches scientific topics, such as cosmology (Q.S. Yāsīn, 36:37–40), meteorology (Q.S. Yūnus, 10:5–6), or biology (Q.S. al-Ḥajj, 22:5), which often accords with scientific discoveries.[7] The compatibility between the Qur'ān and science is expected since the Qur'ān is supposed to permeate human life, including the human quest for scientific discovery.

In line with the preceding view, I certainly believe that scientific and philosophical truth is useful in understanding the Qur'ān. By this, I do not mean to impose scientific truth on the truth of the Qur'ān; rather, scientific findings can be utilized as an alternative explanation of the "scientific truth" of the Qur'ān. Muslims' quest for scientific truth concurs with the Qur'ānic call for humans to use their intellect to comprehend the macrocosm and microcosm as the signs of God: "and among his wonders is the creation of heaven and the earth, and the diversity of your tongues and colours: for in this, behold, there are messages indeed for all who are possessed of [innate] knowledge" (Q.S. al-Rūm, 30:22).

As the primary question of reproduction in philosophy and science centers on the degree to which women contribute to conception, it naturally attracted much attention from the Greek natural scientists and philosophers.[8] The Hippocratic writings, for instance, propose a theory that male and female both contribute their seed to conception; otherwise the child would never resemble either or both of them.[9] According to Aristotle, in animals with red blood, the female provides either egg or menstrual fluid as the matter for generation, and the male provides semen, which conveys the moving cause and form to the matter.[10] Four centuries later, Galen augments the Hippocratic perspective with his interpretation of the ovaries in female reproductive organs as the source of female semen.[11] Certainly, Aristotle knew about ovaries and knew that they produced eggs in birds. However, he could not see the mammalian ovum, and because he could not see it, he did not think that it existed.

The various Greek arguments about the respective parental contributions to conception were generally available to Muslim philosophers by way of translations. One philosopher who availed himself of this information was Ibn Sīnā, who considerably advanced the discussion of the issue. Like Hippocrates and Galen, Ibn Sīnā believes that the female seed, like the male semen, is equally important to the process. However, following Aristotle, he considers the female seed to be the menstrual blood.[12] In *al-Ḥayawān*, section 8 of *al-Ṭabī'iyyāt* of *al-Shifā'*, Ibn Sīnā maintains that what is called semen is the same for men and women in that it comes from blood which is liable to alter. The term "semen" itself, though it was commonly used at that time to refer to both male and female reproductive principles, could not be applied to both of them. If male seed is called semen, the other cannot be called semen in the same sense.

Because Ibn Sīnā identifies the menstrual blood as the female seed, he assigns different parental contributions in conception. He reiterates the Aristotelian premise of generation in that the female seed provides the matter, whereas the male seed functions as the principle of movement.[13] For instance, he depicts how men and women contribute differently to procreation.[14] A similar discussion can also be seen in his *Canon of Medicine*, where he explains the extent to which the origin of human beings comes from both male and female sperm, with each contributing in a different manner:

> The human being takes its origin from two things—1) the male sperm, which plays the part of "factor" [efficient cause]; 2) the female sperm, . . . which provides the matter. Each of these is fluid and moist, but there is more wateriness and terrene substance in the female blood and the female sperm, whereas air and igneity are predominant in the male sperm.[15]

While Ibn Sīnā recognizes the male and female contributions to the process of generation, he fails to articulate the kinds of male and female seed that act upon the creation of human beings.[16] In fact, Ibn Sīnā's theory of human origin, just like that of Aristotle, presupposes the superiority of male to female sperm in that he associated male sperm with the "factor" or "initiator" of the movement, and the female sperm with the matter upon which male sperm acted.

Ibn Sīnā's view of male superiority in procreation should not come as a surprise, since he shares with Aristotle the belief that individual substance is composed of form and matter.[17] Form is the nature of a thing and acts as the principle or initiator of change, whereas matter is what receives the changes.[18] While Aristotle believes that a human being is a combination of form and matter, he again correlates form to man and matter to woman: "... the female always provides the material, the male that which fashions it, for this is the power that each possesses, and this is what it is for them to be male and female."[19] Aristotle assumes that the natural differences between men and women are determined.[20] For this reason, it becomes necessary for the form to come from men, and matter from women.

Like Aristotle, Ibn Sīnā also applies the metaphor of hot and cold to generation. Ibn Sīnā tacitly identifies light and hot with men, and heavy and cool with women. Such contraries should be expected, since Ibn Sīnā maintains that opposition is what constitutes unity and multiplicity. This opposition is also appropriate to the different natures of men and women. Even though Ibn Sīnā does not clearly state that women are the opposite of men, it can be inferred from the way he associates heat to men and cold to women in procreation. Heat never turns out to be cold, even though warmth is removed from that state. It also true for cold. Cold will remain, despite any attempt to replace it. Ibn Sīnā illustrates this opposition as privation—"a condition of a thing which is replaced by another condition to the extent to which the condition of privation leaves the thing."[21] As hot refers to the male nature and cold to the female, woman is the privation of man—in a sense, she is the negation of man.

Ibn Sīnā's primary opposition between hot and cold, in particular, and the contraries in general, has its origin in Pythagorean philosophy:

> Other members of this same school say there are ten principles, which they arrange in two columns of cognates—limit and unlimited, odd and even, one and plurality, right and left, male and female, resting and moving, straight and curved, light and darkness, good and bad, square and oblong.[22]

Moreover, like the Pythagoreans, Ibn Sīnā sees the contraries as the principles of things. The assignment of hot to male and cold to female is essential to explaining the principles of human generation. It is inevitable then that two causes or principles of generation should be framed, namely, matter and the source of movement. This is also the case for Aristotle who classifies men and women as contraries, just like the opposition between hot and cold. Aristotle explains:

> But the male and female are distinguished by a certain capacity and incapacity. (For the male is that which can concoct and form and discharge a semen carrying with it the principle of form... but the female is that which receives semen, but cannot form it or discharge it). And all concoctation work by means of heat. Therefore the male of animals must needs be hotter than the females. For it is by reason of cold and incapacity that the female is more abundant in blood in certain parts of her anatomy.[23]

Aristotle relates cold to female and hot to male. This theory, according to Allen, probably derives from the Hippocratic School, which held that males of all species are warmer and drier and females "moister and cooler."[24]

The premise that "heat is the fundamental principle in the perfection of animals" eventually becomes the center of Aristotle's generation process and his biology in general.[25] The more heat the animals are able to produce, the more they will likely contribute to the process of generation. On this assumption, it becomes necessary for Aristotle to show that males produce more heat than females. The presence of heat and cold relate to the different natures of blood detected in men and women.[26] Blood is circulated to all parts of the body. The residue of blood in its most refined nature is semen and the menstrual discharge.[27] Semen comes from the blood and its color is thick and white.[28] The whiteness and the thickness of the semen is the result of a proper concoction when "the body whence it issues was hot."[29] It also has "a quantity of hot air in it because of the internal heat."[30]

Unlike semen, the menstrual fluid is discharged from the female body. However, since females are naturally weaker animals and their blood is less concocted,[31] they do not produce semen. Women are also weak because they by nature have only a little share of heat. For this reason a woman is like a prepubescent boy in form, as the latter does not yet emit semen. Aristotle states that "The woman is as were an impotent male, for it is through a certain incapacity that female is female, being incapable of concocting the nutriment in its last stage into semen... owing to the coldness of her nature."[32] Aristotle argues that the presence of heat in males is greater than it is in females. Consequently, the male semen becomes the active principle, which is the source of movement, whereas the menstrual blood is the passive principle that provides matter.

Aristotle further explains that menstrual discharge "is analogous in females to the semen in males."[33] He reasons that "the semen begins to appear in males and to be emitted at the same times of life that the menstrual flow begins in females" and that "the generative power fails in the one sex and the menstrual discharge in the other"[34] at about the same time for each as well. Here, Aristotle is right in pointing out that the male's and female's ability to emit "seed" correlates with the fertile period of reproduction.[35] However, he is incorrect in equating the semen with menstrual discharge. Semen (seminal fluid) is produced whenever men ejaculate, while menstruation occurs every month and has nothing to do with sexual intercourse. Instead, Aristotle seems to be assuming here that something analogous to male semen would come out of the female if there were only enough stimulation.[36]

Since Aristotle incorrectly assumes that both semen and the menstrual discharge are similar, he calls both of them "*sperma*," which want "to be this sort of nature: the first 'from what' in the generation of natural constructions."[37] The phrase "from what" implies that the generation process does not come from the parents equally, because the female does not contribute semen to the reproductive process, but provides the matter in the nature of the menstrual flow.[38] Preus simplifies Aristotle's argument as follows: "the female is weaker, and therefore less active; that which is acted upon is matter; therefore is likely to produce the matter for generation."[39]

Ibn Sīnā also treats the issues of semen and menstrual blood in Aristotelian fashion. The semen for him is the final residue of nutriment. It is a well-concocted residue, which becomes white due to its maturity. Like semen, menstrual blood is also a final digestive residue. However, the nature of her semen is not as well-concocted as that of men. It does not reach its maturity, as does the male semen. This theory was readily accepted since women are generally regarded as physically inferior to men. Women, for instance, have fewer hereditary dispositions, have less muscle, and have a slighter physical build. Even if women were fatter and produced more residue, they still could not concoct the nutriment as well.[40]

Like Aristotle, Ibn Sīnā mentions that the generation process, according to philosophical understanding, is comparable to the manufacture of cheese: "Thus the male sperm is equivalent to the clotting of milk, and the female 'sperm' is equivalent to coagulum of milk."[41] Ibn Sīnā's analogy of cheese refers to Aristotle's analogy of milk: "in the coagulation of milk, the milk being the material, the fig-juice or rennet is that which contains the curdling principle, so acts the secretion of the male, being divided into the parts in the female."[42]

Again, Ibn Sīnā reiterates Aristotle's belief that the male element is more important in determining the generation process:

> The generative faculty is two-fold. (i) That which gives rise to the male and female "sperm," the reproductive units, (ii) the formative power (i.e., in the male element) which separate from one another the various faculties in the sperm and rearranges them in such a way that each member (and tissue) receives the temperament appropriate to it—thus, to nerve, its distinctive temperament. The one "sperm," apparently homogenous, open out in all these directions. This is called *primary* transformative faculty.[43]

Ibn Sīnā indicates that while both male and female sperm are the tools of reproduction, male sperm is the more dominant of the two because it acts upon the other sperm. The male element is also a formative power in that it acts upon matter. This faculty is able to transmute the material cause of reproduction from its formal state into an embryo.

One may recall Aristotle's explanation of how the semen acts as the source of movement. If the female provides the matter, then what exactly does the male contribute to generation? Aristotle uses a different analogy to answer it.

> But the female, as female, is passive, and the male, as male, is active, and the principle of the movement comes from him . . . the one being active and motive and the other passive and moved, that one thing which is produced comes from them only in the sense in which a bed comes into being from the carpenter and the wood, or in which a ball comes into being from the wax and the form.[44]

In these passages, Aristotle makes a comparison between works of art and works of nature.[45] In one analogy, he explains that a carpenter may be seen as the form, and the wood on which he works as the matter. Neither the carpenter nor any part of him becomes a material part of the bed as the product; on the contrary, the carpenter's soul and knowledge become tools necessary for causing different movements to produce different products.[46] In a similar way, the male semen functions as a tool, which has "motion in actuality."[47] Indeed, Aristotle at some points acknowledges, "the mixture of the menstrual fluid with the semen will generate the offspring."[48] Nevertheless, he intends to show that the nature of semen is just such a principle of motion, which becomes the tool to act upon matter. The movement that brings the matter as potential being into actual being is "set up by the male parent."[49]

Ibn Sīnā uses a quite different argument to explain Aristotle's statement, according to which the semen neither mixes with the menstrual blood nor becomes part of the embryo.[50] He maintains that the semen mixes with the menstrual blood in the sense that semen functions as the efficient cause that gives a new life its form, while menstrual blood provides the matter to work upon.[51] Following conception, the male semen evaporates and does not become part of the embryo. The parts of an embryo develop on the other hand by virtue of the menstrual blood coming from the mother.[52]

Both Ibn Sīnā and Aristotle believe that the male element is dominant in the generation process, although the former's theory differs in some respects from the latter's. Ibn Sīnā describes women's contribution to the reproduction process in the following terms:

> Just as the beginning of the clotting is in the milk, so the beginning of the clotting of the form of man lies in the female "sperm." Then, just each of the two—the rennet and the milk—enter into the "substance" of the cheese which results, so each of the two—male and female sperm—enters into the "substance" of the "embryo."[53]

Aristotle insists that women do not contribute semen to generation, only the matter of the menstrual flow,[54] whereas Ibn Sīnā correctly assumes that "female organs carr[y] the semen to the site of the conception."[55]

Moreover, while Ibn Sīnā and Aristotle share common ground with respect to the idea of the soul as the source of the nutritive and generative faculty,[56] they have different opinions with respect to the idea of "rational human soul." Mind (*nous*) or the rational power of the soul is Aristotle's biggest problem and he remains ambiguous about it.[57] He questions "when and how and whence" the soul that is required by those animals who share it comes into being.[58] While Aristotle denies that it would be impossible for it to exist prior to the body, to mix with the body, and to enter from outside,[59] he seems to suggest that the rational soul comes from outside "for the reason alone to enter and alone to be divine, for no bodily activity has any connexion with the activity of the reason."[60] Both come from the semen as he notes in the following passage:

> Let us return to the material of the semen, in and with which is emitted the principle of the soul. Of this principle, there are two kinds; the one is not connected with matter, and belongs to those animals in which is included something divine (to wit, what is called reason), while the other is inseparable from matter.[61]

Like Aristotle, Ibn Sīnā understands the soul as constituting "the earthly or corporeal soul, the perfection of corporeal body, which is in its instrument; the source of all those faculties upon which movements and various bodily operations depend."[62] He also believes that the soul cannot exist prior to the body.[63] Nevertheless, Ibn Sīnā has a firmer idea of the origin of the soul (human rational soul). In *Kitāb al-Najāt*, he elucidates the process of how the soul is implanted from outside whenever the body is ready to receive it. After all elements—derived from male and female sperm—are blended proportionately and harmoniously, "other beings also come into existence out of them due to the power of heavenly bodies."[64] Ibn Sīnā further shows how the soul originates from the source outside the body. He states

> the body and the temperament are an accidental cause of the soul, for when the matter of a body suitable to become the instrument of the soul and its proper subject comes into existence, the separate causes bring into being the individual soul, . . . And the being of the soul does in fact emanate from something different from the body and the bodily functions, as we have shown; its source of emanation must be something different from the body.[65]

While Ibn Sīnā's theory of generation is delivered in the terminology of Aristotelian philosophy, he is not able to disentangle himself from the general discussion of the theory of creation of human beings in Islam. Ibn Sīnā's idea of the male sperm as the starting point of the generation process has affinity with the following Qur'ānic verses:

> (37) Was he [*al-insān*] not once a [mere] drop of sperm that had been split.
> (38) And thereafter became a germ-cell—whereupon He created and formed [it] in accordance with what [it] was meant to be,
> (39) and fashioned out of it the two sexes, the male and the female[66]

The above verses illustrate that part of the male sperm constitutes the becoming of a new individual being. Even though Ibn Sīnā admits that male sperm is the initiator of procreation, he argues that male and female are equally important to the process, since parts of the man's and woman's sperm constitute the origin of an individual human being.

Like Ibn Sīnā who regards, to a great degree, both men's and women's contributions to procreation as equally important, Aristotle too believes that both male and female are the principles of generation to the extent that they contribute differently to the procreative activity.[67] This perspective is remarkable because Aristotle's theories of reproduction expressed in *Generation of Animals* Books I and II, which assign the male parent a more significant role than that of the female parent, have become the target of feminist criticism.[68] This criticism finds ample material to object to:

> The form which Aristotle says is contributed to the developing animal offspring by the father, the male parent, is in his view more important and more superior to the matter, which in his theory, is contributed by the mother, the female parent.
> (729a10–12, 730a26–27,732a4–10, 738b20–28)

> The male parent is said to be the source of three of the four causes that contribute to the coming to be of the offspring: the formal, efficient or moving, and the final cause or end. The female contributes only the matter.
>
> (cf. above passages and 641a21–43)[69]

Nevertheless, some scholars argue that Aristotle's *Generation of Animals* is not fully responsible for advocating the female's inferior status in reproduction. Aristotle attempts in this work to "solve a group of problems which are central for biology"—and philosophy as well,[70] because both are concerned with the origins of life. Along the same lines, Tress asserts that in Book I Aristotle demonstrates "male and female are both the principles of generation," especially as they are "anatomically fitted for the work of generating offspring"; their contribution, therefore, should be seen as "causally efficacious."[71] In Book II Aristotle investigates the generation of animals from the standpoint of metaphysical causality, in that he reckons generation to consist of four causes:

> (1) the final cause, " 'that for the sake of which' a thing exists, considered as its 'end' "; (2) the formal cause, the logos of the thing's essence (725a4–5). . . . (3) The material cause is "the matter for the thing" (715a6). . . . (4) The moving cause is "that from which comes the principle of the thing's movement" (715a6).[72]

In his *Metaphysics*, Aristotle offers a more lucid explanation of generation in his metaphysical system:

> When one inquires what is the cause, one should, as causes are spoken of in several senses, state all the possible causes. E.g. what is the material cause of man? The Menstrual fluid. What is the moving cause? The *semen*. The formal cause? His essence. The final cause? His end.[73]

In light of the above passages, it is obvious that Aristotle enhances the way in which a mother contributes to reproduction, especially since in his day "preformation"—the view that the mother does not contribute to generation—was widely held to be true.[74]

While Ibn Sīnā's intellectual debt on the generation of human beings to Aristotle is clear, he creates his own theory of how the generative self comes into being. Ibn Sīnā believes that both partners contribute to procreation. This view is parallel to the statement of the Qur'ān that "We created human [*al-insān*] out of a drop of sperm intermingled [*nuṭfah amshāj*]" (Q.S. al-Insān, 76:2). The intermingled sperm is the combination of sperm and ovum in the female uterus. Yet the procreative process is still not perfect until the soul is implanted into the potential body. Such a formative power is the "soul or nature—that which is in the decree of Allah (*amr Allāh*)."[75] In this sense, Ibn Sīnā echoes the position of Islam: that humans provide the materiality of generative self and God ensouls this new individual. Body and soul become the composite of all humans.

The politics of gender and reproduction in the post-Ibn Sīnān period

Among the philosophers who came after Ibn Sīnā, Ibn Rushd (d. 1198), al-Ghazālī (d. 1111), and Ibn Qayyim al-Jawziyyah (d. 1350) attempt to advocate the complementary roles of men and women in procreation. While Ibn Sīnā and Aristotle accentuate the philosophical import of the material causes, like sperm and egg, the post-Ibn Sīnān philosophers highlight the importance of the mixing generative materials from parents as the starting point of the procreation. Despite these differences, the Greek philosophical views on the generation of human being rejuvenate Muslims' quest to understand the way in which the generative self materializes into being.

Like Ibn Sīnā, Ibn Rushd believes that both male sperm and the menstrual blood are the agents of a new creation. Like Aristotle and Ibn Sīnā, he posits a similar theory respecting the superiority of male sperm. He regards the latter as the originator of generation in that it can potentially act and can be a cause in actuality.[76] In his *Metaphysics*, he asserts that

> For instance we can say that menstrual blood is the matter of the man and that man begets man; we can also say Zayd begets 'Amr, his son, and that menstrual blood of this woman is the matter of this individual person.[77]

As the male sperm gives the form to a new creation, the female sperm provides the matter. The union of the form and the matter produces a new individual being.

Even though Ibn Rushd relies on Aristotle's explanation of reproduction, the former nonetheless emphasizes the equality between male and female in procreation. He suggests that male and female sperm complement each other in the generation process; otherwise it would be impossible to produce a new creation.[78] The significance of both male and female in reproduction is seen in pregnancy, which occurs as a result of the sexual act, even if such an action happens without pleasure and "orgasm."[79] At this point, Ibn Rushd attempts to prove that the conception of an animal takes place in the womb where the male semen and the blood, which are both hot and moist, are mixed.[80] Ibn Rushd's emphasis on the mixing of these fluids is intended to prove that both entities change in quantity and quality into another entity, which in turn forms a new being. For this reason, even though he agrees with the Aristotelian theory of reproduction, he believes that the new individual starts when male and female fluids are mixed in the mother's womb. At the same time, he wants to criticize Aristotle who maintains that woman, unlike man, does not contribute sperm to the procreation process.

Unlike Ibn Sīnā and Ibn Rushd, who lay out their theory of generation in Aristotelian terms, al-Ghazālī (d. 1111) depicts the male and female contribution to procreation as complementary. After a man ejaculates semen, it will be mixed with the female secretion in the uterus. In this sense, both parents produce the generative self that carries human form and its genetic code. The mixing semen and egg will then be condensed to become a clot.[81] The coming of a new life depends on whether the parents decide to mix the male sperm and the female secretion or whether they choose to withdraw before its blending. If they choose the first option, it is clearly their intention to fuse these creative principles. A woman's role here is portrayed as particularly significant in carrying the zygote in the uterus. Therefore, men and women complement each other in the sexual act since such activity requires the instruments of their sexual organs.

Like al-Ghazālī, Ibn Qayyim al-Jawziyyah (d. 1350) sees an equal parental contribution in conception.[82] In his *Tuḥfah*, Ibn Qayyim describes the semen as coming from all parts of the body.[83] Here Ibn Qayyim's opinion is in line with Hippocrates' notion in *On Generation* that "[t]he sperm of the human male comes from all the humours in the body: it consists of the most potent part which is secreted from the rest."[84] At the same time, Ibn Qayyim rejects Aristotle's theory that male semen comes from the residue of the blood.[85]

Ibn Qayyim further notes in his *al-Tibyān* that the female contributes semen to conception, out of which God creates the child.[86] To support his opinion, he reiterates Umm Salamah's discussion with her husband, the Prophet Muḥammad, on the question of whether or not women should take a bath after a nocturnal emission:[87]

> Umm Salama said, "O Allah's Apostle! Verily Allah is not shy of (telling you) the truth. Is it essential for a woman to take a bath after she had a wet dream (nocturnal sexual discharge)?" He said, "Yes, if she notices discharge." On that Umm Salama laughed and said, "Does a woman get a (nocturnal sexual) discharge?" He said, "How then does (her) son resemble her (his mother)?"[88]

This ḥadīth clearly establishes the presence of the female seed from which the resemblance and heredity of the mother is transmitted. With this in mind, Ibn Qayyim's treatment of the female seed has an affinity with both Hippocrates and Galen who argue for the existence of female semen. Conversely, he also disagrees with the Aristotelian principle that the female does not have semen.[89]

Ibn Qayyim's general treatment of an equal contribution to reproduction is in accordance with Islamic teaching. There are two verses of the Qur'ān, as mentioned earlier, showing that a new individual results from the fertilization of sperm and the female secretion. The Qur'ānic verses al-Ṭāriq, 86:6–7 declare that human beings are created "out of a seminal fluid [*mā' dāfiq*] issuing from between the loins [of man] and the pelvic arch of [woman],"[90] whereas the Qur'ānic verse *al-Insān*, 76:2 states that humankind (*al-Insān*) is created out of *nuṭfah amshāj* (the mingled "sperm"). Both verses draw attention to the fact that it takes both the male sperm and the female secretion to create a zygote, which will eventually become a new human being.

Ibn Qayyim's discussion of the equal parental contribution to conception brings up the issue of hereditary traits. The new individuals will at some point inherit hereditary characteristics from their parents. In fact, Ibn Qayyim uses the issue of the resemblance between the child and the parents to prove the equal contribution of parents in conception. Interestingly, he uses Hippocratic writings to explain the idea of resemblance as narrated in the following ḥadīth:

> As for the resemblance of the child to its parents: If a man has sexual intercourse with his wife and gets discharge first, the child will resemble the father, and if the woman gets discharge first, the child will resemble her.[91]

Hippocrates in "On Generation" writes: "If any part of the father's body a greater quantity of sperm is derived from the corresponding part of the mother's body the child will, in that part, bear a closer resemblance to its father . . . ."[92] Similarly, if the female semen is of greater quality than the male sperm, the child will resemble his/her mother.[93] Ibn Qayyim's point of resemblance is to show the parental contribution in reproduction. In his *al-Tibyān*, he argues that the semen is the totality of the humidity and the residue of the body—qualities that belong to both men and women.[94] By virtue of the mix between the male and female semen, a new offspring is formed. If the semen does not come from both parents, how is it possible that the new individual should resemble his/her mother or the latter's ancestors?

Even though Ibn Qayyim's argument on the resemblance issue appears to be very convincing, the concept can also be discussed even if the parents' contribution is unequal. Aristotle, for instance, observes that the transmission of hereditary qualities is expected in that

> Naturally then it is most likely that the characteristics of the male and of the father will go together, whether they prevail or are prevailed over. For the difference between them is small so that there is no difficulty in both concurring . . . Hence, for the most part the male offspring resemble the father, the female the mother . . . But if the movement coming from the male principle prevails, . . . or vice versa, the result is that male children are produced resembling the mother and the female children resembling the father.[95]

This is also the case because Aristotle maintains that the female does not have semen. He believes that the power of movement of the male semen forms and shapes the matter so that it eventually develops as the parts of the fetus. It is very likely then that the fetus will inherit either the hereditary characteristics of one side of the family or the other, or have a resemblance in different ways to both parents.

In the European Renaissance, while Muslims' philosophical inquiry into the generation of human beings declined, European scholars' interest in Aristotle's theory of hereditary traits increased. Harvey, for instance, was among the foremost to discuss the transmission of hereditary characteristics from both parents. Like Aristotle, he studied different embryos, and especially the embryo of the chick, by means of simple lenses.[96] His observations, however, led him to a different conclusion from Aristotle's. While Aristotle proposes that an embryo depends on the male semen for its efficient cause of reproduction and the female menstrual fluid for its matter, Harvey concludes that the original conception comes from both parents equally. His statements specifically refer to the conception of the chick in that the hen and the cock are the necessary principles of generation and are equally efficient in the work of reproduction.[97]

Harvey's discovery of the equal parental contribution in reproduction somehow marks the advent of the study of heredity in modern biology. Heredity usually is understood as a mixture of genes coming from both parents. It was Mendel who introduced the study of heredity in a quantitative, experimental, and analytical form in 1865.[98] While Mendel's experimentation was limited to plants, his observation of the remarkable pattern that reappeared in fertilization demonstrated the transmission of the characteristics of hybrids to their offspring.[99] Mendel's main contribution was his initial step in demonstrating how the germ-cell of the parents becomes an agent in determining hereditary characteristics, with no cause of marked disturbance of the characteristics passed on by the parents to their offspring.[100] The carrier of the hereditary characteristics is then called a gene.[101] Mendel's postulation of the separation of genes led to further investigation of "the parallelism between chromosome behavior and gene segregation" by Boveri (1904), Sutton (1903), and others.[102] Morgan, for instance, demonstrates the linkage by studying sex-linked mutants where the linkage of genes results from being transmitted by the same chromosome. He suggests that genes lying in close proximity to one another in a chromosome would be more often coupled than those at a greater distance from each other.[103]

In contemporary biology, research on heredity is far more advanced. It has reached a stage where the composition of the gene of a new individual is more predictable than ever. The new individual starts at fertilization in which the sperm (spermatozoon) or a male gamete, mixes with an ovum (oocyte), or a female gamete, molding into a single cell or a zygote (*zygōtos*) in the process.[104] This zygote carries the chromosomes and genes that are inherited from each parent. Both father and mother contribute an equal amount of chromosomes and genes to the zygote, even in the case of sex chromosomes (X and Y).[105] The composition of the union of those chromosomes determines the sex of the fetus. Hamilton and Mossman state that

> If a sperm with 22 + X chromosomes unites with an ovum with 22 + X chromosomes the total number will be 44 + X + X, giving rise to female zygote. On the other hand, if a sperm with 22 + Y chromosomes unites with an ovum with 22 + X chromosomes the total number will be 44 + X + Y chromosomes and a male will result.[106]

It is clear, therefore, that the new creation is a union of the heredity of the mother and the father, and of all the ancestors who have come before. The new individual being receives the components of the genetic material of the parent, in particular, and the parent's race, in general.[107]

The discoveries of genes and chromosomes demonstrate the essential process in which hereditary characteristics possessed by each parent are mapped in order to produce the genotype of each individual. And yet, while both chromosomes and genes are modern Western discoveries, Islamic authoritative texts, such as the Qur'ān and the ḥadīth, acknowledge that both men and women are equally important in the formation of a zygote. It should be noted, however, that while Islamic knowledge recognizes the significance of both parents in the generation of human beings, it neither particularly identifies what constitutes the hereditary characteristics nor does it impart the manner in which heredity is transmitted from the parents to their offspring. For this reason, the advanced scientific discoveries on human reproduction are useful when approaching the scientific themes of the Qur'ān as will be seen below.

The stages of fetal development: a Qur'ānic view

This section elaborates the stages of fetal growth in the mother's womb according to the understanding of the Qur'ān and the ḥadīth and in light of relevant biological and philosophical arguments. Following the Qur'ān, I reiterate the nature of a woman's womb as the essential condition for an embryo's development. In this respect, not only is the woman one of the components of the principle of conception, she actually carries the fetus to term. The Qur'ān describes how the fetus develops in the mother's womb (Q.S. al-Mu'minūn, 23:12–4). I will elaborate these verses as a way to highlight the significance of a woman's body, and her role in conception.

The verses that deal with the common origin of human beings as well as the general process of embryonic development in the uterus are found in al-Mu'minūn, 23:12–4, where it is stated:

> (12) Now, indeed, We create man [*al-insān*] out of the essence of the clay,
> (13) and then We cause him to remain as a drop of sperm in [the womb's] firm keeping
> (14) and then We create out of the drop of the sperm a germ-cell [a leech-like structure], and then We create out of the germ-cell [a leech-like structure]an embryonic lump, and then We create within the embryonic lump bones, and then We clothe the bones with the flesh—and then We bring [all] this into being as a new creation: hallowed, therefore, is God, the best of artisans.
>
> (Q.S. al-Mu'minūn, 23:12–14)

Ibn Qayyim uses these verses as his starting point to discuss fetal development. In the chapter entitled "On the Development of The Children of Adam [Human Being] during the Nuṭfah State" in his *Tuḥfah*, Ibn Qayyim depicts the common origin of human beings out of dust (*turāb*) and water (*mā'*).[108] These material substances are dissolved into human bodies and produce "the essence of a humble fluid" (*sulālatin min mā'in mahīn*).[109]

Ibn Qayyim also refers to Qur'ānic and Ḥadīth teachings and those of philosophical discourses, such as the Hippocratic writings, in his treatment of how the fetus grows in the mother's womb. Having mentioned the union between male *nuṭfah* (semen, sperm) and female *nuṭfah*, which is usually called *nuṭfah amshāj* (the mingling of semen), he further demonstrates his scientific knowledge of fetal development when he quotes Hippocrates, as follows:

> The seed, then, is contained in a membrane, and it breathes in and out. Moreover, it grows because of its mother's blood, which descends to the womb.[110] . . . As the semen becomes a fetus several other membranes are formed, and grow within the original membrane, all being formed as the first. Some membranes are formed at the beginning, others after the second month, and others in the third month. . . .[111]

After describing the early development of the fetus growing in the mother's womb, Ibn Qayyim justifies his scientific explanation with the Qur'ānic verse al-Zumar,

39:6, stating that "He creates you in your mother's womb, one act of creation after another, in threefold depth of darkness."[112] He further explains that each of these membranes has its own "darkness," and that one of them is the darkness of the membrane, which contains the embryo.[113] Ibn Qayyim notes that the exegetes interpret the term "darkness" to mean abdomen, uterus, and placenta.[114] While his attempt to shed light on the concept of the uterus is worthwhile, modern biologists, like Moore, argue that the most appropriate interpretation of "the veil of darkness" is probably: (1) the anterior abdominal wall; (2) the uterine wall; and (3) the amniochorionic membrane.[115]

As Ibn Qayyim has already demonstrated, the verses Mu'minūn, 23:12–4 refer to the stages of human development in its embryonic state. For this reason, these verses merit an explanation. In an attempt to discern its fullest meaning, I will explore its ideas thematically. It should, however, be kept in mind that there is a certain degree of difficulty in translating the Qur'ānic terminology into other languages, since the Arabic word has many different meanings and the translator must prefer one meaning over the others.[116] Consequently, any translation of the Qur'ān will necessarily reflect the translator's mind and agenda. In explicating certain biological terminology, I will refer to the contemporary discussion of the Qur'ān and embryology.

Al-Insān (*human being*). The Qur'ānic verse 23:12 mentions the term '*al-insān*.' Most English translations of the Qur'ān interpret the word *al-insān* to mean "man,"[117] but it can also be translated as "human being," "person," and "human."[118] Certainly, the term "man" is often meant as "humanity" in general,[119] but translating *al-insān* as "human being" makes more sense since it conveys a more universal message of ethical equality of human beings. It also supports the idea of equality in origin and the progress of creation in human beings as the Qur'ān consistently employs the word *al-insān* in relation to the commonalities of humans and their common properties as stated in the very first revelation to the Prophet Muḥammad in al-'Alaq, 96:1–5.

Sulālah (*clay*). Verse 23:12 uses the phrase "out of the essence (*sulālah*) of clay," which alludes to the fact that the human body is constituted "of various organic and inorganic substances existing in the earth as well as the continuous transmutation of those substances, through the intake of earth-grown food into reproductive cells."[120] The word "clay" usually coincides with other organic and inorganic substances, like fluid, water (*mā'*), and dust (*turāb*) and their subsequent essential change within human bodies.[121] The use of the term "clay" and its similar substance, "dust,"[122] is reminiscent of the discussion of creation in Genesis, 2:7: "And the Lord formed man of the dust of the ground, and breathed into his nostrils the breath of life; and man became a living soul."[123]

Nuṭfah (*a zygote*). *Nuṭfah* is also mentioned as a further stage of human development. The term "a drop of semen," or *nuṭfah*, is usually connected in readers' minds to male sperm because the Qur'ān repeatedly mentions a drop of semen being ejected from man.[124] And as man produces semen, it is often believed that the ejected male semen is the most important element in reproduction.[125] Such a claim finds its ground in the Qur'ānic verse that states "He has created both sexes, male and female from a drop of semen which has been ejaculated" (al-Najm, 53:45–6).[126]

However, Rabia Terri Harris, a contemporary American Muslim, argues that it is not required to read *nuṭfah* as "sperm," even though that is the way it has been generally translated.[127] In fact, Moore discovers that for the term *nuṭfah*:

> a more meaningful interpretation would be the zygote which divides to form a blastocyst which is implanted in the uterus ("a place of rest"). This interpretation is supported by another verse in the Qur'ān which states that "a human being is created from a mixed drop. The zygote forms by the union of a mixture of the sperm and the ovum.[128]

The zygote, transformed out of the union between the sperm and ovum is also found in the Qur'ānic verse al-Insān, 76.2, which states "Verily, it is We who have created man out of a drop of sperm intermingled, . . ."[129] Asad speculates that the word *nuṭfah amshāj* refers to the female secretion coming from the pelvic arch (*tarā'ib*) of women as "the female ovum,"[130] whereas Albar interprets *nuṭfah amshāj* as "the resultant of mixing and mingling of the male *nuṭfah* (sperm) and the female *nuṭfah* (ovum)."[131]

The ability of men and women to produce the different *nuṭfah* necessary for reproduction accords with the Qur'ānic verse al-Ṭāriq, 86:5, which mentions the word *mā' dāfiq* (a gushing fluid or water) as follows:

> Let Man, then, observe out of what he has been created:
> He has been created out of a seminal fluid (*mā' dāfiq*)
> issuing from between the loins [of man] and the pelvic arch (*tarā'ib*) [of woman]

This verse belongs to the first Meccan period (612–616). It mentions the seminal fluid or water as one of the primary material causes for human creation. This gushing fluid is liquid without the form and measurement that the organs of life would need.[132] The Qur'ānic verse al-Ṭāriq, 86:5 also introduces the role of women in begetting a child. According to Abduh, the term "loins" (*ṣulb*) is part of the male structure, while the pelvic arch (*tarā'ib*) is part of female anatomy, the implication being that the seminal fluid from which human beings are created must come out of both man and woman.[133]

'Alaqah. If the *nuṭfah* is to be understood as the zygote, the word *'alaqah* has two meanings. One refers to something that clings to something else, like the process of the "implantation of blastocyst in the compact layer of the endometrium."[134] The other meaning refers to "a leech or bloodsucker"[135] or germ-cell. Moore explains that

> This is an appropriate description of the human embryo from days 7–24 when it clings to the endometrium of the uterus, in the same way that a leech clings to skin. Just as the leech derives blood from the host, the human embryo derives blood from the decidua or pregnant endometrium.[136]

Moore's account concurs with another verse from the Meccan period stating that human beings are created out of a clot: "Proclaim! (or Read!) in the name of thy Lord and Cherisher Who created; Created man out of a (mere) clot of congealed blood."[137] The word *'alaqah* is sometimes translated as "a clot or congealed blood."[138] Here, it is worth mentioning that Moore, a scientist, and Abduh, a theologian, share a similar understanding of *'alaqah* (the feminine form of the noun of *'alaq*) as the embryonic state. Abduh translates *'alaq* as "congealed blood—a state of a fetus in the first moment of the conception."[139] Bell also mentions that the term "clot" (*'alaq*) "denotes the first stage in the formation of the embryo in the womb."[140] Asad expands our understanding of the aforementioned verse by commenting that it refers to the repeated process of the creation of human beings that "alludes to man's embryonic evolution out of a 'germ-cell'—i.e., out of a fertilized female ovum."[141]

Muḍghah (a chewed lump). While *'alaqah'* describes the process of implantation of the external layer of the blastocyst, *'muḍghah'* captures the progress of the inner cell mass in which a human embryo develops into an embryonic lump.[142] *Muḍghah* refers to the phase of the formation of the primitive tissue that becomes the growth center for the structure of the early embryonic body.[143] Early differentiation of the cephalic and trunk region increases along with the formation of "the series of paired prominences which indicate the location of blocklike masses of mesoderm called somites."[144] Accordingly, the human embryo toward the end of four weeks of fertilization looks very similar to "a chewed lump of the flesh. The chewed appearance results from the somites, which resemble teeth marks."[145]

'Iẓām and *laḥm* (bones and muscles). The continuation of verse 23:14 indicates that the *muḍghah* (the chewed lump) provides the foundation for the development of bones and flesh. This stage of development, according to Moore, accords with "embryological development. First the bones form as cartilage models and then the muscles (flesh) develop around the somatic mesoderm."[146] As all the major organs and systems of the body begin to take shape, the human embryo by the end of the eighth week has acquired an undoubtedly human look.[147] This is what scientists call a fetus.[148]

Having chronicled the stages of embryonic development, God proclaims that He is the Best Artisan (*Aḥsan al-Khāliqīn*). The notion of Best Artisan alludes to one of God's names, the Creator (*al-Khāliq*). The root of the word *'khalaq'* here is to be understood in two senses: (1) to create something based on a previous example and (2) to estimate.[149] God, as the Creator (*al-Khāliq*), always refers to His own role as the Maker of human beings in "the best conformity (*aḥsan taqwīm*),[150] in that human beings continue to share the same humanity or genus. *Al-taqdīr* usually indicates God's power to create something (anything) from what was previously "nothing" or was different from its origin. In this case, God as the Best Artisan refers to Him as the Best Appraiser (*aḥsan al-muqaddirīn*),[151] in that God creates human beings out of "nothing" in the form of organic and inorganic substances, like clay (*sulālah*), fluid, water (*mā'*), and dust (*turāb*), and transforms those material causes into a perfect human being through a complex development in the mother's uterus. This new creation is an independent individual being, which is quite different from its origin.

While the Qur'ān explains in detail God's role in creating human beings, complete with their best qualities, it makes it clear that He in no way becomes part of human creation. God is the Creator, whereas humans are the creatures. This may be seen in the analogy between God as the Best Artisan and the carpenter, which Aristotle—who sees the male as an active principle of movement and the female as passive[152] —provides for us: "the one being active and motive and the other as passive moved, that the one thing which is produced comes from them only in the sense in which a bed comes into being from the carpenter and the wood."[153] From the above passage, it can be inferred that both man and woman are principles of generation, just like the carpenter and the wood are the principles in bringing the bed into being.

It must be admitted, however, even though the above analogy portrays a distinct similarity between them—in that both possess the power to form a new being without necessarily becoming part of the product—they are not analogous at all. The analogy of the carpenter signifies the role of the male semen in generation, whereas God as Best Artisan lies completely outside the principle of procreation. The man, according to Aristotle, constitutes the principle of movement, which initiates the movement in the embryo; the female on the other hand provides the material to work with.[154] As the man contributes the form, his contribution is

> no part of the resulting embryo; just so no material part comes from the carpenter to the material, i.e., the wood in which he works, nor does any part of the carpenter's art exist within what he makes, but the shape and the form are imparted from him to the material by means of the motion he sets up, it is his hand that moves his tools, his tools that move the material; it is his knowledge of his art, and his soul, in which is the form, that moves his hands or any part of him with a motion of some definite kind, a motion varying nature of the object made.[155]

The carpenter analogy shows that the carpenter makes the bed. However, neither the artisan nor any part of him becomes part of his product.[156] Likewise, the male semen functions as the tool whose role is to pass on the principle of movements and to transform the matter from the potentiality into actuality.[157] The male semen, therefore, does not become part of the generated matter, but it does transfer the soul from the procreator to the new individual.[158]

In contrast to Aristotelian philosophy, the Islamic intellectual tradition perceives God as playing the role of Best Appraiser, Who creates human beings in their best form from "nothing" in the sense that sperm and egg are human disposals. Several verses indicate how God gives shape and form to human beings according to their proportions:

> Verily, it is We who have created man [*al-insān*, human being] out of a drop of sperm intermingled, so that We might try him [in his later life]: and therefore We made him a being endowed with hearing and sight.
>
> (Q.S. al-Insān, 76:2)

> (6) O man [*al-insān*, human being]! What is it that lures thee away from thy vountiful Sustainer, (7) who has created thee, and formed thee in accordance with what thou art meant to be, and shaped thy nature in just proportions, (8) having put thee together in whatever form he willed [thee to have]?
>
> (Q.S. al-Infiṭār, 82:6–8)

> And God has brought you forth from your mothers' wombs knowing nothing—but He has endowed you with hearing, and sight, and minds, so that you might have cause to be grateful.
>
> (Q.S. al-Naḥl, 16:78)

In the process of generation, while men and women produce the generative self in the form of the male sperm and the female egg, respectively, as material causes for reproduction, God alone individualizes each new individual with proper senses, mind, and soul (Q.S. al-Naḥl, 16:78 and Q.S. al-Insān, 76:2). Even though human beings play a significant part in conception, several verses point to God's unlimited Omnipotence over the microcosm (human beings), in particular, and the macrocosm (the world), in general. In fact, the logic behind the verses, such as Q.S. al-Mu'minūn, 23:12–14 and Q.S. al-'Alaq, 96:1–2, is to demonstrate the Omnipotence of God and the created nature of human beings. As human beings are God's creatures, there is no one among them who is superior to others.

After all, the created nature of humans is best explained by the Qur'ān, which envisions the development of the fetus and entails substantial knowledge about procreation. Muḥammad conveys the divine knowledge of "the microscopic development of the human embryo in the 6th century AD without a microscope, technical training, a laboratory of any kind or even the ability to write his own name."[159] Haas argues that Muḥammad's knowledge of the embryo's development marks his "independence of direct Biblical influence," just as it is "quite unique to the Qur'ān, and finds no parallel in the Genesis account."[160]

While the development of the fetus in the Qur'ān reminds Muslim readers of how each individual comes into being, it is not conclusive as to whether life begins at conception and whether or not it can be aborted. The term abortion is medically defined as "the intentional termination of a pregnancy at any stage in the pregnancy."[161] This is also called induced abortion, which differs from spontaneous abortion or miscarriages referring to "the unintentional or accidental loss of pregnancy prior to viability (about twenty-four weeks)."[162] There are three types of abortion: selective, elective, and therapeutic abortions. Selective abortion refers to any abortion because of the unwanted sexuality of the fetus; elective abortion refers to the termination of pregnancy because the woman and/or the couple do not want the pregnancy; and therapeutic abortion refers to any abortion performed to save the mothers' life or because of the fetal abnormalities and rape.[163]

Islamic law (*Sharī'ah*) rules out the possibility for abortion if pregnancy endangers the mother's life. The abortion could take place in the first four months or 120 days of pregnancy.[164] The abortion occurred during the first 120 days of pregnancy is equivalent *'azl* (*coitus interruptus*), which is used as the prevention of pregnancy. Well-known Muslim jurists have different opinions on its legitimacy of *'azl* (*coitus interruptus*):

> The Shāfi'is, for example, consider *'azl* as undesirable (*makrūh*). Ḥanafīs, Zaydīs and Shī'is consider *'azl* permissible only if the wife approves (*mubāḥ*). The Ḥanbalīs consider it undesirable or permissible only with the wife's approval. Mālikīs range between those labeling *'azl* "undesirable," and those labeling it "forbidden" (*ḥarām*).[165]

Despite these diverse opinions, the majority of scholars use *'azl* reasoning as the basis for allowing the family planning, even if it is by way of abortion as declared by Sheikh al-Azhar, Jād al-Ḥāqq 'Alī Jād al-Ḥāqq.[166] The permissibility is understood since the first 120 days of pregnancy is what Ibn Qayyim calls the stages of human development in its embryonic state, starting from *nuṭfah* (a zygote). *'alaqah* (a leech or bloodsucker/germ-cell), *muḍghah* (a chewed lump), *'iẓām* (bones), and *laḥm* (muscles) as stated in Q.S. Mu'minūn, 23:12–14.[167] After the fetus receives God's Spirit (*rūḥ*) (Q.S. as-Sajdah, 32:9), the fetus becomes a full person.

In spite of this acknowledgment of abortion as a woman's reproductive right, Muslim countries in general ban abortion, except to save the mother's life. Abortion is forbidden for fear that it would foster promiscuity and is seen as equivalent to infanticide. In Indonesia, even though abortion has reportedly been performed at a rate of more than a million each year since 1994, it is considered a felony and is equal to killing a newborn. This kind of felony is punishable by a sentence ranging from 4 to 15 years.[168] In Egyptian law, abortion constitutes a misdemeanor or a felony,[169] depending on the degree of criminal aspect of the abortion. With the gate to a safe abortion closed, many women undergo unsafe abortions to end their unwanted pregnancies. At risk are the reproductive organs and even lives of women. Women's lack of access to reproductive healthcare is one of the many problems faced by Muslim women in Muslim countries.

Conclusion

The preceding discussion has shown that Islamic philosophy is not alone responsible for de-essentializing women's role in reproduction, since the different Qur'ānic interpretations of the way in which male and female contribute to conception also relegate women to inferior status. While both Islamic philosophy and the interpretation of the Qur'ān are potential in generating the contradictory claims regarding women's inferiority in conception, Muslim women do not look at the philosophical discourses on conception and reproduction with the authoritative command. I have argued that it is the pervasive power of the interpretation of the Qur'ān that has been dissolved with the local cultures nurtures and perpetuates the Muslim patriarchal perception of the truth of the women's roles as reproducers, wives, and/or mothers.

While unfolding the social, cultural, political, and religious construct of the mystification of women as reproduces remains challenging, women should celebrate their reproductive potential. Without women producing the ovum necessary for procreation, reproduction would never take place. This assertion remains true even in the modern era of reproductive technology. The sexual act can definitely be reduced to the different forms of assisted reproduction, like *in vitro fertilization* (IVF) or *gamete intrafallopian transfer* (GIFT) and other techniques.[170] This is distinct from cloning—a procedure designed to produce a genetic replica of individuals by way of asexual reproduction—which is now theoretically possible.[171] Yet at this particular time, when people still debate the ethical and theoretical dimensions of cloning, it generally takes both sperm and ovum to procreate a new human being. This process highlights the importance of women's bodies and their reproductive potential.

Indeed, women's reproductive potential, coupled with the advanced technology can be very commercial, especially if the pregnancy involves "surrogate motherhood,"—where a woman who agrees to carry the embryo of a couple or an individual to term and give the baby up after birth to that family.[172] However, while the phenomenon of surrogate motherhood proves that a women's body, wherein the fetus develops, is irreplaceable, its practice often oppresses women. Surrogate motherhood usually involves money being exchanged for the service, while compensation might be claimed for the time she carries the baby or for any discomfort that she might experience during the pregnancy and delivery. The problem with such payment is that surrogate motherhood can potentially be used as commodities to produce babies for better off families. Certainly, some women may volunteer to become surrogate mothers. Their choices are not free of all the discomfort, pain, loss of the time, and worries during and after the pregnancy.

The bottom line is the female reproductive potential as a regime of power not only invites repression, but also conveys the duality of subject and object, masculinity and femininity, blame and responsibility, virtue and vice, pleasure and pain, and other distinctions which, *again*, bestow on men with superiority, power, and authority in both the private and public spheres. These dualities, regrettably, continue to separate men and women as humans and their feminine and masculine traits, as we will show in Chapter 4.

4 The embodiment of masculinity and femininity

The making of material self

This chapter explores the nexus of religious knowledge, power, and cultural practices that shapes masculinity and femininity and its impact on the making of material self. I argue that the way the self is represented in the cultural intelligibility, religious narratives, religious opinions (*fatwā*), and authoritative legitimacy fosters the masculine and feminine constituent of the material self. The masculine and feminine construction gradually accumulates and creates a pattern of material self that is loaded with the fixity of the masculine and feminine physical appearance and morality. This popular construction of masculinity and femininity is channeled through multiple powers of social institutions, legal system, norms, and local cultures, which, successively, foster the perpetuation of the patriarchal system in Muslim societies.

The appropriation of masculinity and femininity takes place in many different forms at different stages of a human's life. This is true even when a new individual still resides in the womb of the mother. Many expectant parents choose colors appropriate to the sexuality of the unborn fetus. While sexual organs mark the biological difference of a new individual, the masculine and feminine constructs are appropriated along with the embodiment of the specific norms associated with male and female sexuality. This engendering process of masculinity and femininity in the context of a Muslim's life is a lifetime project that is promulgated by Muslim legal scholars, preachers, and mystics through religious media such as the *ḥalaqah* (religious meeting), literature, and speeches (*da'wah*) accentuating the masculine expectation of what is appropriately feminine. This concept of femininity, according to Hassan, is derived from the interpretations of Islamic texts done by "Muslim men who arrogated to themselves the task of defining the ontological, theological, sociological, and eschatological status of Muslim women."[1] The basis of such an act stems from gender thinking that the politics of sexual difference entails different moral, social, and political responsibilities.

With this in mind, the Qur'ān and *aḥādīth* are used to justify the different constituents of feminine and masculine material self, instead of the commonality of the self as humans that complete each other. The embodiment of religious narratives and pronouncements outlined in the Qur'ān and *aḥādīth* goes along with the sexual dichotomy that has its theological basis in that humans are created male and female; it is the making of sexual difference as the site for the materialization of attitudes, characteristics, behaviors, and morality associated with each sex, which usually shapes the material self-becoming. What I mean by the materiality of the self is "what constitutes the fixity of the body, its contours, its movements, will be fully material, but materiality will be rethought as the effect of power, as power's most productive effect."[2] For this reason, the feminine constituent of the material self is loaded not only with characteristics suitable for the feminine self, but also the corporeality of femininity in the case of veiling, virginity, and circumcision.

The making of the masculine and feminine material self is linked to the identification of woman with body and men with spirit. The fundamental distinction here is that spirits are luminous, lofty, knowledgeable, and alive, whereas bodies are dark, low, and ignorant.[3] Beyond the confines of ideology, these attributes are applicable to any human being, to the extent that one can have different degrees of knowledge (more or less intellect), different degrees of power (strong or weak), and other similar characteristics. The making of feminine material self, however, is most likely to be designated as having less knowledge, lacking in strength, tending to emotion and disobeying reason. In this sense, the feminine self-becoming is defined in terms of what the male material self is not and what it lacks. The variations of these identifications have been fixed providing one of the many different means by which women's bodies are controlled.

Because women's bodies have been policed to enforce the ruling ideologies of what are men's and women's accepted and expected characteristics, I propose to depict various ways in which the making of "embodiment" that is conceptualized in Islamic intellectual tradition and expressed in Muslims' daily lives constitutes the material self-becoming. I argue that Muslims' expressions and embodiments of religious narratives and opinions (*fatwā'*) and their subsequent authoritative legitimacies adhere to the gender thinking of the female material self as sexed and gendered. The gendered material self is constructed through the citation of the narrative self in religious narratives and the imposition of the authoritative reading of religious texts and its variations, which are often reinforced in different localities throughout the Muslim world.

Hierarchical gender-minded Muslims often cite the Qur'ānic narratives to justify the masculine and feminine construct of the material self. The two favorite Qur'ānic narratives, already mentioned in this study are the stories of Adam and Joseph. The story of Adam portrays man as superior and woman as inferior, whereas the story of Joseph suggests that Joseph was "the prototype of rational, pious, and reserved man," and Zulaykhā "the prototype of female temptation." The stories of male prophets, scholars, mystics, jurists, and religious leaders become so ingrained into daily conversations and religious meetings that Muslims are accustomed to hearing them. Among Indonesian Muslims, the narratives of Eve and Zulaykhā become a feature of everyday life: they are preached at religious meetings and taught to students of religion to show honorable masculine characteristics and shameful feminine traits.

In this chapter, I discuss the making of the masculine and feminine material self in Muslim societies drawn from the religious narratives and pronouncements depicted in the Qur'ān and *aḥādīth*. The first section discusses narrative of the self in the account of Joseph as "the prototype of rational, pious, and reserved man," and Zulaykhā, as "the prototype of female temptation." The making of material self through the depiction of "the prototype of female temptation" has a ripple effect that constructs the lives of Muslim women. I then examine how numerous practices, such as veiling, virginity, and circumcision—practices widely believed to originate from Islamic teachings—contribute to the constitution of the material self.

The narrative of the self and the making of material self

The narrative of female self as temptress and its repetitive material practices becomes a powerful means of reinforcing the different categories of masculinity and femininity in Muslim societies. Examples of common masculine concepts include "men are superior to women," as inferred from the story of Adam or "men are more able to control their lust," as illustrated in the story of Joseph. I use these two stories because of their popularity among hierarchical gender-minded Muslims. In this section, I focus especially on the masculine and feminine traits delineated in the story of Joseph.[4] I argue that the interpretation of this narrative has been marshaled and used to perpetuate the ideal and popular concept of masculinity and femininity. The impact of this and other narratives has not only been to construct a gendered narrative of the material self, but also to foster and perpetuate the dominant hierarchical gender system in the Muslim world.

The narrative of the masculine self centers in the male figure of Joseph who is portrayed as a man of dignity, rationality, and spirituality. Such traits are usually also attributed to men in general, in the sense that men are seen to have more potential for rationality, spirituality, and superiority than women. Accordingly, masculine traits are built on a positive image of men, while feminine traits are based on characteristics that are the antithesis of the male images.

By contrast, the narrative of the feminine self is derived from "the prototype of female temptation" that is constructed as the eternal cursed image of Zulaykhā. The Qur'ān portrays the duality of the female narrative self: of temptress having the vicious attributes of cunning and madness[5] and of a self-speaking truth who took refuge in God (Q.S. Yūsuf, 12:51). Even though the narrative of Joseph and Zulaykhā shows humankind's inner tension of good and evil and truth and falsehood, the traditional Muslim depiction of Zulaykhā's narrative (presented later in this chapter) is usually embellished with a misogynistic tone. Because Zulaykhā is constantly portrayed as a temptress, hierarchical gender-minded Muslims assume that women are full of unruly desires that incite men to evil. This natural disposition is allegedly extended to all women and becomes part of material practices reiterated through the religious authority of male exegetes, narrators, mystics, theologians, and legislators.

The contradictory portrayal of Zulaykhā's persona in Muslim scholarship brings to mind the diverse legitimacies that offer differing views of how masculine and feminine self is constructed. Because the narrative of the female self in the 12th *sūrah* of the Qur'ān contributes to the making of the appropriation of the material self, it is absolutely important to consider the Qur'ān as the primary reference for its authentic and truthful meaning. The Qur'ān uses not only vicious adjectives, such as alluring, captivating, and enticing, but also the positive attributes such as repentance, integrity, and trustworthiness.[6] Stowasser even suggests that the story of Zulaykhā provides a complexity of characteristics revealing the best and worst in a woman's nature. Regrettably, its overall impact has been frequently reduced to "woman's transgression" because of the exegetical emphasis on its depiction "as [a] symbol of the sexually aggressive, destabilizing, and dangerous nature of women as a whole."[7]

The portrayal of the feminine material self as a sexual being remains the most prevalent stereotype in Muslim society. Woman is consistently described as sexually dangerous because "[t]he nature of her aggression is precisely sexual. The Muslim woman is endowed with a fatal attraction, which erodes the male's will to resist her, and reduces him to a passive acquiescent role."[8] Women are depicted as sexually "active," while men are innocent and the victims of female temptation. Rarely do men acknowledge as Joseph did that he too desired Zulaykhā (*hamma bihā*) (Q.S. Yūsuf, 12:51). Even though mutual admiration and longing exist between Joseph and Zulaykhā, the constructed narrative of the self produces the misogynistic images of women as inferior and unequal in every respect in comparison to their male counterparts.

Zulaykhā, whose name was Rā'īl, according to Ibn Ḥumayd, was Potiphar's wife. Potiphar bought Joseph and brought him into his own house.[9] Potiphar was a man of power, an *'azīz*, but he never had any sexual encounters with women—not even with his wife, whose beauty was well-known.[10] Humphreys calls Potiphar the "unobservant husband" who worried neither about his own affairs, nor those of his "licentious" wife.[11] Zulaykhā is sometimes even portrayed as having been unable to control herself from the moment she saw Joseph.[12]

Zulaykhā and Joseph were often in each other's company. Nor did she hesitate to express her feelings to her adopted son. But her adopted son was a prophet. The question, as Bouhdiba asks it, is "[C]an a prophet fall in love with women who already have husbands?"[13] This inquiry is intriguing because it not only asks about the nature of prophecy, but also demands an explanation of the mutual relationship between the sacred and the sexual. Joseph's prophecy is challenged by his ability to maintain his purity from the most condemnable of behaviors, one of which is to commit adultery or *zinā*. Mutual relations must be lawful, because the unlawful cannot result in an honorable outcome.

> "O Joseph, I love you with all my heart. Lift up your head and look at me in the fullness of my beauty!"
>
> "Your master has more right to that than I do."
>
> "Come close to me, Joseph!"
>
> "But I fear lest my portion of Paradise be lost."
>
> "I have discretely veiled my affair from the people, so come close to me!"
>
> "But who will veil me from God, the Lord of the Universe?"
>
> "If you do not do as I wish," she screamed, " I shall kill myself this very instant, and you will be put to death on my account!" And she put her hand on a knife as if to kill herself (but it was just a ruse on her part to trick Joseph). Hastening toward the knife, he snatched it from her hand and threw it aside. Then she

> threw herself upon him and untied seven of the knots in his trousers, one after the other. *She resolved within herself to enjoy him and he would have resolved to enjoy her.*[14]

In the midst of Joseph's encounter with the master, the search for truth begins. In Kisāʾī's account, it is Joseph who starts to explain what just happened,[15] while Ṭabarī contends that both Joseph and Rāʾīl met their master on their way to go out of the door.[16] In tears, Zulaykhā says that Joseph had tempted her into an evil act and that he should therefore be imprisoned (Q.S. Yūsuf, 12:25). Hearing his wife's account, the master turns to Joseph and expresses his anger. In reply, Joseph sobs and explains:

> Everything that Zulaikha told you is nothing but lies; her lies are as black as an unlit lamp. Woman was created from a rib on Adam's left side; that is why there is never any righteousness to be seen in her! Anyone who can tell left from the right can understand that.[17]

The mystery of the truth remains mysterious until Rāʾīl's cousin says that if Joseph's garment was torn from the front, it would be Joseph who had lied, but if it was torn from behind, he was right and she had lied (Q.S. Yūsuf, 12:27).[18] When the shirt is presented to Potiphar, and he sees that it was torn from behind, he turns to Rāʾīl and says "This is [typical of] the guile of you women. Your guile is very great" (Q.S. Yūsuf,12:28).[19]

There are two consistent descriptions of the feminine traits in Kisāʾī's account of Joseph's story, one of which is dishonesty, and the other, seductiveness. When Joseph defends himself to the master he uses misogynistic reasoning. He restates what most Muslims believe to be the truth: that women cannot be trusted because they were created from Adam's rib. Because Adam's rib was crooked, crookedness becomes a "feminine" trait. Once crooked, it remains curved forever. This material construct of feminine traits differs from masculine ones. Masculine traits are independent, rational, honest, and superior, while the feminine character is dependent, emotional, dishonest, and inferior.

Along the same lines, women are not only depicted as being crooked in nature, but also as seductive in character. The phase "innahū min kaydikunna, inna kaydakunna ʿaẓīm" (Behold, this is [an instance] of your guile, O womankind! Verily, awesome is your guile!)[20] becomes the theological basis for establishing women's slyness. The hierarchical gender-minded Muslims utilize the idea of women's slyness as a powerful machinery along with other dominant patriarchal stereotypes to place limitations on women's rights. As women live in a male-dominated society, they often become the victims of the structure of domination, a situation that has been described as one where "men [have] robbed women of their confidence and then have thought that women [are] devil's helpers...criticizing women's natural dispositions, belittling their minds, and warning other men of their slyness."[21] Although men or women can be slyness—depending on what triggers it, this characteristic is more frequently attributed to women rather than men.

With women's inborn potential to deceive men a fixture in the female mind, the hierarchical gender-minded exegetes interpret the phrase "kaydakunna 'adhim" as "the eternal condemnation of women.... Zulaykhā certainly constitutes the prototype of the female temptress, intriguing, false, lying. But how sly and playful she is!"[22] Exegetes like al-Zamakhsharī and al-Bayḍāwī go into great detail about women's slyness, attributing a cunning nature to Zulaykhā and all women.[23] Indeed, women's cunning's is considered enormous. It is believed that women are more delicate in trickery and more prolific in making excuses than are men. Women bring their charming and lenient nature to the task of overcoming men.[24] Woman's slyness is also useful in inciting a man to seek sexual and emotional pleasure, which, in turn, becomes the basis for Satan's ability to corrupt his behavior.[25]

The cunning nature of women can also be seen in the manner of the Egyptian women, among whom the rumor of Zulaykhā's scandal of seducing Joseph was spread. In the story, a group of women attend a gathering in the house of the 'Azīz. Witnessing Joseph's beauty makes them forget what they are doing, so that they hurt their own hands (Q.S. Yūsuf, 12:30–33). Their presence in the gathering embellishes the core of the story, in which behaving irrationally and gossiping are considered part of female characteristics. When the women were exposed to temptation, the story argues, they by and large lost their reasoning power and could not resist. Therefore, Zulaykhā's allegory is seen as an accurate depiction of female characteristics such as "cunning," aptness in provoking evil, irrational, and open to other evil-doers. Such traits are dangerous not only to men, but to the social order itself in the long run.[26]

The question remains: does Zulaykhā really represent the "prototype of female temptation" in this story? Is she really seductive? Or is Joseph really sinless? To what extent did he follow his own desire? The Qur'ān depicts the emotional states of Joseph and Zulaykhā as desiring each other: "And, indeed, she desired him and he desired her" [wa laqad hammat bihī wa hamma bihā] (Q.S. Yūsuf, 12:24). So both of them were filled with certain unruly desires. In one account, Ibn 'Abbās writes that Joseph "loosened his waistband and sat with her as one who possesses would sit."[27] He also states that "she lay on her back for him and he sat between her legs removing his clothes."

Since the Qur'ān depicts that Joseph and Zulaykhā voluntarily follow their desire, it is a grave mistake to blame only Zulaykhā, especially if such a one-sided assignment of blame is intended to justify mistrust of female sexuality in general.[28] As strange as it may seem, Joseph was considered sinless by virtue of his good intention in avoiding temptation. But he only succeeds because God comes to him, in the vision of his father, and saves him from evil-doing (Q.S. Yūsuf, 12:24). Joseph is said to be fully aware that "man's inner self does incite him to evil" (Q.S. Yūsuf, 12:53). However, a Prophet cannot be a sinner; therefore his willingness (*irādah*) is initiated by God's Grace in order to attain the Truth.

Zulaykhā, for her part, is depicted as riddled with grief over her error. She regretted her previous deed and saluted her evil-doer with an awesome utterance: "Now has the truth come to light! It was I who sought to make him yield himself unto me—whereas he, behold, was indeed speaking the truth!" (Q.S. Yūsuf, 12:51). With her integrity and fidelity for Joseph at the back of her mind, Zulaykhā transforms her desire for her beloved into a quest to regain union with the Beloved.[29] Zulaykhā's solitude and servitude merit forgiveness from God, who grants her a physical union with her beloved Joseph.

Considering the full narrative of Zulaykhā, it seems rather dubious to use such an account to portray the material constitution of the self as a sexed being along with its gendered feminine construct. While this generalization stems from limited information or scattered accounts, such as the stories of Eve and Zulaykhā, hierarchical gender-minded Muslims have used these narratives of the self as guides in dealing with and controlling women.

Along these lines, the gendered narrative of the material self as a sexed being is drawn from the interpretation of the prophetic account of the "Night Journey" (*al-Isrā'*) and the "Ascension" (*Mi'rāj*). This narrative is cited on many different occasions, especially in the month of Rajab, when Muslim societies celebrate the event. This account provides a rich description of a constant reminder of the female material self, devoid of spiritual import, as the source of temptation for those who are in search of spiritual journey. Such a reading effectively sustains the politics of sexual difference, which nourishes male desire for the perpetuation of their supremacy and superiority over women.

It is said—in the tradition recorded by Ibn Ḥajar in his *Fatḥ al-Bārī* upon the authority of Anas—that the Prophet was called out by an old woman, who, according to Gabriel, symbolizes the temporal world (*al-dunyā*).[30] A similar account is given by Ibn Sīnā, as follows:

> A woman, alluring in her (beauty), called from behind me, "Stop! So I can reach you." Again Gabriel said, "Go on, don't stop!" When I went on, Gabriel said "If you had waited for her until she reached you, you would have become the lover of the world.[31]

Ibn Sīnā alludes to the old woman as a symbol of the faculty of imagination, which usually captures the desirable image and is able to transfer desire onto pleasurable things. He goes on to reason further why the imagination is likened to a woman:

> ... because most natures incline toward it, and most people are in its grasp. Furthermore, whatever it does is baseless and is tainted with deceit and fraud, and this (like) the doings of women are known. And the faculty of imagination is also deceitful, lying, and treacherous. In this way it allures, haunting human beings with its representations then not fulfilling its promises, for how quickly become false.[32]

These quotations show that Ibn Sīnā makes use of the metaphor of the "old woman" for a twofold purpose: (1) to demonstrate the imaginative faculty, with which both men and women are endowed and (2) to convey women's nature as being alluring, tempting, and untrustworthy.

Echoing this line of thought, al-Ghazālī gives a more candid account of how female sexual desire is stronger. In Book III of his *Iḥyā'*, he restates again and again the stories of how beautiful and young women incite sexual intercourse.[33] Of course, al-Ghazālī attempts to show that sexual desire is experienced by both men and women. However, he considers women to be more capable of provoking and looking for sexual enjoyment than men. Here, al-Ghazālī can hardly be faulted for his opinion that women are more prone to deceive men into their arms. He is not to be blamed, since his account of the danger of female sexuality only reiterates what had been said in the Prophetic sayings:

> Allah's Apostle (peace be upon him) said: I have not left after me turmoil for the people but the harm done to men by women.[34]
>
> Allah's Apostle (peace be upon him) said: The world is sweet and green (alluring) and verily Allah is going to install you as vicegerent in it in order to see how you act. So avoid the allurement of women: verily, the first trial for the people of Isra'il was caused by women. And in the ḥadīth transmitted on the authority of Ibn Bashshar the words are: "So that He should see how you act."[35]

Again, women are portrayed as sexual beings with an irresistible charm, a danger about which men need to be cautious. If it is necessary, men should renounce both women and the world, as do ascetics, in order to attain unity with God.

The preceding discussion has shown how the narrative of the self as sexual being contributes to the fixity of the material self. The appropriation of sexuality and its subsequent masculine and feminine construct are molded onto men's and women's self-concepts. Men are, therefore, not only in charge in the production of knowledge of the concept of "woman," but they are also responsible for reviving and reinforcing the particular gendered tenets and practices into engendering material self. Men's active participation in theorizing an ideal and virtuous woman has gone for centuries; indeed, the masculine concept of masculinity and femininity has been passed down through countless generations. In this sense, the masculine and feminine concepts and practices become the material practices that foster and sustain the hierarchical gender system. Even a modern Egyptian Islamist thinker, like Sayyid Quṭb (1906–66), was able to relate to the masculine concept of an ideal woman as part of the grand plan of his utopian Muslim community.[36]

Hierarchical gender-minded Muslims can easily materialize this ideal woman when they begin looking for suitable and marriageable candidate. They often use their portrayals of ideal women to screen "Mrs. Right" who would be most likely to be receptive to their desires, sensitive to their feelings, and appreciative of their thoughts, along with other feminine characteristics, such as motherly, loving, caring, and understanding. More importantly, they often make the condition of staying at home and quitting any job after getting married before proceeding with their marriage proposal. Muslim parents, both conservative and moderate, are involved in the screening process in order to assist their sons, daughters and/or female relatives to find suitors.[37]

The existing mechanism of the gendered process in the production of material self reflects not only the frequent citation of religious narratives, but also the profound materialization of religious legitimacies attached to them. Muslim scholars, mystics, theologians, and jurists generate various legitimacies that are inextricably bound to the perpetuation of the sexual division of labor, spheres, and social order in Muslim societies. In other words, the orderliness of Muslim societies depends on women's full conformity to what is regarded Islamic by Muslim standard, even though this standardization may actually only reflect the embodiment of a particular Islam. Included in the cost of maintaining "social tranquility" is the control of the material self through the multiplicity of powerful mechanisms such as veiling, circumcision, and virginity.

The formativity of material self

I elaborate on the multiple religious, social, and cultural powers that constitute the fixity of material self. I argue that the embodiment of religious, cultural, and social practices subject female bodies to the performance of a gendered construct. In particular, I propose to examine how certain practices, such as veiling, circumcision, and virginity, are used as means to constitute the material self. While veiling is external to women's bodies, it is central to the constitution of the material self because it measures the materialization of modesty and morality internalized into women's cultural bodies. This is also true for circumcision and virginity in that both practices shape the material process of the self-becoming.

Biological and cultural bodies

The goodness of female and male material self is central to Islam in that it emphasizes "the meaning and comportment of the body in everyday life. Islam prescribes in minute detail how the body in its myriad activities must be presented."[38] While the ethical message of Islam promotes a balanced well-being of male and female bodies, women's bodies, their contours, suppressions, and concealments reveal good and bad, truth and falsehood, virtue and vice, honor and shame, and blame and responsibility. I argue that the duality of the materiality of the female self is not cut off from the prevailing norms and culture around her existence. This constructed material self is what I call a "cultural body" in the sense that this body internalizes both the popular masculine concept of femininity and what she imports from religious culture into her life. In this way, she learns and observes what is appropriate for a woman. By "real body" on the other hand, I mean the physical body, which is composed of visible and invisible parts. The visible parts are what everyone sees, or can see, whereas the invisible parts are inside the body and control the mechanism and dynamics of her physical movements.

Even though women are identical with body, they have not been perceived as owners of their "physical" bodies. In fact, the abjection of a female body is reinforced through "*the regulation of identificatory practices*."[39] Women's bodies have been conquered and controlled by men in the sense that the husbands have mighty rights to regulate women's bodies and enjoy their pleasure anytime, anywhere as they please. Muslim governments extend their power over women's bodies by means of state policies, like family planning or "happy family" program where the burden falls mostly on women, not men. The religious establishment controls women's bodies by regulating their dresses in public as is the case in Iran, Saudi Arabia, and formerly in Taliban-ruled Afghanistan. The cultural exposition marks bodies with the "curse" to be weak, to menstruate, to get pregnant, and to give birth and to be seductive.

Perhaps the only time that physical bodies function independently is in the context of caring for bodies as a medium to perpetuate the endless forms of prayer to the Creator. Even though the formality of prayer is often limited to five occasions a day, the activities of prayer extend to laboring, working, and acting insofar as the individuals intend to do these actions out of duty.[40] Ritual cleansing is one of the pre-conditions before any religious observance. It comes as no surprise, then, that Muslim religious education usually centers on the body, its secretions, fluids and orifices.[41] Similarly, a large number of legal (*fiqh*) books focus on the purity of the body. God expects bodily cleanliness because He is the Lover of Cleanliness.

While bodies are endowed with material and sexual differences, their fixity is, as mentioned earlier, determined by and formatted through the materialization of different norms, texts, and practices. The materiality of the self occurs through the repeated repetitive narrative of the self, norms of "what is proper for women" and practices such as genital mutilation, veiling, and virginity. These norms and practices are materialized, reiterated, and repeated through multiple powers that operate within society. The multiple powers that channel the perpetuation of norms and practices that disempower women often run in the family, religious institutions, and state regulations, so that cultural intelligibility engenders a multiplication of signs and dominations empowering the body and mind.[42] This power, in Foucault's sense, constitutes the multiplicity of force relations, which manifest themselves through the language of cultural and social norms.[43] This power is dynamic because it is "produced [from] one moment to the next"[44] and it is "something that circulates," so that there is a constant attempt to engender the state of power.[45] At the practical level, such as when the state makes veiling obligatory; this instituted call becomes so powerful so that different religious, social, and cultural institutions produce and reproduce the powerful regulations to be executed up on women.

The power also takes on different forms on different occasions. The power that circulated in pre-Islamic culture, for instance, was not always welcoming to the female self. At one point in time, pre-Islamic Arabian society even perpetuated the barbarous practice of burying female offspring alive, as the Qur'ān records:

> (17) For [thus it is:] if any of them is given the glad tiding of [the birth of] what he so readily attributes to the Most Gracious, his face darkens, and he is filled with suppressed anger: (18) "What! [Am I to have a daughter—] one who is to be reared [only] for the sake of ornament?"—and thereupon he finds himself torn by a vague inner conflict.
>
> (Q.S. al-Zukhruf, 43:17–18)

The irony is that pre-Islamic Arab women enjoyed a number of freedoms in their family life. They could live within their own tribes, even though married to husbands from different tribes. They could travel freely within the towns, without having to be veiled or to live in seclusion (*purdah*). They could demand a divorce and they divorced their husbands as they pleased. Similarly, they could choose their mate or suitor freely. Such freedom can be easily understood within a social structure where female kinship is prioritized.[46] What is interesting from the observation of such phenomena is that scholars often jump to the conclusion that, in pre-Islamic Arabia, women enjoyed more freedom than Muslim females.[47] Such a claim is not, however, in accordance with the facts that these matrilineal values were upheld within patriarchal milieus. As the formal authority circulated among men, women's freedom is subject to male power.

Even though the early nature of Islam continued to be strongly patriarchal, it brought about the fixity of the cultural bodies that were friendly to women. Muslim women received more rights and protections. Female children had the right to exist as humans and were protected from being buried alive. Females as daughters were given rights to inheritance, education, and property. They were protected from abusive parents who would take them for granted in the event of marriage. Virgins had to be asked prior to the marriage contract. Women's rights to education were granted by the God and the Prophet, who included them, especially his wifes 'Ā'isha b. Abī Bakr, in the transmission of ḥadīth or knowledge. Husbands could not prevent their wives from seeking knowledge and performing religious observance. Women's rights to finance were protected, especially if they were orphans. Their former husbands had to give divorced women with children the right to economic security for taking care their children. Polygamous marriage was limited to four. Women and children's life were protected in times of war and peace.

Have Muslim women received God's granted rights as the constituent of the materiality of the self? Do Muslim women receive their rights and protections from their families and societies the way the Prophet Muḥammad wanted women to be treated? Fewer Muslim women have received education because the male members usually have greater rights to education than women. Educating women, especially at the level of higher education, may be at no use because women do not always go to work after they get married. Even if they go on to the higher education, it only provides the chance to boost their marketability to a suitable family. Fewer women have access to economic stability since most wives do not work, but rather take care of the family. Fewer women are protected from crimes of honor since men usually set the law in such a way that women have no escape, while men can get away freely with murdering a sister in an honor killing.[48] Fewer women receive protection and right after divorce since men turn their backs on them and their children as soon as they set their mind on such an option. Fewer women seek for divorce from abusive husbands because they often do not have safe places to go. If they decide to go back to their parents, the punishment from the family and society is often unbearable. Fewer women have rights to property and wealth since most women who are wives are economically dependent on men. The variations of these social realities wherein women live contribute not only to the making of cultural bodies, but also to constitution of the materiality of the self.

Veiling women's bodies

In this connection, the issue of veiling is relevant to mention because it originally functions to empower the materiality of the female self in the public sphere. Along with the establishment of Islam, veiling became one of the many mechanisms that repress not only women's bodies, but also the fixity of the material self. As veiling remains a controversial issue, I propose to discuss the historical and contextual context of veiling as a regime of power that contributes to the fixity of the material self. While Islam attempted to depart from the patriarchal system in place at the time of its birth, it was not void of its reminiscent. Veiling falls into this snare. Assyrian law (1200 BC), for instance, reflected the patriarchal mode of controlling women through close male relatives, such as the husband and the father.[49] It imposed veiling upon eligible women. Assyrian law determined who was to be veiled and who was not. The wives and daughters of upper class families and the slaves who accompanied them, as well as former prostitutes, had to wear veils, whereas regular slaves and active prostitutes did not.[50] Here veiling was used to distinguish between women of the elite and common folk. Veiling functions as class category and the social status of the women in the society. If the latter group disobeyed the law, they were liable to have their ears cut off.

Indeed, the prevalence of the veiling practice in other cultures and religions prior to Islam raises many questions about the present-day debate over veiling.[51] The most intriguing question is whether or not veiling has an Islamic origin or has nothing to do with Islam at all. Muslims' answers to this question will be divided between its advocates and its critics. The only thing that both advocates and the critics of veiling agree on is that modesty is important in the dress code. In an attempt to contribute to the complexity of the veiling discourse, in what follows I will discuss how veiling is used to measure a woman's body and her morality.

Ḥijāb: spatial dimension (seclusion)

I argue that seclusion in Islam is a social fact and its practice during the Prophet's period was contingent upon the social and political context of a given time. Its practice dates from the early period of Islam during the year 5 of Hijrah (627 AD).[52] Seclusion becomes permanent in Islam as an embodiment of the interpretation of al-Aḥzāb, 33:53. The word '*ḥijāb*,' according to anthropological and Islamic feminist analyses, refers to space or dimension, which usually stands for "a sacred divide or separation between two worlds and two spaces: deity and mortals, good and evil, light and dark, believers and nonbelievers, aristocracy and commoners."[53]

Seclusion derives from one of the meanings of the word *ḥijāb*, which, in its original sense, refers to the curtain used to divide the public and private spaces in one's household.[54] Another meaning of *ḥijāb* refers to "Islamic" personal dress. This twofold understanding of the veil (*ḥijāb*) stems from al-Aḥzāb, 33:53:

> O you, who have attained to faith! Do not enter the Prophet's dwellings unless you are given leave; [and when invited] to a meal, do not come [so early] to wait for it to be readied: but whenever you are invited, enter [at the proper time]; and when you have partaken of the meal, disperse without lingering for the sake of the mere talk: that, behold, might give offence to the Prophet, and yet he might feel shy of [asking] you [to leave]: but God is not shy of [teaching you] what is

> right. And [as for the Prophet's wives,] whenever you ask them for anything that you need, ask them from behind a screen [*ḥijāb*]: this will but deepen the purity of your hearts and theirs. Moreover, it does not behove you to give offence to God's apostle—just as it would not behove you ever to marry his widows after he has passed away: that, verily, would be an enormity in the sight of God.

The two meanings of *ḥijāb* are well-explained in the exegetical interpretation of al-Rāzī. He holds the view that the phrase '*min warā' ḥijāb*' has a twofold interpretation.[55] One interpretation refers to the fact that men's communication with women should be from behind the curtain, except for those who have a socially sanctioned relationship, that is, marriage or blood relationship; otherwise, men could fall into transgression. Second, the words '*min warā' ḥijāb*' are interpreted to instruct women to wear the veil. In this respect, veiling is seen to be synonymous with Islamic teaching, which commands Muslim women to don the veil. Therefore, if Muslim women comply with the rule on veiling, they are doing good, are serving God, and are following the example of the wives of the Prophet who were considered among the elite of the early Muslim community.

While seclusion has been conveniently used by Muslim men as a mechanism to domesticate women in their private domain, there are specific accounts for which al-Aḥzāb, 33:53 was revealed. The first account maintains that the Prophet recited this verse on the occasion of the celebration of his marriage to Zaynab b. Jaḥsh. As the guests prolonged their stay, the Prophet had to stand between Zaynab's chamber and the living room so as to keep anyone from entering. Hence, verse 33:53 was revealed ordering the installation of a "cloth curtain" (*ḥijāb*)[56] separating the private chamber from the meeting room. Assuming that the curtain was drawn to mark out the chamber of the Prophet's wives', Muslims were forced to communicate with the Prophet's wives from "behind the curtain." This interpretation makes sense because none would want to have a visitor go directly into their private rooms.

The second account asserts that al-Aḥzāb, 33:53 was delivered after 'Umar Ibn al-Khaṭṭāb urged the Prophet to command his wives to draw a veil or seclude themselves so that their piety would not be distracted by either the pious or the immoral guests who often visited the Prophet's house.[57] It is also said that the Prophet legalized the *ḥijāb* after 'Ā'ishah's hand accidentally touched the hand of one of the companions, while they were enjoying a common meal. Along with the *ḥijāb* regulation, the Prophet's wives were ordained not to remarry after the death of the Prophet. 'Umar's concern for the purity of the Prophet's wives is seen in this case as the primary cause for the appearance of the verse.[58] With this reason in mind, seclusion does not necessarily represent God's divine ordain; rather, it was culturally, socially, and politically needed for the situation at that particular time. In view of this fact, Mernissi comments that seclusion represents the triumph of misogynistic demands over the Prophet's dedication to advancing women's rights.[59]

The last reason for the occasion for the verse's revelation was to introduce the notion of privacy as an integral part of family and public life. Al-Aḥzāb, 33:53 regulates the etiquette of the host and the rights of the company or guests in the Prophet's household.[60] This household, as we saw earlier, was an extension of the mosque and was open to public access. To maintain the privacy of both the Prophet and his wives, a cloth screen to divide rooms was ordained. In a broader sense, however, al-Aḥzāb, 33:53 stipulates the ethics of gathering with "a genuine feeling of brotherhood, mutual consideration, and respect for the sanctity of each other's personality and privacy."[61] Privacy, therefore, denotes spatial dimension in the household as well as in the public domain. Within the private sphere, Islam highly advises equal respect for one's own and others' rights. In the public sphere, one has moral duties to others, just as, vice versa, others have duties to their fellow being as well. Privacy, in other words, stands for respect for each other, whether male or female, so that any human being counts equally. This ethical norm is universally appropriate to cultivate a just gender relationship.

Even though the revelation of al-Aḥzāb, 33:53 provided the ethical grounds for human equality in both private and public domains, the embodiment of this verse marked the beginning of the materiality of the self as secluded body through a series of exclusions of women from public life. Initially, this seclusion was directed primarily toward the wives of the Prophet, based on several reasons: (1) the Prophet's wives' quarters were located very close to the Mosque wherein public activities took place, so the seclusion provided familial comfort and privacy for these elite Muslim women; and (2) the political and social situation in Medina was not fully secure. Women, regardless of their social status, were humiliated in public life and targeted with the *ta'arrud*—a violent practice of the pre-Islamic age, which consisted in taking "up a position along a woman's path to urge her to fornicate."[62] For these reasons, the Prophet took 'Umar b. al-Khaṭṭāb's advice to seclude his wives.[63]

Since then, the tradition of seclusion has been part of the daily life of Muslim women. It has become a justifiable means to preserve women's righteousness. Its practice becomes more practical as Islam was spread to Mediterranean regions where seclusion was common. This arrangement has lent women privacy and honor with the establishment of harem. Yet, because of the earlier presumption that women posed a danger to men and society, with its reiteration of the masculine conceptions of feminine traits (such as sexual allure, cunning, irrationality, and slyness), seclusion becomes a necessary institution to control women. At the same time, men feel more secure because women can no longer tempt them to do evil. Seclusion is, therefore, considered by men to be mutually beneficial to both men and women.

With the social order preserved at the expense of women's suffering, women have remained out of the public eye for centuries. Women have been shut out of the world and society. They are deprived of their fundamental rights to pursue religious, intellectual, cultural, and social advancement. Women are alienated from their potential to be autonomous and social beings. Ahmad Amin, the famous Egyptian thinker, portrayed the phenomenon of seclusion in Egypt by 1890s as physically and mentally damaging to women's health because it forced women to stay inside the house and took away their enjoyment of sunlight.[64] From society's point of view, these sufferings do not even count for the imaginary harms that women can cause are of greater concern.

The emphasis on the use of the veil in the sense of seclusion and its implication as the primary point of al-Aḥzāb, 33:53 often oversimplifies the complexity of the verse. One forgets, however, that al-Aḥzāb, 33:53 also teaches Muslims the excellence of the

Prophet Muḥammad morally, spiritually, and socially. The Prophet is described as "a witness [to the Truth], and a herald of glad tidings and a warner."[65] In al-Aḥzāb, 33:53, the Prophet's relationship with his followers is to be characterized in two ways: (1) respect for the Prophet's household privacy and (2) veneration (*ta'ẓīm*) of the Prophet.[66] At this point, it was plausible for the Qur'ān to establish rules that would maintain the Prophet's distinct individual moral, and spiritual qualities. These qualities were extended to his wives, so that it became necessary for them to maintain their purity and morality.

The Prophet's speech, behavior, and intentions became a perfect example to Muslims after his death. The same applied to the Prophet's treatment of his wives. Because the Prophet ordered his wives to abide quietly in their homes, it seems to be implied that Muslim women should be secluded. With this interpretation in mind, the verse al-Aḥzāb, 33:53 became the foundation for segregating women not only because that seclusion followed the tradition of the Prophet, but also because it was seen as being socially, culturally, and morally desirable for women. As a consequence, seclusion has been a widespread practice in Muslim communities for centuries.

The question remains: To what extent would the practice of seclusion make women morally equal to the wives of the Prophet? Al-Aḥzāb, 33:32 indicates that the Prophet's wives were at any rate not equal to ordinary women:[67]

> O wives of the Prophet! You are not like any of the [other] women, provided that you remain [truly] to God. Hence, be not over-soft in your speech, lest any whose heart is diseased should be moved to desire [you]: but, withal, speak in a kind way.

The above verse clearly assigns the Prophet's wives special status. It implies that the, rules contained in al-Aḥzāb, 33:53 were to be applied specifically to the Prophet's wives and household. The practice of seclusion is not, after all, in accordance with the universal Qur'ānic pledge to allow women the right to own property and to stand as equals before the law. If women are allowed to own property, to engage in trade, serve as eyewitnesses or be prosecuted, they are presumably permitted to immerse and participate in public life. For this reason, the institution of seclusion as drawn from al-Aḥzāb, 33:53 calls for reinterpretation.

The practice of seclusion generally alienates Muslim women from the rest of the world. The purpose of seclusion may be thought to be generous and benevolent because it aims at protecting women's chastity and morality. However, the institution of seclusion is clearly sexist because women's honor and morality are secured and secluded on the grounds that they are women. This practice assumes that female sexuality is a constant threat to society, so that women's social life should be confined to their private spheres. On this basis, countless women have lived their lives without full access to knowledge, religion, economy, politics, culture, society, and civilization.

Jilbāb and khimār: personal covering

Additional Qur'ānic verses to that of al-Aḥzāb, 33:53 affecting personal covering include al-Aḥzāb, 33:59 and al-Nūr, 24:30–31. In al-Aḥzāb, 33:59, the use of *jilbāb* (outer garment) was expanded to apply to Muslim women believers and their daughters (all slaves were excluded). Al-Aḥzāb, 33:59 states:

> O Prophet! Tell thy wives and thy daughters, as well as all other believing women, that they should draw over themselves some of their outer garments [when in public]: this will be more conducive to their being recognized [as decent women] and not annoyed. But [withal,] God is indeed much forgiving, a dispenser of grace.

Wearing the *jilbāb* thereafter became obligatory for any eligible and free Muslim woman. This reading is in fact put into practice everywhere in contemporary Muslim societies, even though the specification of the form of *jilbāb* varies considerably from place to place.

While the *jilbāb* connotes Muslim women's submission to complete covering, the term *khimār* (covering) is treated in a different tone in terms of its appropriation onto women's bodies. Al-Nūr, 24:30–31 introduces the *khumur*—(plural of *khimār*)—which often functions in a way similar to the *ḥijāb*, as follows:

> (30) Tell the believing men to lower their gaze and be mindful of their chastity, this will be the most conducive for their purity—[and,] verily, God is aware of all that they do.
>
> (31) And tell the believing women to lower their gaze and to be mindful of their chastity, and not to display their charms [in public] beyond what may [decently] be apparent thereof, hence, let them draw their head-coverings over their bosoms. And let them not to display [more of] their charms to any but their husbands, or their fathers, husband's fathers, or their sons, or husband's sons, or their brothers, or their brothers' sons, or their sisters' sons, or their womenfolk, or those who rightfully possess, or such male attendants as are beyond sexual desire, or children that are as yet aware of women's nakedness; and let them not swing their legs [in walking] so as to draw attention to their hidden charms.

The word *khimār* really stands for head covering, which was usually worn by Arab women before and after the arrival of Islam. In conforming with their culture at that time, women wore a tunic with a wide opening, which allowed the bosom to be widely exposed. In this regard, the phrase "draw their head-coverings over their bosoms" does not always entail the use of the *khimār*, but it indicates that the breasts are not included in "what may [decently] be apparent."[68]

Another interpretation is that it obligates women to practice veiling. This view is in accordance with the conversation between Asmā' and the Prophet.[69] In this case, the phrase *illā mā ẓahara minhā* or except for "what may [decently] be apparent," is to be understood to exclude the face and hands. Al-Qiffāl, as quoted by al-Rāzī, interprets the phrase *illā mā ẓahara minhā* as suggesting what a person may display in accordance with customary culture.[70] According to the prevailing custom, what is considered decent for women has been to display only the face and hands, and for men as well, the face, hands, and feet.

Al-Qiffāl's interpretation of the phrase *illā mā ẓahara minhā* points in two directions. On the one hand, women may choose to practice veiling (except for their face and hands), because this practice concurred with the existing culture when it was instituted. This is to say that veiling was not unique to Muslim women, that they did not invent it.[71] After all, adherents of other world religions, like Judaism and Christianity, and members of such world civilizations as the Persians, Greeks, and Byzantines observed veiling as religiously recommended.[72] On the other hand, it allows for the possibility that women may display more than just the face and hands if it is considered "decent" to show hair, face, hands, and feet in their own culture insofar as the personal dress accords with the Qur'ān's notion of modesty. These two different interpretations of veiling show that while the Qur'ān is inextricably bound to the historical context; its ethical message of such modesty is ethically universal.

Situating the Qur'ān within its historical and cultural contexts has become the core of the feminist discourse on the veil. Muslim feminists interpret the veil as a historical, social, and political phenomenon, rather than a religious requirement. Mernissi's analysis of the linguistic, social, and historical contexts of al-Aḥzāb, 33:53 shows that "the descent of the hijab" in Medina was an instant solution to "the web of conflicts and tensions," during the military defeats in the year 5 of Hijrah.[73] The verse regulates the etiquette of the Prophet's relationship to his wives and to his Companions. It also regulates the separation of the public and the private. In other words, the above verse suggests neither the segregation of the sexes nor the covering up of women's bodies.

In a similar tone, Ahmed argues that the veil is a cultural phenomenon, rather than a religious obligation. The Greeks, Romans, Jews, and Assyrians commonly veiled their women in order to distinguish the latter's female social status.[74] Pre-Islamic women veiled in order to differentiate the respectable from the available,[75] whereas Muslim women drew their cloaks so that they were socially recognized as believers and not "available" for harassment.[76] In view of this fact, the use of veiling by Muslim women represents a synthesis of the assimilation of different cultures and civilization, rather than the embodiment of religious teachings since "[it] is nowhere explicitly prescribed in the Quran;[77] it only instructs women to maintain their chastity and wear a scarf over their bosoms (24:31–32)."[78]

Like Mernissi and Ahmed, Barlas argues that veiling as a personal dress code removes the historical context and the specificity of the verses 33:59 and 24:31–32.[79] First of all, the specific context of the two verses was the Prophet. While this Qur'ānic injunction was addressed to the Prophet, it authorizes neither the Prophet nor Muslim men to force women to comply with the use of the veil. The Prophet was reported to have neither forced any of his wives to abide by the rule of veiling, nor punished women who had failed to wear the veil. Second, both Qur'ānic verses 33:59 and 24:31–32 do not suggest any form of veiling as a proper personal dress code. Linguistically, the words *jilbāb* (cloak) and *khumur* (shawl) used in the Qur'ān do not mean to cover head, eyes, hands, and feet, but bosom and neck. Moreover, the purpose of both verses is different. In the Qur'ānic verse 33:59, *jilbāb* functions as a form of "recognition/protection" for women (as a member of community) in "*a slave-owning Jāhili society*;" hence, there is a close connection between the use of veiling and the *Jāhili* society. In the Qur'ānic verse 24:31–32, "the veil" is generalized for both men and women in a sense that both are required to cover their private parts. This verse does not concern with the veil as a cloth of the veil; instead, sexual modesty is extended to both men and women. Finally, the Qur'ānic verses 33:59 and 24:31–32 do not frame the use of the veil in terms of "women's sexually corrupt/ing bodies or nature."[80]

Even though the use of the veil is inextricably linked to the historical context, Muslims generally view the veil as an epitome of Islamic teaching. This view has become the departure point of how the veil, in its contemporary form, is used.[81] Göle discusses this discourse within the framework of "the cultural Islam" and "the political Islam." "The cultural Islam" advocates "Muslim personality and identity" at the individual level so that both men and women can become "the conveyor of a new value system."[82] In this context, the veil is used as an affirmation of the identity and functions of women as a social requirement in order to maintain the polarity of the sexes and order in the Muslim society.[83] "The political Islam" endorses "the re-Islamization of society,"[84] and uses Islam as a political instrument to defend "Islamic identity and independence" from the Western "imperialist" forces.[85] In this context, the veil functions as "a discursive symbol [that is] instrumental in conveying [Islam's] political meanings."[86] The veil serves as an active reappropriation of Muslim women's engagement collectively and publicly in political Islamist movements.

Veiling as part of women's experience, thus, carries multiple meanings. For some women, veiling becomes a powerful force that subjugates women.[87] In Iran, for instance, veiling during the Iranian revolution was initially seen as an expression of religious, social, and political identity; however, it soon became obligatory in the Iranian Islamic state. Veiling was then channeled through the apparatus of political institutions and accompanied by the enactment of certain punishments. Penalties varied from expulsion from their occupations to criminal sentencing. This kind of force violated the rights of women to choose what was best for themselves, rather than what was best for male relatives or the government. This was also the case with Afghani women who were forced to wear the veil by the former Taliban government and now, a similar endorsement of veiling began to appear in Kashmir by the militant Muslims.

Because veiling is assumed as a means to exert men's power over women's bodies, the practice of veiling is considered as by some as the cause of the subordination and the backwardness of women.[88] Hekmat, for instance, portrays how pitiful it is for women to submit their life to the Qur'ānic rule of veiling without protesting it. However, this assumption is not fully accurate, since what women experience with their veil is often quite different from what secular Muslims and Westerners believe. In fact, though Muslim women do not deny the fact that veiling has operated within the network of the patriarchal system that regulates and controls women, they also use this institution to liberate themselves from male dominance and to gain freedom and agency.[89]

The overstatement of female veiling overlooks the ethical message of the verse al-Nūr, 24:30–31, in which God regulates chastity for men and women equally.[90]

Muslims themselves often use a double standard to define morality for men and women. As this chapter attempts to demonstrate, female sexuality is often a mark of the honor of the men and the family. In fact, the practices of veiling, virginity, and circumcision are all functions associated with the masculine Muslim vision of feminine chastity. I do not mean to deny the religious import of the rules on veiling and virginity, but what I disagree with is that the freedom to exercise personal religious beliefs is politicized for the interests and needs of men. Virginity and circumcision are often demystified to meet male pleasure rather than to provide mutual enjoyment.

NB

Circumcision and virginity: control over sexuality

While veiling is only external to women's bodies, there have been certain practices materialized onto women's bodies, such as the notion of virginity and the need to go through a circumcision. While both virginity and circumcision have to do with women's bodies, they are two different issues. Virginity symbolizes the honor of the family, and it is even the pride and prize of women. If a woman fails to prove herself to be a virgin on her wedding night, it can result in shame to her and her family. In contrast, men are "virgin by default," because they are not commanded to be virginal by the honor system.[91]

Every Arab girl, according to Nawal El Saadawi, an Egyptian feminist, is expected to have the fine membrane, called the hymen, intact. It is the most essential part of the female body.[92] Having this hymen can mean ultimate happiness or abject bitterness. Happiness can occur if the girl proves her virginity during the wedding night, but it can also lead to rejection, humiliation, cruelty, or even death if the girl is found not to bleed during that night. In Arab society, the defloration of the bride by the husband with his finger, such that red blood appears on their white sheet is considered to be one of the primary marriage rituals. If this happens women achieve honor within the family. Interestingly enough, however, this standard of honor is imposed only on women. Men are not subjected to any such notion. This double standard of morality shows how masculine concepts shape women's lives and bodies.

Second, circumcision is a much more radical form of control of female sexuality. El Saadawi gives her own account of this experience:

> I was unable to see and somehow my breathing seemed also to have stopped. Yet, I imagine the thing that was making the ripping sound coming closer and closer to me... Somewhere below my belly, as though seeking something buried between my thighs. At that very moment I realized that my thighs had been pulled wide apart, that each of my lower limbs was being held as far away from the other as possible, gripped by steel fingers that never relinquished their pressure... Then suddenly the sharp metallic edge drops between my thighs and they cut off a piece of flesh from my body.[93]

This story shows how the violence of circumcision is sustained in girls' memories. This practice educates the female child about the masculine expectations of what it means to be a woman growing up within the Muslim patriarchal system.

The practice of female genital mutilation (FGM) can be divided into four different types, namely *circumcision proper*, *excision*, *infibulation*, and *introcision*.[94] These practices vary from place to place depending on how it is customarily done in particular villages. However, FGM consists of a series of genital operations performed on children as young as newborns, and on children, teenagers, and grown women.[95] It is a cross-religious and cross-cultural practice, which is practiced globally. Muslims, Catholics, Protestants, and even non-believers in all countries, have observed FGM.[96] Culturally, FGM is as old as ancient Egyptian and pre-Islamic customs in numerous parts of the world.[97] Nowadays, it is practiced in Asian, African, and even Western cultures by immigrants from the countries where FGM is prevalent.[98]

What is circumcision for? It presumably functions as a preparatory stage that gives women the fullest possible right to have sexual pleasure, even though the current research finding in Sudan shows that 91 percent of newly married females reported the negative experience of the sexual intercourse, 82 percent expressed negative desire for it, and 74 percent of their husbands "reacted aggressively with complaints about the negative attitudes of their wives during intercourse due to FGM acute health complications."[99] Generally, in the countries where FGM is prevalent, many men do not want to marry uncircumcised, even though the finding also shows that the "sunnah" form is more desirable.[100]

Currently, FGM and its various forms are not simply practiced to improve female sexual gratification. It has been done rigorously and violently to the extent that female genitalia and reproductive organs fail to function for sexual purposes. FGM has become an act of violence and a matter of life and death.[101] It has been used to provide "a series of continuous warnings about things that are supposed to be harmful, forbidden, shameful, or outlawed by religion."[102] This reminder is not only regulated by Muslim preachers and jurists in the ruling ideologies such as through the reiteration of the saying, narrative, literature and religious speeches, but is also imposed on women's bodies.

The prevailing practice of genital rites among Muslim families has generated a heated debate over the claim that clitoridectomy and infibulation circumcisions originate in the Muslim world.[103] This claim has no basis in Islamic teaching, since the Qur'ān does not preach the necessity of the female circumcision. The *aḥādīth*, of course, refer to several occasions in which the Prophet addressed the issue. In one instance, the Prophet said that circumcision (*khitān*) is obligatory for men for hygienic reasons and optional for Medinan women (*ḥifẓ*) who had practiced it.[104] Moreover, while the Prophet did not forbid female circumcision, he strongly advised that it should not inflict harm on women. Because the Prophet did not forbid Medinan women to have circumcisions, however, it is claimed that the practice of circumcision has its roots in the tradition of the Prophet. But it is also true that Muslims often exaggerate the Prophet's sayings, so that they lose their moderation and original meaning. Thus, one can postulate that he would have disapproved of total clitoridectomy and infibulations of female genitalia, because these procedures reduce the female capacity for sexual pleasure. Anees argues that any attempt to deprive a woman of her basic right to sexual rapture, either through total clitoridectomy, circumcision, or infibulations, is to act counter to Islamic teaching.[105]

As noted earlier, circumcision is a practice that makes the control of female sexuality possible. The control of women's sexuality, as El Saadawi observes, accompanies patriarchy:

> When patriarchy started, monogamy was forced on women. If women marry two husbands, the whole patriarchal system will collapse because the man will never know with certainty who his father is, or if he is a father. To force monogamy on a woman, she has to be satisfied with one man, her husband. So they have to diminish her sexuality. They have to cut her clitoris, either physically or psychologically. Because clitoral orgasm is very strong, and it resembles somehow the male orgasm. So if the clitoris functions really normally then the orgasm in the woman is great and big and she will have a lot of pleasure .... Because the clitoris is a male organ in a female body.[106]

Indeed, circumcision that includes excision of the clitoris is physically damaging.[107] Psychologically, women even become afraid of their sexuality; they do not feel free to talk about it because it is taboo. Even if women were to begin talking about it, they would be easily punished by the society, the government, and possibly the family. El Saadawi argues that women's issues are political, social, economic, and psychological in nature, and unless women's issues are addressed in these modes, women's circumcision will continue to be justified through social norms, religious beliefs, and cultural barriers.

Since circumcision is ingrained in the locality of the Muslim world, its eradication should be able to unfold the assumed common thread that upholds its status quo. The confluence of the consciousness raising and the social and cultural changes toward FGM should be seen as the need and the interest of the local men and women. Along with this strategy is the acknowledgment that the practice of FGM is "a violation of the human rights of women and girls."[108] Parents, the local non-governmental organizations (NGOs), and the governments are crucial in advocating women's freedom from the practice of FGM and offering the strategies that would work in the locality. Coupled with this process is the state's enactment that outlaws the practice of FGM, just like "Egypt's highest court upheld a 1996 ban on FGM stating that the practice is not sanctioned in Islam and is subject to Penal Code."[109]

The absence of stick punishment for parents who endorse circumcision and/or of FGM and the correct interpretations of it show the resilience of the gendered moral dimension of feminine traits and practices as a way to maintain female chastity. Here, femininity refers to the way in which the authoritative texts and the cultural practices are used to construct the appropriate traits, behavior, and virtues for women simply, because of their biological nature. In contrast to femininity, masculine traits are constructed in opposition to what is appropriate to women. The construction of masculinity and femininity has gradually strengthened the dichotomous distinction between male and female, even though what are claimed to be masculine or feminine traits do not always correspond to either gender, respectively. Masculine traits, such as rationality, independence, resistance to temptation, and autonomy are equally applicable to women, in as much as feminine traits, such as irrationality, dependency, and sexual allure also belong to men.

However, as men have more authority and privilege to interpret Islamic texts, they are responsible and more involved in the production of masculinity and femininity. The interpretation of Islamic teaching, together with the local practices that Islam has encountered, has led to the creation of the social, religious, and cultural categories of femininity and masculinity. The masculine concept of femininity is more often invoked than the male concept of masculinity; and it is embodied in and generally inscribed on women's bodies. As a result, the materiality of Muslim female's status, roles, identities, and behaviors are constructed along with traits of submissiveness, irrationality, ignorance, cunningness, and sexual allure.

Conclusion

I have argued in this chapter that while Muslim women have undergone different degrees of internalizing and experiencing masculine conceptions of femininity, they share a similar experience in the way in which fixity of the material self is constructed. Gender hierarchy, which emphasizes the appropriateness of both men's and women's roles on the basis of sexual difference and their perceived complementarity in everyday life, has its religious justification as the following: "Islam has thus made woman an honored partner of man in raising family. A chaste and virtuous woman is a blessing to her household, and makes her children virtuous in the way of Allah."[110] The mythologizing of the divine role of women as a partner in reproduction (with all its attendant household responsibilities) is seen as ideal for every woman. It also places men in charge of women's well-being and their best interests,[111] since they know better. The mythologized image of women is reiterated through numerous institutions ranging from the family, society, and state regulations, and are often magnified and politicized by the Islamist movements that are interested in embodying the Prophet's practice and in preventing the invasion of women's liberation from the West.[112]

It is "safer" for a Muslim woman growing up in the Muslim community to embody the fixity of the material self—which means acting timid and obedient in order to maintain a harmonious relationship with the male and female members of the family and society. Assertive and talkative women are stereotyped as descendants of Zulaykhā. Similarly, disobedient and unruly women are labeled as being as "crooked as Eve." Because of these stereotypes, submissive, docile, and timid are the ethical qualities that women desire to achieve. Even familial and religious educations are, in some ways, designed to construct subservient Muslim women. The male religious teachers, shaykhs, jurists, intellectuals, preachers, colleagues and friends, and fathers and husbands frequently reinforce these masculine conceptions of femininity on both formal and informal occasions.

The lives of Muslim women represent the fact of how the popular authoritative legitimacy embodied in women's "real/physical" bodies becomes the constituent of the material self and reflects public perception of the truth. These bodies are socially, culturally, and politically constructed by the male's interpretations of religious teaching and the cultural values, whereas women have internalized these processes within their own lives. The majority of Muslim women neither question the validity of that interpretation nor analyze them, because doing so would require religious authority and training. This pattern repeats itself from generation to generation. Yet, this everlasting construction is only a small segment of the patriarchal system, for femininity and masculinity are becoming more complex within the web production of the performance of gender, the self-process, pleasure and truth at the personal, familial, and societal levels, as will be seen in Chapter 5.

5 The performance of the self

Engendering dependency and pleasures

The dominant and hierarchical gender system in Muslim communities is what Butler calls "performative—that is constituting the identity it is purported to be."[1] It is sustained by "a theological tradition that fosters and sustains images of women and practices by men that deny women their full worth as human beings created by God and as carriers of the spirit of God."[2] The performance of gender is profoundly socialized and politicized through different theological, biological, social, and political mechanisms that are rooted at the heart of personal, familial, and social institutions in each locality. Hierarchical gender-minded Muslims justify the systematic schemes of engendering process with the reiteration of interpretation of the Qur'ān, the ḥadīth and established religious legitimacies that are embodied at personal, familial and societal levels. For many Muslims, there is nothing more religiously appealing than saying something that is Qur'ānicly or prophetically sound, regardless of whether the Qur'ānic verses and/or the ḥadīth are taken out of context. Not many Muslims would do a background check on the validity or the historical and contextual contexts of the quoted sources of Islamic teaching since lay Muslims and scholars are respectful of the religious scholars (*'ulamā'*). Daring to be ill-mannered to religious scholars (*'ulamā'*) is tantamount to being disrespectful to Islam and that would reduce the chance of receiving the blessing (*barakah*) of the *'ulamā'*.

As the material self is constructed to fit into the existing gender system, the lived experience of the self faces inconsistency, contradiction and biased appropriation. The hierarchical gender-minded Muslims' understanding of how the material self is supposed to behave in both private and public life is often in opposition to what the Qur'ān advocates in regard to the equality of the self before God and fellow humans as inviolable subjects and morally responsible on their own account (Q.S. al-An'ām, 6:164, Q.S. Ghāfir, 40:17, and Q.S. Ṭāhā, 20:15). The equality of the self at the ontological level attests to commonalities of human form regardless of gender, race, and ethnicity. The diverse self-expressions and other accidental categories are environmental and relative to the localities where men and women live and interact with one another.[3]

However, the ontological self and one's moral responsibility are not considered the most important parameters—at least not in the case of the personal choices, actions, and lives of women—since the embodied social, ethical, psychological constructs measure the different male and female moralities. What measures a woman's morality is her superficial relationship to the male members of her family and often the extended family, kinship, and ethnicity because a woman's honor is the epitome of familial and social standing. The family's reputation depends on her behavior and contour in the private and public spheres. If a woman betrays the family's wishes and reputation, the male members of the family have every right to humiliate and punish her.

On the personal level, the female's self-becoming is affected by those with whom she is related. The extensional relationship with family members not only shapes her existing marital and/or familial relation to the family, but also carries with it the familial and social expectations of what is appropriate and inappropriate. This appropriation is multifaceted and complex depending on seniority, authority, gender, and class. Ingrained in this multiple level of relationship is the self's encounter with the world outside him/her that somehow contributes to the self-perception, identity, determination, religious commitment, knowledge, and public perception of the self.

Given that what constitutes the material self is his/her active/inactive encounter with God, macrocosm, and microcosm, I argue that the hierarchical gender system not only constructs a unified multiplayer performance of the self, but also the pleasures that the self produces. Among the constituents of the self that I deal with in this chapter is the construction of an ethical and psychological self, as will be seen in the first section. Embedded in the construction of the self is the existing extensional dependency among family members and the alternative reciprocal dependency that will promote equality, respect, and responsibility, as discussed in the second section. Finally, I discuss the constitution of the self through the interplay between the way the embodied self is cited and the truth of pleasure it produces.

The construction of the ethics and psychology of the self

The concept of the self is multifaceted and is constructed within the framework of Islamic teaching. In Islam, God is the center of worship and veneration.[4] As God's creatures, humans accept and submit to His Guidance, according to which they are required to utilize their reason and deliberation on every aspect of their life. Islam guides human conduct and determines all ethical and moral decisions. Similarly, a human's psychology guides his/her conscience to act with good intention in order to create a good community. A balanced self's relation to God (*ḥabl min Allāh*) and to other humans (*ḥabl min al-nās*) is ethically desirable and psychologically fulfilling.

In its subsequent analysis, the concept of the self is classified into traditional, theological, philosophical, and mystical categories.[5] The traditional concept of the soul is rooted in the Qur'ān and the ḥadīth. The theological concept (that of *kalām*) maintains the Qur'ānic view of the soul, but formulates it in a rational manner, and defends it dialectically.[6] The philosophical conception of the soul is the one formulated by philosophers, like al-Kindī (d. 870), al-Fārābī (d. 950), Ibn Sīnā (d. 1037) and Ibn Rushd (d. 1198). The mystical concept of the soul refers to "those of man's characteristics that are afflicted with illness and his blameworthy actions," to ways of purifying the soul, and to the soul's intimate relationship with God.[7]

In this regard, I discuss the notion of the self (*nafs*) in Islamic and philosophical accounts. Both disciplines identify the self as common to each individual in that men and women share a single humanity, regardless of race, gender, class, sexual, and religious differences. The multiplicity of the self is what marks humankind as human. According to the Qur'ān, each human being shares a common origin, namely, "self" (*nafs*).[8] This self is translated as living entity that constitutes the common origin of both men and women. As the self is the essence of humanness, what constitutes the corporeal self originates out of earthly substances, which are consumed and then internalized as a part of human tissues and fluids. This human flesh is transmitted from parents to their progeny by virtue of the generative self in the reproduction process.

The embodied self carries within it an inner and an outer construction. In particular, I analyze the construction of ethical and psychological self as the constituent of self-becoming that is constructed with a certain social, religious, philosophical, and cultural worldview. This paradigm measures what is ethical and acceptable in one specific culture and is not in another. It also validates and/or invalidates one's intentions, actions, behavior, and responsibilities. It is, therefore, expected that the ethical and psychological self is not static since it is influenced by constant exposure to what is religiously ethical and psychologically acceptable in one's immediate environment and society.

The psychological dimension of the self (nafs)

I propose to discuss Ibn Sīnā's theory of the self to show how the self's psychological construction is gendered. Articulating his theory of the self, to some extent, in line with Aristotle's *De Anima*,[9] Ibn Sīnā defines the soul as "the first entelechy (or the first actuality) of a natural body having in it the capacity of life."[10] Like Aristotle, Ibn Sīnā qualifies and divides the soul into vegetative, animal, and rational categories.[11] He, like Aristotle and the Stoics, also regards the soul as the source of life, "a 'particular,' material, terrestrial principle" which continues to exist even after the decay of the body.[12] Seen from this perspective, the body is less significant than the soul because the body will cease after death, while the human rational soul will return to its origin.

As Ibn Sīnā's theory of the soul largely mirrors an Aristotelian legacy, his theory is generally viewed as being completely Aristotelian. Rahman, however, argues that Ibn Sīnā explores the theory of the soul in a different manner from that of his predecessors by inserting the idea of a "Divine intelligence" as the peak in the hierarchy of the human rational soul and its search for knowledge. Certainly, Ibn Sīnā shares a view similar to that of Aristotle regarding the nature of the soul, but he also attempts to systematize various theories at his disposal and reconcile them into one of his own.[13]

In fact, Ibn Sīnā's theory of the soul reflects the development of his ideas. In his first work, *Compendium on the Soul* (*Maqālah fī al-Nafs 'alā Sunnat al-Ikhtiṣār*), he contends that there are five divisions of the faculty of the soul.[14] Nonetheless, in his *al-Najāt* and *al-Ishārāt wa al-Tanbīhāt* (*Remarks and Admonitions*), Ibn Sīnā rejects his earlier fivefold scheme. His later and more mature theory of the soul can be found in his *al-Najāt*, where he divides the faculties of the soul in the following manner.[15]

The first faculty is the vegetative soul, which is "the first entelechy of a natural body possessing organs in regard to reproduction, growth, and nourishment."[16] The function of this soul is to preserve the parts of the body and to refine the latter in order that it remain healthy and in a proper balance.[17] The source of its strength is taken from food, drink, and breath. In these sources lies the pleasure of the vegetative soul. Given its physical nature, there will be no reward for this soul after the death of the body. Once the human body dies, it will never be called to life again.

The next faculty is the animal soul, which is the "entelechy of a natural body possessing organs so far as it perceives individuals and moves by volition."[18] This soul is connected by God to the heart and governs two types of movement: active (*fā'il*), which is "distributed through the nerves and muscles," and impulsive, including desire and anger.[19] Added to these motive faculties are those of the perceptive faculties, which are twofold: external senses and internal senses. The external senses include sight, hearing, smell, taste, and touch, while the internal senses form abstract conceptions, that is, the meaning underlying the data perceived by the five external senses. Among these internal senses is "common sense" (*al-ḥiss al-mushtarak*),[20] which serves as an intermediary between "the brain and the senses."[21] Other faculties that are included in the hierarchy of internal senses are "the compositive imagination (*mukhayyilah*)," "the cogitative (*mufakkirah*)," "the estimative (*wahm*)," and "the preservative (*ḥāfiẓah*) or collective (*dhākirah*, *mutadhakkirah*)."[22] The function of the animal soul is to manage all movement and imagination and to protect the body from any injury or harmful action through the faculties of anger and appetite.[23] This type of soul likewise cannot expect any reward after the death of the body, as its existence and happiness have ceased.

The final faculty is the human rational soul, which is the "entelechy of a natural body possessing organs insofar as it acts by rational choice and rational deduction, and insofar as it perceives universals."[24] This soul embodies two elements, that is, the practical and the theoretical intellect.[25] The practical intellect functions to control the lower souls, that is, the animal and vegetable souls, in order to stimulate them to perform virtuous deeds and to resist bad behavior, which is their natural tendency.[26] This faculty also causes all movements of the body and is capable of directing one's practical life.[27]

Theoretical intellect functions to conceptualize particulars, and is derived from the animal soul's understanding and the practical intellect's inclination toward universal concepts.[28] It also works to conceive of the universal proceeding from the celestial intelligence and to use it as a means of studying the cosmos and human kind; hence, this faculty is seen as being able to produce knowledge (*'ilm*).[29] The theoretical intellect has different levels of manifestation, whether it be in the state of the material intellect (*'aql hāyūlānī*), which is shared by all human beings, in the state of the habitual intellect (*'aql al-malakah*), as a human learns the basic principles of knowledge, in the state of actual intellect (*'aql al-fi'l*), where he/she is able to postulate his/her own knowledge, or in the state of acquired intellect (*'aql mustafād*), as he/she wins the privilege of gaining knowledge through illumination from the Active Intellect.[30] The theoretical faculty also has its source in the Translunar Higher Principles (*al-mabādi' al-'āliyah*), that is, the Celestial Intelligence, which is reached after starting at the Active Intelligence, then ascending to the Celestial Intelligence, and finally, by achieving unity with the Necessary Existent. In this respect, Ibn Sīnā's notion of union with the Necessary Existence, that is God, suggests the ultimate goal of Islamic mysticism.

The unique characteristic of the human rational soul is that it is capable of performing good deeds (*ḥusn al-khuluq*) and is able to seek knowledge. This soul plays a role in such religious actions as remembrance, humble petition, and worship, leading men and women to lead virtuous lives and to be mindful of God. In this sense, prayer, to which the Prophet refers as "the foundation-stone of religion," is one of the paths to human perfection, achieved through purifying the human soul from corruption and worldly interests.

While Ibn Sīnā's theory of the psychological state of the soul demonstrates that each element of the soul works to sustain the bodily mechanism, he seems to attribute less ability to the female psychology when it comes to exercising human rational soul. He depicts women as controlled by sexual desire, easily deceived, inclined to emotion and to disobey reason.[31] Women's inability to obey reason justifies the Muslim male's total control, protection, guidance, and leadership over women. If women are not guarded and controlled they may entertain sexual freedom with many men as a result. This kind of freedom can cause calamity to the family and promiscuity in the society.

Ibn Sīnā's image of the potential harm of female sexual freedom is justified within his theory of psychology. Women generally have no authority to exercise sound reasoning. Since women are less rational and more emotional, they need to be protected from acting on vicious desires and impulses. By contrast, men are endowed with reason and the resulting ability to make rational choices so that they can handle as many as sexual relations as they wish. Such an implication is perpetuated in polygamous marriages, even though, in reality, sex does not involve reason as much as one would like to think.

Central to Ibn Sīnā's sexist attitude toward women is the tradition of inequality between the sexes. This attitude is widely shared by hierarchical gender-minded Muslims. Among these inequalities are the female's lower status in giving testimony and her disqualification from religious observance while menstruating and suffering postpartum bleeding. While the slur on women's reliability in court remains controversial, the easing of religious obligations due to physical discomfort has been a blessing and reflects compensation for women since many women cannot always endure the hardship of either condition. Abdul-Aziz argues that the recognition of these disadvantages does not imply any inability to understand matters of religion.[32]

Even though Ibn Sīnā's psychology is not gender sensitive, he demonstrates how each soul materializes in a human's body. The vegetative soul facilitates the growth, the maintenance of the body and reproduction. Here, Ibn Sīnā speaks of reproduction in terms of its growth to maturity. While reproduction belongs to animal soul, the act of procreation entails religious, ethical, legal, and social implications. The animal soul makes the human body and life vibrant and vital. Equally important is the human rational soul, which allows the human soul to reach the utmost celestial sphere and even achieve union with the Necessary Existent. I certainly believe that the psychological capacity of the soul is equal in both men and women in that, as humans, they are endowed with the capacity of the vegetative, animal, and rational souls. However, the extent to which each soul develops from potentiality to actuality depends on whether each exercises its fullest capabilities.

The ethical feature of the self

Islamic ethics calls attention to the individuality of the self and its mutual relations with others. The Qur'ān highlights individual responsibility regardless of sexual and gender differences. It assures the believer: (1) that the "self" (*nafs*) will not be charged, save to its capacity (Q.S. al-Baqarah, 2:233 and 286; Q.S. al-Mulk, 65:7); (2) that each "self" will be responsible for its own account (Q.S. al-An'ām, 6:164, Q.S. Ghāfir, 40:17, and Q.S. Ṭāhā, 20:15); and (3) that any good deed will return to one's "self" (Q.S. al-Baqarah, 2:272). These verses indicate that each self is responsible for its own intentions, actions, and wills. Any good deed will become the individual's investment in the hereafter.

The individuality of the "self"/person (*nafs*) serves as "the locus of autonomous agency and responsibility and, hence, is the subject of praise and blame."[33] This role operates in an individualistic and communal sense,[34] for the Qur'ān posits each individual "self", be it male or female, as equals before God's judgment. Yet, Islam also perceives the "self"/person as part of a community where mutual respect for each other is the condition for human flourishing. In this sense, Islamic ethics is conducive to fostering healthy community that offers recognition, respect, and protection for individuals.

The establishment of a good social order goes along with the duty (*farḍ*) to become a good member of the Muslim community. The role of the individual "self" as a member of a community is immediately bestowed following the birth of a new individual. His/her participation as part of a family and, at the same time, as part of a larger community depends on his/her right to live regardless of sexuality. It is through and within the community that the individual self flourishes and becomes who he/she is. Every member of the community is urged to take part in maintaining or creating the best community, one which will invite people to call that "[which] is good, and enjoin the doing of what is right and forbid the doing of what is wrong" (Q.S. Āl 'Imrān, 3:104 and 110). In this regard, both individual and communal selves are called to benefit society and restrict themselves from condoning evil-doing, which may cause harm to each member. When a corruption occurs, the communal selves are advised to change their inner selves and moral quality so that the orderliness of the community can be sustained.

Given that "righteousness" is open to individual and communal selves regardless of sexual, gender, ethnic, or racial difference, both men and women have the opportunity to compete in a positive way to better the society. In this respect, what is important is that their personal intentions and actions have the right cause. Similarly, communal "righteousness" is common for both men and women, since doing what is good is the foundation of the community (the *Ummah*), as expressed in the Qurānic verses of Āl 'Imrān, 3:114–115 as follows:

> They believe in God and the last Day, and enjoin the doing of what is right and forbid the doing of what is wrong, and vie with one another in doing good works: and these are among the righteousness (114). And whatever good they do, they shall never be denied the reward thereof: for God has full knowledge of those who are conscious of Him (115).

As men and women are equally capable of performing "right" actions, the performance of gender should in some ways complement human equality.

Not only is "righteousness" the backbone of personal and gender performance, it is also the condition for mutual and participatory process in the community. Each self should look after its peers. This mechanism operates just as the body works. If one part of the body is sick, the other parts should engage in battling disease and getting healed. This reciprocal dependence, however, does not suggest in any way that Muslims ought to collaborate in order to bring about mass destruction, damage, or evil-doing. Relationality and participation are means of maintaining the communal interests that benefit society. In this regard, all individual selves should come together and work with each other to bring justice into being.

To this end, the embodiment of "righteousness" at a personal level is a top priority. The individual self is judged based on individual investment in doing what is "right" and preventing the doing of whatever oppresses other people. Having the right intention (*niyyah*) is tantamount to doing what is good since such an intention is highly regarded in Islamic ethics. In the process of attaining the good, however, it highly recommends that nobody harms or oppress others because the plea of the oppressed person is counted. Since each human being is sovereign in himself or herself and he/she is entitled to the rights God has ordained, it is the responsibility of Muslim communities to act in compliance with what Islam demands in regard to gender equality.

Overall, Islamic ethics requires actualization in order to bring into being the good life for individuals and communities. A good community, certainly, requires both men and women to actively participate in doing what is good with good intention and in order to produce a good end. A balanced embodiment of good individual and society is achievable if every individual acts as an autonomous agent and makes use of reciprocal dependency on each other. To embody ethical qualities at personal and communal levels in daily life is to engage with one another justly in diverse expressions of Muslim families.

Extensional and reciprocal dependency

The multiplicity of Muslim families in different localities throughout the Muslim world is a constant reminder of the diverse beliefs and practices that characterize it. Ingrained in the locality of Islamic culture and society are the assumptions, values, philosophies, norms, and traditions that produce the gender system against which both men and women seek to be measured. This everyday life event shapes the making of the self to the point that one's existence is enmeshed within a web of relationality determining with whom one relates and interacts. While the interior self shapes the gist of his/her own becoming and the way he/she carries his/her being in public, the exterior self is constructed through self-relationality with others, public perception of the self and the way the self wants to be perceived in the family and societies.

I argue in this section that the hierarchical gender system fosters the self-relational dependency to the family and society and this dependency has impact on the self-perception. I propose to call this relation an extensional and reciprocal dependency. "Extensional dependency" refers to the way the self is constructed as an extension of family that carries with it the rights of certain family members over others, such as the parents' rights over their children or the children's obligation toward parents. "Reciprocal dependency" promotes mutual and equal gender relationship with everyone involved in such a relation.

Extensional dependency and the making of the self

Extensional dependency not only bestows the female self, especially mothers, wives, and daughters as extension of the family, but also becomes the site of social, psychological, cultural, and religious construction. I argue that extensional dependency means more than the legal aspect of heredity, blood relation, lineage and inheritance, for which reason it is often perceived as giving legitimacy to authoritative figures, who are usually the male members of the family, that is, father, husband, and sometimes older sons. These figures often define the female's moral status and see themselves as responsible for upholding the family's social standing and the social order by means of excessive protection, scrutiny, and control.

The use of extensional dependency as a means to establish marital and familial relations is not new to Islam. In the pre-Islamic period, the patriarchal agnatic clan to which the first generation of Muslims belonged bestowed on the male members of the family and the members of the tribe the power to be in charge of the well-being of female members of the family and its extended membership. Islam not only maintains the extensional dependency of women, but also introduces love, respect, responsibility, and care to be embedded in that relationship. While Islam adopts the pre-Islamic model of the patriarchal agnatic clan, where the family descended from a male lineage, it paves the way for

> ...moral and spiritual reform and introduced a new freedom and dignity to individual family members. In particular, it enhanced the status of women and children, who were no longer to be considered merely chattels or potential warriors but individuals with rights and need of their own. For the benefit of women, marriage was recognized as having important spiritual and religious values...In marriage women were recognized as persons to be respected.[35]

The Qur'ān's transformation of the patriarchal family was, indeed, revolutionary in that it provided an avenue to recognize each member of the family as humans. It tranformed the family so that it becomes "the crux of a social and metaphysical revolution"[36] and includes women as humans. The equal and mutual importance of men and women in marriage plays down the assumed male superiority. Traditionally, Eve is seen as an extension of the male Adam, because this theory regards Eve as having been created out of Adam. As the ancestor of women was derived from the male entity, the female existence is, therefore, of second-class status in the family and society. While this kind of theory is widely accepted among hierarchical gender-minded Muslims and becomes the condition on which the self-evolving being flourishes, the Qur'ānic ideal of the male and female complementarity as inviolable subjects is the backbone of humanity.

The complementarity of men and women in reproduction, as discussed in Chapter 3, without a doubt tumbles into the trap of the assumption that a woman's existence is essentially an extension of a man. This assumption would be true if women were seen as reproducers having no role in conception. This assumed theory of reproduction is gendered since the idea of family marks the importance of how generative self materializes into existence. The human element in reproduction is central to passing down the generative self from parents to a new individual being. As parents are crucial to conception, Islam declares parents deserving of respect, love, devotion, and care out of duty (Q.S. Luqmān, 31:14 and Q.S. al-An'ām, 6:151).

The constructed extensional dependency renders the "more superior" members of the family (especially husbands over wives and children, mothers over children, and brothers over sisters) the power to become the moral police and to regulate the way the self carries himself or herself in the private and public spheres. Irigaray argues that,

> while the form of domination is exercised by men over women but also, in another form, by women over their children. Even if the way it operates and their effects are different, this double form of domination does exist, and one form can explain the other: the woman, subjected to her husband, transmits her alienated state to her son, and the son to his wife.[37]

The moral authority to regulate female morality, in certain locations, is exercised through an extended family, tribe, and kinship.[38] If the female is accused of immodest behavior or of violating the honor of the family or the tribe, the woman herself, her family members and her extended tribe will face the consequences. Women are also subjected to punishment for the crimes that the male members of the family commit, as in the famous case of Mukhtaran Bibi in Pakistan.[39] The inferiority of women in the family and society causes women to remain silent about rape crimes inflicted on them, with the result that "women who have been raped routinely killed themselves."[40]

The embodiment of a male's authorized role in disciplining women by virtue of extensional dependency is often justified by reference to the familial model in the Qur'ān, especially al-Nisā', 4:34, where it is stated:[41]

> Men are in charge of women by [right of] what Allāh has given one over the other and what they spend [for maintenance] from their wealth. So righteous women are devoutly obedient, guarding in [the husband's] absence what Allah

> would have guard. But those [wives] from them you fear arrogance—[first], advise them; [then if they persist], forsake them in bed; and [finally], strike them. But if they obey you [one more], seek no means against them. Indeed, Allah is Exalted and Grand.

Even though the literal meaning of this verse seems to suggest that, within the familial context, husbands are in charge of wives due to their financial support, this verse has become the backbone of males' claim to superiority over females and the hierarchical gender system. Since husbands represent men in general, the contractual relation in marriage is constructed in such a way that wives ought to be "wholly" obedient to their husbands. If wives disobey their husbands and persist in their disobedience (*nushūz*), they deserve to be punished depending on the level of their rebellion, that is, through advice, withdrawing from the bed, or even physical punishment.

While the syntax of this verse (Q.S. al-Nisā', 4:34) needs further explanation and consideration of the context in which it was revealed, Muslims often taint this verse with their gender thinking by saying that if wives disobey them, they should be punished by a beating. This logic yields to the widespread violence against women in its fiercest forms as religiously condoned in the Muslim world.[42] However, to blame Islam as the primary agent of increasing domestic violence in the Muslim family and community is misleading. Although hierarchical gender-minded Muslims read that particular verse (Q.S. al-Nisā', 4:32) as the religious grounds for striking a wife, the Prophet Muḥammad viewed it as something not recommended. He could have said that wife-beating is my "*sunnah* (practice)," as he had in regard to marriage,[43] should he have wished to institute it as a means of disciplining women. Instead, he strongly objected to wife-beating, saying that "could any of you beat his wife as he would beat a slave, and then lie with her in the evening?"[44] Based on the example and sayings of the Prophet, Barlas argues that *ḍaraba* signifies some kind of restriction rather than actual wife-beating.[45]

The popular construct of wife-beating as the means to discipline and punish wives represents the embodiment of a particular Islam and the failure to implement reciprocal dependency in the institution of the family. Such a practice assumes the relativity of wives to husbands and condones the inequality between them. This social reality which Muslim women faced in the family is more often characterized by unchecked domestic violence. The endorsement of violence in the family is not Islamic at all since the early Muslim paradigm of the familial model has always sought to inculcate respect and recognition of women as individuals.

Wife-beating as a form of discipline happens when the wives fail to completely comply with their husbands' desire for obedience and they rebel "against the male authority" (*nushūz*).[46] Obedience is often defined as a wife's total submission and obedience to her husband. Ṭūsī illustrates obedience among the characteristics of a wife as follows:

> The best of wives is the wife adorned with intelligence, piety, continence, shrewdness, modesty, tenderness, a loving disposition, control of her tongue, obedience to her husband, self-devotion in his service and a preference for his

> pleasure, gravity, and the respect for her own family. She must not be barren, and she should be both alert and capable in the arrangement of the household and in the proper allotment of expenditure. In her courteous and affable behaviour and her pleasantness of disposition, she must cultivate the companionship of her husband, consoling him in his cares and driving away his sorrows.[47]

A wife's obedience to her husband is the condition for the enjoyment of his companionship. Her intelligence, love, caring and devotion mean nothing, if she disregards or disobeys her husband's wishes for satisfaction. Al-Ghazālī lists the wife's first duty toward her husband as being that "if the husband wants to enjoy her body, she should not refuse."[48] The wife is expected to be "there" for her husband twenty-four hours a day or whenever he needs the fulfillment of sexual satisfaction or other personal needs. If a woman refuses to obey his request, she is judged disgraceful and even sinful for the whole night. Her salvation lies in her husband's sincere forgiveness.

Embedded in women's obedience as a virtue is that obedience is used as an institution to control women's bodies and their mobility. It becomes the resilient power whose effect is used to maintain the status quo of the patriarchal and dominant norms in family and society. It reinforces the existing hierarchical gender relations between men and women. Obedience is also seen as a condition to maintain the familial and marital relationship, as if marriages would not work without wives' subservience to their husbands.

For women, obedience is the most fundamental virtue, regardless of any religious conviction. If women do not obey rules set by men, they are guilty of vice that will inevitably lead to misery. In Hinduism, a wife's obedience to her husband, whether he is dead or alive, is her guarantee to go to heaven.[49] If it happens that she is married to an abusive husband, a wife should perceive it as "paying her debt of her previous life and thus her sins are being destroyed and she is becoming pure."[50] Since obedience and purity preoccupied Indian culture,[51] Buddhism also teaches a wife to be obedient to her husband by "ordering her household well; by showing hospitality to their relatives; by demonstrating fidelity; by taking care of his wealth; by her industry."[52] In Confucianism, a wife's obedience to her husband is a condition for harmonious relation in the family that is part of a well-ordered society.[53]

The religious and cultural expectation of a wife's total obedience to her husband shows that marital relations in Muslim societies are not necessarily based on mutual partnership or enjoyment. This unequal power relationship shapes the way wives relate, not only to their husbands, but also to other men. A woman's experience of this unequal relationship is not new at all because she is accustomed to being obedient and compliant to her parents, to her immediate male relatives in their extended family, and then later to her husband. What women do is basically to extend the degree of obedience from the familial to a marital relationship. Women see this pattern of obedience as natural. They really have no alternative or even the courage to choose not to accept it. In fact, parents and those outside the family revere an obedient woman, because obedience is a woman's pride and price. In this sense, obedience, along with other virtues, like docility, sense of duty, respect, and submission are well-woven into the institutions of marriage and family.

Given that obedience is at the heart of the moral, social, and cultural construct of women's status and roles in Muslim societies, the ideas of honor and dignity become important issues "not just of personal commitment, but an elaborate social, legal and moral code."[54] Muslims justify their wariness of the dignity of their wives and daughters on the basis of an eschatological verse which counsels that "[you] who believe shield yourself and your families from a fire whose fuel will be [human beings (*al-nās*)] and stone" (Q.S. al-Taḥrīm, 66:6). The fear and the hope of ease in the Day of Judgment along with the view that the male members of the family, especially fathers or husbands are "in charge" of each member of the family cause them to be overprotective of the female members of the family, especially wives and daughters. The fathers or husbands feel morally responsible for making their wives and daughters obedient by all means, fearing punishment in the world and hellfire in the hereafter.

The Prophet Muḥammad's life provided several examples of how extensional dependency shapes individual dignity in the Muslim family. The slander against 'Ā'ishah's chastity in AH./627 AD. affected the Prophet's dignity and honor. 'Ā'ishah accompanied the Prophet on the occasion of the raid against the Banū Musṭaliq.[55] She explained that she slipped from her covered camel litter because she had lost her necklace when she went out for the call of nature. As she wandered alone in the desert, a young Muslim man named Ṣafwān ibn al-Mu'aṭṭal al-Sulamī passed by. He helped her to catch up with the rest of the army the next morning. The accusation against 'Ā'ishah spread at a rapid pace and became the public perception of the truth. In the face of a personal that became a communal rumor, 'Ā'ishah "refused to lie as a defense against the falsehoods being spread about her."[56]

The magnitude of the event is recorded in the Qur'ān, al-Nūr, 24:11, where God reveals 'Ā'ishah's innocence without mentioning her or the context in which the verse was revealed, yet in the process sows "the seed of conceptual conflict regarding issues of honor and shame, belief and unbelief, truth and falsehood."[57] The extensional dependency of the male's honor through the female's shame puts the Prophet Muḥammad's personal dignity, social standing, and religious commitment to the test. His male honor depends on 'Ā'ishah's chastity as a female. This means that "[w]omen are not active in promoting and attaining honor, but demonstrate only passive proof of its maintenance in the public vigilance of male control and protection."[58] This conceptual construct of honor was to shape the faith of billions of Muslim women to come.

The archetype of honor becomes the foundation stone of how female morality is policed in Muslim communities. While "[t]he female role in the pre-Islamic definition of honor was tied to male maintenance of the purity of the male tribal lineages, the masculine construct of the female misconduct and shame represent not only the individual disgrace but also 'an affront to her entire family.'"[59] For this reason, men are responsible for making sure that *their* women do not bring disgrace upon the family, since the family's dignity is constructed on the purity of female members. In this sense, the notion of honor killing, which has been practiced in Muslim societies, especially in the Middle East and South Asia, demonstrates that the family's reputation for chastity depends heavily on women's behavior and contour, while men's behaviors, however bad these might be, are not subject to this tradition.[60] In Pakistan, honor killings reportedly occur every day and "are carried out by men who assume that their wives, daughters, or sisters have in some way contravened rules of behavior of men which reflect on and damage a man's honor."[61] The popular practice of honor killing has certainly no basis in Islamic teaching; instead, it violates the dignity of each individual member of the family.

Embedded in the masculine concept and practice of honor is the notion of female chastity and decency. The materialization of this notion within the early Muslim community is not devoid of a context. The genesis of Islam took place against a background of enduring war that did not simply end with the death of the Prophet Muḥammad in 632.[62] Beginning with the war of al-Aqraba in 633, Abū Bakr, subsequent caliphs and the various Muslim empires waged wars for religious, economic, political, and geographical reasons. Despite the lasting warfare during the Prophet's lifetime, the Qur'ān and the Prophet's example convey the importance of liberty, dignity, and decency of the self. In this sense, what is decent in regard to modesty—that is, what to show and what to hide in regard to the female body—is bound by a set of rules designed to protect the self's interest and recognition. The phrase *illā mā ẓahara minhā* meaning "except for what may [decently] be apparent" (Q.S. al-Nūr, 24:31), shows what could be excluded, like the face, hands, or feet, within seventh-century Arabian culture and what could not be revealed at all.

Despite the Qur'ān's rich understanding of decency, Muslims generally share one understanding of it in common: that to be Muslim is to cover the whole body, without exception. This endorsement of Islamic modesty is regulated within the self-extensional dependency to the family and politicized by states like Iran, Saudi Arabia, and the former Taliban in Afghanistan. In these countries, dignity and decency clash with the liberty of the individual self. The question is how the self maintains the Islamic concept of dignity and decency, without losing the rights and liberty that the Qur'ān grants to women as human beings.

From the preceding discussion, we have seen how the constructed extensional dependency subdues women through such institutions as family, marriage, autocratic law, theocracy states, and the household. The constructed extensional dependency confines women to what society approves as the most fitting roles for each sex. Regrettably, the construction of extensional dependency violates women's integrity as persons because their fundamental rights are often neglected. Wadud-Muhsin argues that the role of a woman "represents social, cultural, and historical context in which that individual woman lived;" that it coincides with their biological function; and that it meets a non-gender specific that sustains human endeavor to replenish the earth.[63] In this sense, women as individuals and as members of their communities can perform what is good insofar as they are mindful of their existence as God's vicegerents: "[God is aware of] those who keep their bond with Him are consciousness of Him: and, verily God loves those who are conscious (Q.S. Āl 'Imrān, 3:76).

While extensional dependency bestows a legitimate relationship among family members, constructed extensional dependency shapes women's relational and participatory process with others through the social, cultural, religious, and political construct of what is appropriate for them. The existing construction produces a "partial" self in that the self is constructed by "interrelationship with and dependence on other persons from whom they 'acquire the essential art of personhood,' and with whom they remain in relationship of interdependence and 'reciprocal influence.'"[64]

As the self in Muslim culture is never devoid of encounters with the family and society, the essential composite of the self "is constructed not by a single element but by interacting participants, within local community."[65] Even though the composite of the self is "partial," this self as individual actively engages in negotiating her autonomy and agency at the personal and familial levels. This mode of self-determination definitely needs to be maximized. It may work effectively if the notions of female ownership and male leadership disappear. This move is possible if women actively engage in empowerment process by way of inserting their existence as the speaking subjects with the power to decide and act upon their own decision.

Reciprocal dependency and the production of the self

This section proffers an alternative model to the constructed extensional dependency in order to promote equal gender relation at the personal, familial, and societal levels. I call this relationality reciprocal dependency. It advocates the individual self as a speaking subject with a balance of responsibility and rights. In particular, I look at the participatory engagement of the performative self that promotes the individuality and agency within the web of relationality in the family and diverse communities.

Reciprocal dependency at the personal, familial, and communal levels demands the recognition of each member of the family as human with physical, mental, intellectual, and spiritual needs, regardless of sexuality, race, ages, and seniority (Q.S. al-Nisā', 4:1). The Qur'ān instills mutual respect in the family by prohibiting the killing of the children (Q.S. al-An'ām, 6:151). As humans are inviolable beings, Muslims in their capacity as husbands, wives, daughters, sons, neighbors, brothers, sisters, mothers, fathers, employees, employers, subordinates, and other labels are to withhold themselves from violating the rights of other individuals. This is to say that the extensional dependency does not confer rights on the authoritative members of the family to withhold women's growth and becoming, which they deserve as individuals.

Respect for each individual in the family and society stems from the equality of human becoming. Like a man, the female self exists by virtue of the generative self coming from both parents, which is shaped (*ṣawwara*) in the womb of the mother (Q.S. al-Qiyāmah, 75:39). While Muslims may have preferences regarding the sex of their children, Islam abolished female infanticide in recognition of a woman's right to life (Q.S. al-Naḥl, 16:58–9). In fact, to be embarrassed at having a female child is an act of *jāhiliyyah* (ignorance). Similarly, to deprive one's daughter of the rights to education, personal morality, property, and various opportunities—when they are available—simply because she is biologically female is tantamount to burying her alive.

The equality of human generation conveys the significance of female reproductive potentiality. While a woman's body is endowed with the reproductive potential of childbearing, this is only relevant to her insofar as it involves her reproductive organs. The Qur'ān acknowledges women's ability in childbearing in Q.S. Luqmān, 31:14:

> And [God says:] "We have enjoined upon man [*al-insān*] goodness towards his parents: his mother bore him by bearing strain upon strain, and his utter dependence on her lasted two years: [hence, O man,] be grateful towards Me and towards thy parents, [and remember that] with Me is all journeys' end."

Yet, neither of these functions in any way reflects the fundamental characteristics of women.[66] The Qur'ān only mentions the biological function of "mothering," but not the "psychological and cultural perceptions of 'mothering'."[67] Certainly, many Muslim women, individually or collectively, believe that reproduction and care are their main roles.[68] However, these roles are not innate since women need to deliberately decide and to exercise their reproductive potential and its consequence.

Being a wife is an avenue toward materializing one's reproductive potential. Yet, this avenue should not in any way diminish the self's individuality. Reproduction is a potential innate to the biologies of both men and women, should there exist reciprocal and mutual interest in both parties, as indicated in the Qur'ān, al-A'rāf, 7:189:

> It is He who has created you [all] out of one living entity [*nafs wāḥidah*], and out of it brought into being its mate [*zawjahā*], so that man might incline [with love] toward woman. And so he has embraced her, she conceives [what at first is] a light burden, and continues to bear it.

If couples are unable to conceive, some means of reproductive technology may be an option as long as it falls within the bounderies of marriage. Islam emphasizes marriage as the only institution that legalizes the union between a male and a female who have consented to be married in order to sustain heredity and genealogy of a family.

Central to the individuality and partnership of men and women in the family is the need for the couple to be responsible for the family's growth and happiness. This need is natural to both men and women since the underlying reason for the creation of male and female out of the "self" is that they are created for each other. The Qur'ān consistently portrays this mutual love in al-Rūm, 30:21, as follows:

> And among His wonders is this: He creates for you mates [*azwāj*] out of your own kind (*anfus*), so that you might incline toward them, and He engenders love and tenderness between you: in this behold, there are messages indeed for people who think.

The preceding verse operates on three different levels. On the metaphysical level, it declares that both men and women are ontologically the same since the self (*nafs*) is one of the constituents of human beings. The sheer equality of ontological self in both men and women demands that they recognize commonalities and respect differences. On the level of the marital relationship, the verse emphasizes that love and tenderness operate as the norms, which bridge two different personalities and backgrounds. This principle binds humans within the family as the smallest unit of the society, in which democracy and gender justice begin. On a societal level, the verse declares that the equal relationship between men and women is the most important element on which gender relationship is contingent. This contingency is not only biologically necessary, but is politically, culturally, socially, and morally required.

As for the reciprocal dependency of the couple as parents, it is important to acknowledge that loving, nurturing, educating, and properly taking care of their children are the prime duty of a husband and a wife. Parents are nevertheless blessed by this responsibility in that children are one of the primary delights of life. At the same time, parents should not feel burdened in caring for, educating and loving them (Q.S. al-Baqarah, 2:233). In the case of divorce—however disliked it is—parents need to decide in a fair manner (*ma'rūf*) the best interests of the children. By mutual consent, the divorced mother may opt to breastfeed the baby for a total of up to two years at the husband's expense. The parents may also choose to have foster-mothers (wet nurses) nourish and breastfeed the baby, provided that the husband pays for the expense. In the same way, the father must continue to provide sustenance and everyday expenditure for the child from his until he/she is mature enough to be responsible for his/her own, even if the child should stay with the mother, other family members or foster parents.

Certainly, Muslims do not generally endorse child support and alimony. However, the everyday well-being of the children is the parents' moral responsibility toward God, themselves, the children, and society. If children are left abandoned and uneducated, this has the potential of creating a disoriented generation that will not value marital, familial and social institutions. In any case, being responsible for children is a duty laid upon parents. It is part of one's devotion to God if done intentionally for the love of God.

In Islam, loving and worshipping God are innate in the human consciousness since human beings are, as it were, a microcosm and because God's creatures are created to worship Him (Q.S. al-Dhāriyāt, 51:56). The act of worship is implicated in everyday life and carries with it moral responsibility to one's self, others, and God. The self-responsibility toward God is in harmony with the ethical concept of the self, as expressed in the Qur'anic admonitions: that the self is responsible for his/her own self (Q.S. al-An'ām, 6:164, Ghāfir, 40:17, and Ṭāhā, 20:15); that the self's responsibility will be based on his/her capacity (Q.S. al-Baqarah, 2:233 and 286, 65:7); and (3) that the self's good deed is for herself/himself (al-Baqarah, 2:272). The family member's relational and reciprocal interactions function to center the self's moral responsibility to God, not to the authoritative figures who are acting in the name of God. To this end, a woman's body is not to be regarded as derivative—as commonly held by hierarchical gender-minded Muslims—in reaching bodily or even higher pleasure.

The "Embodied Self," the truth of sex and pleasures

Having discussed the constituents of the self at the personal, familial, and communal levels and their impact on the perpetuation of the patriarchal and hierarchical gender system in Islam, I will investigate the way the embodied self is encoded with the quantitative and qualitative categories and the truth it produces. While humans are endowed with quantitative measures, such as male, female, and other categories, the hierarchical gender system does not recognize humans as possessing equal qualities such as rationality, intelligence, agency, and autonomy since these qualities are reserved to men. Humans are, therefore, assigned qualities according to the criterion of gender: women are personified with qualities such as sexually dangerous, intellectually deficient, inclined to passion, dependent and cunning; whereas men are knowledgeable, sexually controlled, reserved, independent and rational. In effect, the different qualities predicated to the self tend to the subordination of the female self.

The opposition between the respective male and female qualities, traits, and predicates shows that men's and women's bodies receive different engendering processes. The female self is embodied with every kind of "less" in quality: less autonomy, less rationality, less agency, and less independence. These constructions have definitely become the essential elements of the ways in which the embodied self develops its self-identity and personality. Along the same lines, these identities become the fundamental constituents of "who and what we are."[69]

As male and female bodies have been inscribed with totally opposite qualities, I argue that such constructs affect the way in which the truth of sex is cited. Pleasures, as a corollary of the truth of sex, are gendered in that men and women do not equally reach higher pleasure. For this reason, I discuss how the embodied self makes use of the body to realize the truth of sex. Sexual difference is unfolded, materialized, and reiterated as a way to produce the truth of sex in the sense that that truth of sex can reveal sensation, pleasure, law, taboo, and truth and falsehood in a general sense.[70]

Foucault characterizes the truth of sex in Muslim societies as *ars erotica* rather than *scientia sexualis*. *Ars erotica* connotes the religious implications drawn from the physical forms of sexual expressions, whereas *scientia sexualis* implies the production of sexuality based on the scientific discourse.[71] Unlike *scientia sexualis*, *ars erotica* indicates not only the physical pleasure achieved at a certain moment, but also the production of higher pleasure. Foucault defines *ars erotica* as follows:

> In the erotic art, truth is drawn from pleasure itself, understood as a practice and accumulated as experience; pleasure is not considered in relation to an absolute law of the permitted and the forbidden, nor by reference to criterion of utility, but first and foremost in relation to itself; it is experience to itself, evaluated in terms of its intensity, its specific quality, its duration, its reverberations in the body and the soul.[72]

Foucault maintains that the truth in Islam, at least in al-Ghazālī's view, derives from pleasure. According to al-Ghazālī, one of the sources of pleasure is sexual passion, which has a twofold benefit: (1) to satisfy the desire for sexual intercourse and (2) to preserve humankind.[73] While sexual passion results in true excitement in this worldly life and fosters procreation, it also alludes to the pleasure awaiting humankind in the next life. This is to say that if humans experience the utmost bodily pleasure one can imagine, they can expect that the greatest pleasure awaits in the Hereafter.

Al-Ghazālī depicts the way in which sexual pleasure produces the truth of pleasure in this and the next life in the following words: "God created pleasure of the world with this object: that if the people have pleasure, they will be eager to have lasting pleasure in the next world. To get this pleasure divine service is necessary."[74] In a similar tone, al-Ghazālī reiterates his point that sexual pleasure signifies the truth of the next life:

> The pleasure that is felt in sexual intercourse between a man and his wife is a little sign of next worldly pleasure. If it were lasting, pleasure would have been strong as physical pain inflicted by force was great. The fear of Hell fire and the greed for pleasure and happiness of paradise lead a man towards guidance.[75]

Both passages explain that having known the gratification of sexual pleasure, one would desire to gain the pleasure awaiting him/her in the next life. In order to attain pleasure in the next world one must channel the inclinations of one's organs and sensations into a quest for spiritual pleasure.

The guidance that spiritual pleasure makes possible is obtained through opening oneself up to what is called "intellect" or "the light of certainty of faith."[76] Al-Ghazālī further maintains that the nature of intellect has the potential to receive the spiritual knowledge of God (*ma'rifah*), which is regarded as the greatest pleasure, for it is not found in any other knowledge. In his view, the pleasure in spiritual knowledge extends to:

> . . . knowledge of the reign of angels and heaven and earth. The more is the honor of the acquainted thing the more is the taste and pleasure. A man gets great pleasure in getting the secret information of the emperor. God is the most high and the most honorable. So the pleasure gained by the pursuit of His attributes is the greatest. So divine knowledge is best of all kinds of knowledge. It is thus proved that the best and the highest pleasure can be obtained by the pursuit relating to God and His attributes.[77]

The pleasure in knowledge of God and His attributes is unveiled only to the mystic knower (*al-'ārif*) "who searches for such a paradise as covers the whole earth and heaven."[78]

A similar idea is also conveyed in *The Niche of Lights* (*Mishkāt al-Anwār*), where al-Ghazālī mentions that the true knowledge of God is revealed to those mystic knowers who have attained the peak of their spiritual ascent:

> Then they [the Gnostics] see—witnessing with their own eyes—that there is none in existence save God and that "Everything is perishing except His face" [The Qur'ān 28:88]. [It is] not that each thing is perishing at one time or at

> other times, but that it is perishing from eternity without beginning to eternity without end. It can only be so conceived since, when the essence of anything other than He is considered in respect of its own essence, it is sheer nonexistence. But when it is viewed in respect of the "face" to which existence flows forth from the First, the Real, then it is seen as existing not in itself but through the face adjacent to its Giver of Existence. Hence, the only existence is the Face of God.[79]

Here al-Ghazālī delineates the "Face of God" as the one entity from which all the multiplicity of the universe overflows.[80] This perspective is rather interesting because al-Ghazālī, in his *The Incoherence of Philosophers*, denies any form of Neoplatonic import, while the emanation of the One to the whole of existence is a trademark of Neoplatonism.[81] However, both *The Niche of Lights* and *Iḥyā'* are consistent in showing that the knowledge of God is the highest knowledge for mystic knowers. Landolt also contends that

> The final message is that the true "Attainers" are not only unable to "see" anything but the divine "Essence" in its "Beauty" (*jamāl*); they are, as the "Veils-tradition" itself suggests, literally "burnt" by the "Splendors of His Face." The "Power of the Majesty" (*sulṭān al-Jalāl*) overwhelms them in their own essence, in such a way that only the "True One" (*al-Waḥīd al-Ḥaqq*) "remains" and "everything but His Face" is, indeed, "perishing" in their "taste" (*dhawq*).[82]

Like al-Ghazālī, Ibn Sīnā depicts the Truth (*al-Ḥaqq*) as the source from which the world emanates and as the goal to which all existence desires to return. In his *Tis' Rasā'il fī al-Ḥikmah wa al-Ṭabī'iyyāt*, Ibn Sīnā describes Necessary Existence as being perfect and the factor by which all the multiplicity of the universe overflows from the Essence which is "Absolute Existence, True, Good, Knowledgeable, Powerful and Life."[83] A similar point is also introduced in *al-Ishārāt wa al-Tanbīhāt* where Ibn Sīnā argues that one may wonder why there is no need to cosmologically prove the argument for the existence of the First (*al-Awwal*) and Its Unity.[84] If one meditates upon existence, one shall witness the emergence of existence from its existence. One would then afterwards witness all the multiplicity of existence. Ibn Sīnā supports his point by using the chapter Fuṣṣilat (Q.S. 41:53), which reads as follows: "In the time we shall make them fully understand Our messages [through what they perceive] in the utmost horizons [of the universe] and within themselves so that it will become clear unto them that [*He is the Truth*]."[85]

Ibn Sīnā employs the above verse to show that one may derive proof for the existence of the Truth (God) "from existence itself."[86] This "nobler" proof belongs to the "saints" (*al-ṣiddīqūn*).[87]

Al-Ghazālī also uses the term "saints" (*al-ṣiddīqūn*) to designate those people who witness nothing except "The Face of God." He renders the stage of the "saints" (*al-ṣiddīqūn*) in *Iḥyā'* as one of the highest stages of *tawḥīd*:

> The third stage consists in witnessing it (i.e. *tawḥīd*) by way of unveiling (*kashf*) thanks to the light of the truth (*nūr al-ḥaqq*). This is the stage of "those brought

> near" (*al-muqarrabūn*). At this stage, (the *muwaḥḥid* still) sees many things, yet he sees them despite their plurality, as emanating from (*ṣādiratan 'an*) the "Unique Prevailing" One (*al-wāḥid al-qahhār*).
>
> At the fourth stage, (however), he sees nothing in existence (*fī al-wujūd*) but One (*wāḥidan*). This is the witnessing the "saints" (*al-ṣiddīqūn*). The Ṣūfīs call it 'annihilation in *tawḥīd* (*al-fanā' fī al-tawḥīd*) because (such a *muwaḥḥid*), not seeing anything but One, does not see himself either,... which means that he is annihilated from both the vision of himself and of (all other) creatures (*al-khalq*).[88]

Prior to the third stage, the *muwaḥḥid* (pl. the *muwaḥḥidūn*), that who is being annihilated with the One reaches the preparatory stage of certainty by the light of Islam. By the third stage, the *muwaḥḥid* is overwhelmed by way of *kashf* (unveiling), which results in gaining knowledge of God and His attributes. The fourth stage is the utmost limit of *tawḥīd* in which the *muwaḥḥid* witnesses nothing but God.

Ibn Sīnā's notion of "saints" (*al-ṣiddīqūn*)[89] seems to concur with the mystic knowers (*al-'ārifūn*) in the last part of *al-Ishārāt wa al-Tanbīhāt*, which is known as a mystical work. There Ibn Sīnā opens up the way to attain the Truth. While in the "Metaphysics" section of *al-Ishārāt wa al-Tanbīhāt* Ibn Sīnā demonstrates the way "saints" (*al-ṣiddīqūn*) attain the Truth by witnessing nothing but the Truth, in the '*Taṣawwuf*' section he probes how such a state (*ḥāl*) is possible. Like a Ṣūfī master, Ibn Sīnā, writing on the Ninth Class in the chapter titled "On the Stations of the Gnostics," directs the adept (*murīd*) first of all to have "willingness" (*al-irādah*) and "spiritual exercise" (*al-riyāḍah*).[90] The first preparatory stage is "willingness," that is, the state of overwhelming desire that derives from demonstrative certainty or the tranquility of the soul due to faith. The second preparatory stage is "spiritual exercise" in that the adept exercises a number of practices, like worship, listening to a guidance or soft tone, or other means aimed to improve the quality of the soul. Having undergone the preparatory training, the adept is ready to proceed through the nine different steps that will finally culminate in union with the Truth.[91] While the adept engages in the spiritual exercises appropriate to those stages, he encounters different degrees of pleasure looking at the light of Truth, seeing the Truth, acquiring the knowledge of the Truth and being without the Truth. In the last two steps, the mystic knower (*al-'ārif*) would finally reach the intermediate state between attaining knowledge of the Truth and attaining the Truth Itself:

> Following this, he abandons himself. Thus, he notices the side of sanctity only. If he notices his self he does so inasmuch as it notices the Truth, and not inasmuch as it is ornamented with the pleasure of having the Truth. At this point, the arrival is real.[92]

Both al-Ghazālī and Ibn Sīnā further agree that the mystic knowers (*al-'ārifūn*) should not impart their secret mysteries of the spiritual world to the "common people."[93] To disclose the knowledge of the invisible things, according to the mystic knowers (*al-'ārifūn*), amounts to infidelity.[94] This was exactly the case of Ḥusayn b. Manṣūr al-Ḥallāj (d. 922), who was accused and denounced as an infidel for revealing the secret of the divine love and saying *'anā al-Ḥaqq.'*[95] In his *Ṭawāsīn*, al-Ḥallāj enters into an imaginary conversation with Iblīs and Pharaoh. In response to Iblīs, who says "I am better than him" (7:12), al-Ḥallāj criticized Iblīs in that he could not be possibly any one other than himself. In response to Pharaoh's claims that "I know not that you have any other divinity than me" (79:24), al-Ḥallāj argues that Pharaoh is ignorant in recognizing his people's ability to determine right and wrong.[96] Al-Ḥallāj further says "If you do not know Him, then know His signs, I am His signs (*tajallī*) and I am the Truth! And this is because I have not ceased to realize the Truth."[97] Al-Ḥallāj's experimental expression of the doctrine of *'anā al-Ḥaqq'* is not surprising because he availed himself of many of the terms used by his predecessors. Such an utterance as *'anā al-Ḥaqq'* has its precedent in the sayings of Abū Yazīd al-Bisṭāmī who says, *'anta al-Ḥaqq, wa 'annī al-Ḥaqq narā . . .'*"[98]

In this respect, both Ibn Sīnā and al-Ghazālī are more prepared to declare that mystic knowledge (*al-'irfān*) should remain within the circle of the elect. Even if the testimony of this experience were possible to explain, it should only be done on the basis of intellectual considerations. Al-Ghazālī, for instance, explains how the many—the phenomena of the multiplicity of the world and God—can conceivably become "one." He points, by way of example, to how the body can be seen as a multiplicity of different organs, but also as a single unit or "one" man composed of many things as well.[99] This approach applies to the case of macrocosm and microcosm: on the one hand they are many, but at the same time they are also one as God's creatures.

As the embodiment of pleasure is gendered, Muslim society adopts a binary system of attaining the Truth. While the truth of sex functions as a means to produce sexual pleasure, the truth of attaining the Truth belongs only to mostly the mystic knowers. Such truth needs to remain undisclosed to the "common people"; otherwise, calamity will result. For this reason, the truth as such should only be conveyed in an appropriate manner. Foucault beautifully depicts the secrecy of the truth of such knowledge as follows:

> . . . there is a form of knowledge that must remain secret, not because of an element of infamy that might attach to its object, but because of the need to hold in the greatest reserve, since, according to tradition, it would lose its effectiveness and its virtue by being divulged. Consequently, the relationship to the master who holds the secrets is of paramount importance; . . . The effects of this masterful art . . . are said to transfigure the one fortunate enough to receive its privileges; an absolute mastery of the body, a singular bliss, obliviousness to time and limits, the elixir of life, the exile of death, and its threats.[100]

After all, mystical experience, either in the form of knowledge of the Truth or the attainment of the Truth reflects the most inward personal experience of the mystics, which is ineffable and esoteric in character. Such mystical experience is incommunicable because language would limit the way in which the mystical experience would be explained.[101]

This is also true for the archetypal model of the attainment of the Truth drawn from the example of the Prophet's "Night Journey" (*al-Isrā'*) from "the Inviolable House or Mosque" (*al-Masjid al-Ḥarām*) to "the Furthest House of Worship" (*al-Masjid al-Aqṣā*) in Jerusalem, and his subsequent "Ascension" (*al-Mi'rāj*) to Heaven.[102] The Qur'ān records this journey in al-Isrā', 17:1 as follows:

> Limitless in His glory is He who transported His servant from the Inviolable House of Worship [at Mecca] to the Remote House of Worship [at Jerusalem]—the environs of which We had blessed—so that We might show him some of Our symbols: for verily, He alone is all-hearing, all-seeing.[103]

This verse is often regarded as the basis for mystical experience, by which the Prophet gained the knowledge of the invisible world and attained the Truth. Widengren demonstrates that Muḥammad's ascension to heaven established two important corollaries: the Qur'ān offers knowledge which is accessible to the whole community, and it also contains a secret divine knowledge that Muḥammad sometimes chose to conceal and sometimes not.[104] The latter has to a certain degree become the foundation for the Ṣūfīs' claim that their practices are inspired by Muḥammad's secret knowledge, and that their practices are part of Islamic teachings.[105]

The teaching of Ṣūfism is inspired by the Prophet Muḥammad, who was seen as embodying the perfect man (*al-insān al-kāmil*), whose attitude and spiritual journey have thus become a model for all Muslims. The Ṣūfīs' expressions are also akin to the language and the doctrine of the Qur'ān. Schimmel confirms that the origin of Ṣūfism can be traced back to Muḥammad, the prophet of Islam, and that Ṣūfism was inspired by the divine word which was revealed to him in the Qur'ān.[106] Schimmel also points to the Ṣūfī practices of Muḥammad's companions, such as Abū Dharr al-Ghifārī (d. 635), and Salmān al-Fārisī (d. 656) who were the 'spiritual' ancestors of Ṣūfism. Another early ascetic figure was Ḥasan al-Baṣrī (d. 728), whose ideas about the Day of Judgment were influential among his contemporaries and have remained so for succeeding generations of Muslims.

If mystical experience lends itself to the production of truth, we may wonder "to what extent does the sexual difference play a role in unfolding the truth?" As the mastery of the truth circulates mostly among the male mystic knowers (*al-'ārifūn*), it should be expected that women do not fully partake in the way in which the truth is produced. Indeed, exceptions must be made for the fact that there have been Muslim women who have excelled in their piety, like the virtuous Mary, the wealthy Khadījah, the learned 'Ā'ishah (d. 678), the devout Fāṭimah (d. 633), and the mystic Rabī'ah al-'Adawiyyah (d. 801). However, they are limited in number, while male jurists, mystics, theologians, rulers, exegetes, intellectuals, and philosophers have been countless. This comparison reveals the truth that women have systematically been precluded from the task of discovering the truth.

The current hierarchical gender system virtually excludes women from the pursuit of the truth, even though they in principle have the same potential, like men, to achieve biological, intellectual, spiritual, and mystical pleasure. This goal is viable as long as women equip themselves with such qualities as rationality, knowledge, autonomy, and independence. With these qualities in hand, women's dispositions will succeed very well in engaging in personal, familial, and communal participation.

This politics of inclusion will make women better persons and enable them to live their lives in a more meaningful way. In this milieu, the individual self, whether male or female, can put himself or herself forward to be God's vicegerent, that is one who promotes the doing of what is good and the prevention of what is evil, regardless of the roles they choose for themselves. Similarly, gender relationship between the individual self and others should be governed by mutual respect, interdependency, and coexistent partnership, so that each other's rights are respected and protected.

Conclusion

The existing hierarchical gender system nurtures and perpetuates the performance of the material self's expressions, which are limited to what men consider appropriate for women's femininity, morality, and pleasure. The multifaceted constitution of self, whether ontological, ethical, psychological, or extensional, is diluted with a construct of religious legitimacy and local culture that belittles women's worth as human beings. The equality of the ontological self evaporates in the self's bodily performance so that embodied self is cited with gendered truth and pleasure that are rooted in the Muslims' particular interpretation of Islam.

Since ideal Islam strives for egalitarian gender system that highlights individuality and his/her moral responsibility, Muslims, especially women, should be held accountable for improving and transforming women's lives in better social, economic, political, and cultural conditions. In this sense, women as speaking subjects have the capacity to improve their socio-politico and cultural conditions. To this end, every family could become a major force to eradicate the hierarchical gender system by having reservations about the constructed extensional dependency on the basis of sexual difference and by supporting reciprocal dependency among family members. In a broader sense, Muslims can extend this reciprocal dependency as an avenue to recognize each others rights, commonalities, duties, and responsibilities, while being respectful of sexual and gender differences in the society.

Engaging with the question of sexual difference and its impact on gender and self's construct is one of the most pressing queries of Muslim history.[107] It extends across the boundaries of location, culture, nationality, language, and tradition. Muslim women around the globe have channeled their consciousness raising through indigenous women's movements, feminist movements and gender activism.[108] Women's consciousness and organizing are precisely the opportunity for recognizing the religious, social, cultural, and political roots of the deep-seated oppression in their personal life, immediate family and societies.

The self-personal experience can become political when women altogether voice their concerns of social, cultural, psychological, and political realities that oppress them and care for transforming the current conditions by bringing women into the frontpage of humanity. These changes would be more effective to be initiated from within its locality so that womanists, feminists, and male egalitarianists would find the best possible way to transform their condition without much suspicion from the hierarchical gender-minded Muslims. The transformation should produce a new epistemic production of an egalitarian system that reinstates women's ontological self as human and the ethical transformation that cares for gender justice and for a good community (*ummah*).

Conclusion

The multifaceted explorations of gender and self share in common the fact that the epistemic paradigm of what Muslims perceive and conceptualize as religious legitimacy, knowledge, and power revolves around gender thinking that assumes and maintains the status quo of sexual difference and its politicized construct of the male superiority and female inferiority. This systematic and mechanism sees the embodied self as the site for the materialization of the religious, social, cultural, and social constructs. The embodiment process is reinforced by the citation of the gendered self as a producer of the conditional and particular truth that accords with masculine notions of human origin, reproduction, morality, femininity, and pleasure.

The epistemic perception and practices that shape the public perception of the truth of being a woman and man in Muslim communities are nurtured through the reiterations of: (1) gender thinking in the construction of sexuality and gender system and its cohesive impact on self-becoming; (2) the interpretation of the creation theory so as to establish a male humanity; (3) the greater regard accorded to the male role in matters of reproduction; (4) the grafting of popular masculine concepts of femininity onto women's bodies, resulting in the subordination of women's autonomy, independence and agency; and (5) the construction of self-becoming through the constructed extensional dependency that is prevalent in the current hierarchical gender system.

This book has attempted to trace the seamless thread of the diverse elements that foster and perpetuate the existing hierarchical gender system and that affect the construction of self-becoming. It not only deals with the roots of gender inequality that undermine women's worth as humans, but also examines Muslims' embodiment of Islamic authoritative legitimacies and its powerful corollaries at the theoretical and practical levels that have underpinned the establishment of the hierarchical gender system. The roots of the patriarchal and hierarchical gender system are ingrained in the deep-seated cultural, social, political, legal, and psychological constructs. This profound materialization of a dominant gender system has constructed the materiality of the self so that unfolding the key operatives of the fixity of the self at the theoretical, practical, and institutional levels, including family, cultures, and societies, sounds nearly impossible.

Nevertheless, uncovering the conditional and particular truth at the basis of hierarchical gender system is the moral responsibility of Muslim men and women, if they want to create a new reality that is friendly to human flourishing. Part of this process involves liberating women from the psychological, social, religious, and political barriers that shackle their lives, bringing women's issues to the center of humanity and empowering them with the skills, knowledge, power, and authority necessary for decision-making and survival in the male-dominated world. With this in mind, I propose strategies for the inclusion of women as individuals and as members of the community. I am particularly interested in revolutionary changes to the gender system through an epistemic, ontological, and ethical transformation that will contribute to an egalitarian gender system and a better constituent of self-becoming.

A new epistemic paradigm in Muslim societies commences with deconstructing what hierarchical gender-minded Muslims perceive and understand as the legitimate sources of knowledge, authority, and power. Muslims generally embrace the Qur'ān and aḥādīth as their inspiration for everyday life, even though the embodiment of the particularism of the Qur'ān and aḥādith is anchored within local cultures and societies. The interpretation of the Qur'ān and aḥādīth and the socio-cultural setting, together with what Muslims consider as the public perception of Islam, truth, knowledge, and power, inform Muslims' belief system and practices.

While hierarchical gender-minded Muslims exercise assumed religious legitimacies to influence human behavior, their guidance with regard to women is directed at every level of women's lives, ranging from their ontological origin, biology, sexuality, morality, familial, and social relationships, to their constructed role in the private and public spheres. This emphasis on shaping women's behavior, attitudes, beliefs, and wishes within Islamic boundaries leads them to believe that it is their duty to save women from indecency, immorality, and their potential threat to social disorder. Muslims' excessive protection, control, and safeguarding of women not only perpetuate the hierarchical gender system, but also permeate female self-becoming.

While variations of women's realities exist in the Muslim world, these social, political, and cultural conditions are environmental. Embedded in this conditional construct is the embodiment of Islamic teaching at the local level, where the multiplicity of Islamic expressions and practices is as diverse as the regions that make up the Muslim world. It is believed, however, that to deconstruct what constitutes the existing reality of the perceived Islamic expressions and practices that uphold the hierarchical gender system there must be a return to the Qur'ān. This call for renewal is not novel since Muslims, revivalists, feminists, fundamentalists have availed themselves with the Qur'ān for their purported agendas.

The Qur'ān and aḥādīth are, without doubt, central to Islam, whereas the authoritative legitimacies of these sources are human interpretations of the Qur'ān and aḥādīth that should be subjected to scrutiny. Indeed, the Qur'ān is divine and immutable, but the interpretations of them are bound up with human experience and limitations. In this sense, Qur'ānic interpretation can be fallible and biased depending on what Muslims perceive as the truth. One may argue that the vast scholarship on the Qur'ān reflects the best deliberation of the exegetes in an attempt to elaborate the Divine Will. This is true to the extent that all exegetes, especially those of the early generation, have had direct access to the Qur'ān and aḥādīth. However, they were also responsible for the absorption of local practices and sayings into their interpretations.

Since the interpretations of the Qur'ān and aḥādith generate diverse and sometimes contradictory claims of what is called Islam, it is important to put these sources into their respective contexts. This is necessary because the hierarchical reading of the Qur'ān only emerges strongly in the areas of male economic responsibility (Q.S. al-Nisā', 4:34), the reduced value of the testimony of a female, divorce (Q.S. al-Baqarah, 2:233) and the half share inheritance (Q.S. al-Nisā', 4:176). Even though these cases are exposed in the Qur'ān, they are inextricably bound to the specific historical context. This conditional particularism cannot be used to construe universal Islam since it is founded on the particular interpretation of Islamic teaching. In truth, the cases in point show the legal reform that Islam introduced into a society in which women had been debased. The Qur'ān reforms the social, political, and cultural contexts at that time by way of introducing women's rights into economy, inheritance, divorce, and the like.

Central to reinterpreting the Qur'ān is the task of separating the conditional and particular expositions of Islam from its universal messages. The formulated Islam, as we know it, was assimilated with the existing cultures in seventh century Arabia and its surroundings. In this pre-Islamic period, women were seen as the source of disgrace and dishonor. Islam, when it came, transformed the local belief systems. Gender egalitarianism, however, appears to have been systematically neglected. Women in almost every Muslim culture continue to suffer oppression at the hands of the patriarchal and hierarchical gender system. Even after exposure to Islam, local cultures and practices not only maintained a mode of gender thinking and a worldview in which men and women stood in binary opposition, but also withheld acknowledgment of women's worth as men's equals.

To transform Muslims' minds, theories, and practices, I propose the ontological model of *tawḥīd* (the Oneness of God) as a means to promote an inclusive humanity. Ontologically, God explains that He is the One, the Eternal Absolute: He does not beget, nor is He begotten (Qur'an, 112:1–4). Theologically, God is One in His Personhood (*dhāt*), His Attributes (*ṣifāt*) and His Works/actions (*af'āl*). Cosmologically, God is One by virtue of the multiplicity of His signs in macrocosm and microcosm. God's plurality in terms of Divine Attributes and Creative Activities lies in the fact that they are inseparable and should be seen as complementary to one another.

The concept of God's unity in His Person (*dhāt*) conveys a lesson of unity in humanity that endows humans with a multiplicity of personhood, attributes, characters, skills, individual freedoms, and responsibilities. The ontological self, the stable constituent of human being, is descended from one self (self/*nafs wāḥidah*), which is the original entity of Adam and Eve. What constitutes humans is, therefore, the blend of human form, the material substances, such as fluid/water (*mā'*), clay (*ṣalṣāl*)/clay (*ṭīn*), and dust (*turāb*). In the course of its development, however, this blended being is acted upon its environment. In this sense, while at a metaphysical level, the self is genderless, and of an identical nature in men and women, its social, cultural, political, psychological construction is environmental.

As the metaphysical self is deeply immersed in races, ethnic groups, and tribes in diverse localities and traditions, the self is sexed, embodied, gendered, and coded with different social, cultural, and legal constructs. While the biological difference is innate, the politicization and construction of sexual difference is justified by the assumption that embodied female self is generated out of a male ancestor, Adam, and that women's existence is derived from him for whom they were created. Since Adam is primary and Eve is secondary, it follows that men are more superior to the females. This logic leads to existing humanity that encompasses one singular subject, whereas women are *other* creatures, who are reducible to other subjects.

In the "othering" process, women are subjected to multifaceted power, authority, and religious legitimacies that maintain women as the other. The commonality of women's othering process throughout human history, their oppression, their constructed outcome and their emancipation are philosophical issues. I have argued throughout the book that the plurality of accidental human quantities, such as maleness and femaleness, and the multiplicity of human qualities, such as attributes, behavior, and skills, constitute a mosaic. These different quantities and qualities are conditional, but they comprise the universal. This universalism encompasses particular and conditional differences in the plurality of sexes, tribes, races, ethnicities, religions, languages, nationalities, ideologies, and other categories that enrich the mosaic of humanity. The notion of inclusive humanity conveys a unity that embraces various human differences, teaches humans to co-exist and helps them to cohere as members of a family, society, country, and planet, ready to respect each other and to protect each other's rights and responsibilities.

Humanity's diverse attributes may be seen as a unity, but its efforts (*af'āl*), comprised as they are of different occupations, skills, and career choices, are essential to human plurality. These activities are environmental. People do what they do out of personal interest, economic necessity, and social demand as a means to personal, familial, and community survival and commitment. However, human activities should not become the barriers to an inclusive humanity that embraces differences in sexuality and competence, since for every accumulation of humans' works (*af'āl*) there is a share to be distributed among the needy, the poor, the unfortunates so that justice is served. Nor should human works (*af'āl*) be used as sexual, gender, and social divides of what is appropriate for men and women, since the plurality of humans' works (*af'āl*) complements the perpetuation of humanity.

The embodiment of human personhood (*dhāt*), attributes (*ṣifāt*), and works (*af'āl*) as the mosaic of humanity will prevail if Muslims transform the present hierarchical dominant gender system into an egalitarian one. Part of the cohesive theological, social, cultural, and psychological transformation involves uncovering the prevailing thinking on gender, examining the male superiority in creation, reproduction, family, and society, identifying popular masculine concepts of femininity, affirming self-becoming through the constructed extensional dependency, instituting a legal system friendly to women, and fighting unfair sexual divisions of labor. Along with these revolutionary endeavors is the abolition of violent, aggressive, and vicious practices at the personal, familial, and societal levels that are detrimental to women's sexuality, bodies, and lives and opportunities. At the very least, Muslims should refrain from using the Qur'ān and aḥādīth as a means to justify the end, if the end is to humiliate, demean, and oppress women.

At the communal level, the ontological model of unity in personhood (*dhāt*), attributes (*ṣifāt*), and works (*af'āl*) can be utilized as the common ground of what constitutes humanity. A more community-minded expression would include the recognition of those individual differences that negate uniformity, while granting them the rights and actualization of their potential. Included is this communal actualization is the enactment of a legal system that metes out harsh punishment to personal, familial, and societal violators and that at the same time protects the vulnerable, especially women and children, who can easily be subjected to domestic and sexual violence, negligence, and trafficking.

Centering and empowering women as individuals are what Islam has proposed fourteen centuries ago during the time when women were seen as the source of dishonor, social disorder and weakness, disposable property, sexual objects, and other demeaning labels. Following the abolition of female infanticide, Islam acknowledged women's worth as individual human beings enjoying rights equal to men at the personal, familial, and communal levels. Islam grants each woman rights to pursue personal goals, financial security and knowledge, religious authority and observance, and public participation, without any discrimination. Personal realization and perfection are highly encouraged in Islam, because each individual has the same potential to attain the state (*ḥāl*) of the perfect person (*al-insān al-kāmil*) regardless of gender difference. Female self-realization in religion, politics, knowledge, power, and authority is possible if women are given proper trainings and opportunities to actualize their potential.

Giving women the skills, training and education necessary to become good individuals was exemplified by the Prophet Muḥammad, especially in his attitude towards 'Ā'ishah, who enjoyed considerable autonomy with his blessing. 'Ā'ishah is in fact a good model for the empowerment of contemporary Muslim women who strive for gender justice and peaceful resolution in enfolding the hierarchical and patriarchal gender system. Muslim women deserve the power, knowledge and authority necessary for their personal survival as individuals and members of families, society, and the world. This is at least what Muslims owe them. At the practical level, Muslim scholars, activists, feminists, and local governments are called to put forward working strategies that empower women and center their being in the world of humanity.

As Islam advocates the unity of humans at every level, men and women as God's vicegerents are required to govern every aspect of their lives in accordance with the Qur'ān, since it provides the ground for moral integrity for individuals and community. As morality constitutes the primary interest of the Divine, the Qur'ān assumes that the characters of human beings are always in tension; that they have to seek to exhibit themselves with creative actions, thus promoting justice among people in particular and cosmic justice in general. This moral dimension of the Qur'ān is definitely the backbone of an egalitarian gender system.

Embodying Islam in daily life requires not only the epistemic and ontological reform, but also the ethical transformation. The spirit of Islamic ethics lies in one's ability to promote what is right (*ma'rūf*) and forbid what is wrong (*munkar*) (Āl 'Imrān, 3:104 and 110). This maxim is the universal principle, the one that governs the self as an individual and as a member of family and community. Islam not only recognizes equality of men and women as partners and individuals in humanity and society, but also governs the individuality of a person and his/her relationship to God, others, and the world. What differentiates one self from others is intention, deed, and God's conscience. The individual self, whether male or female, is invited to partake in the materialization of righteousness in every aspect of human life. Individual and communal righteousness is the basis for the establishment and maintenance of the best community.

Even though Muslims would not communally agree to violate the call for "good," personal interest and experience are often involved in the production of what is good. This has been the case with the politics of the interpretation of Islamic teachings and its attempt to actualize its interpretation in practice. The call for promulgating what is good does not discriminate against any self. This is to say that, to be part of a good community is to become good individually: this is to be achieved by habituating oneself so that one has the potential to become a good member of society. On the contrary, if one excludes himself/herself from becoming good individually, society would want to exclude and eliminate such an individual, so that the unity of the community would belong to the good.

However, Muslim societies have established the notion of a "good community" based on the male concept of what is "good." They believe that the mechanism that maintains a good community depends on controlling the imagined harms that can lead to the corruption of society. As these imagined harms potentially come from women, it is assumed that female sexuality equals defectiveness and imperfection; hence, the control of female sexuality becomes the only means of safeguarding women from their presumed fate. With this in mind, the control of women by means of excessive religious norms and practices, like extreme veiling, seclusion, and exclusion from public prayer. In this conjunction, religious guidance, veiling, and seclusion are considered benevolent treatment of women because these opinions and practices are aimed at protecting women's morality, dignity, and righteousness. Muslim women, for their part, have embraced this religious praxis for the reason that they believe in it as their truth; hence, the actualization of beliefs, rules, and practices becomes indispensable.

Despite the male concern to control female sexuality, bodies, and contours (for the sake of women's righteousness), this benevolent protection can result in a woman's denial of humanity. Women are deprived not only of their worth as human beings, but also of their social, political, and psychological constructs that are closely associated with their natural and sexual disposition. Women's lives attest to the binary opposition of sexual and gender difference and the system it produces. The resiliently constructed hierarchical gender system is still dominant, regardless of what Muslims have been through during the challenging eras of colonization, post-colonization, modernization, nationalism, democracy, gender activism and feminism, and modern education.

However, the production of an egalitarian gender system is on the way, however long it may take. Feminists, womanists, and male activists/egalitarianists as individuals and members of the global community are actively engaged in a discourse that contributes to egalitarian gender system by way of uncovering the roots of the hierarchical gender system and its oppressive effect on self-becoming. They call upon hierarchical gender-minded Muslim men and women at every level of society to transform the social, cultural, and political realities, to diminish the degree of oppression and to recognize different avenues for human emancipation from the shackles of religious, psychological, cultural, and social traditions.

Glossary

'Ā'ishah the daughter of Abū Bakr, one of the Prophet Muḥammad's wives, and leader of the forces opposed to 'Alī at the Battle of the Camel in 656.

'alaqah a blood-clot in the shape of a leech, used in the Qur'ān to denote the zygote.

aḥādīth plural of the word *ḥadīth*, that is, a recorded action, wish, or saying of the Prophet Muḥammad.

barakah the blessing that is granted by Allāh to those who interact with flawless Muslim scholars.

bashar a term denoting the physical human being and his power as God's creature.

al-bashariyyah humanity, with special reference to the common traits of the human being's physical form and his/her role as God's creature on earth.

da'wah Islamic preaching aimed at teaching Muslims about Islam.

al-dhakar the male; the Arabic term denoting the biological phenomenon that is a man.

farḍ an act obligatory for all Muslims, the omission of which will result in punishment.

fatwā' a religious opinion that is a product of the *Ijtihād* process.

fiqh "understanding"; used especially in reference to the process of understanding God's Divine Law.

ḥabl min al-nās a human being's relations with other humans.

ḥabl min-Allāh a human being's relations with God.

ḥalaqah a religious meeting.

ḥaqīqah referring to the esoteric meaning of the teaching of Islam.

al-hawā the human being's inner self that aspires to materialize base desires.

ḥijab a screen; it also refers to spatiality (seclusion) and "Islamic" personal dress.

al-ḥiss al-mushtarak one of the internal senses that function as a bridge between the brain and the senses.

Iblīs Satan.

ijtihād exertion, effort, and endeavour. It refers to the jurists' best effort to apply his legal knowledge in order to produce legal opinions.

al-insān the Qur'ānic term denoting human beings in their created natures, human forms and their properties.

Islam peace, purity, submission, and obedience—the religion revealed by God to the Prophet Muḥammad beginning in AD 610.

isrā' the Night Journey of the Prophet Muḥammad from Medina to Jerusalem; part of the event of *Al-Isrā' wa-al-Mi'rāj*.

Jāhiliyyah the age of ignorance that occurred before the rise of Islam.

kalām also called *uṣūl al-dīn* (the principles or the roots of religion), it is the science of Islamic doctrine and serves to defend the truth of the Qur'ān and the faith of Islam.

khalīfah vicegerent; it denotes the human being's superior role in creation and his/her mission as the Prophet's successors on earth.

kimār head covering worn as Islamic personal dress.

malā'ikah angel; created out of light, it executes God's orders with full obedience.

ma'rifah knowledge of God.

mi'rāj The Prophet's "ascension" to Heaven from Jerusalem.

Mu'āwiyah The self-proclaimed caliph who founded the Umayyad dynasty (661–80).

Muḥammad the Prophet and founder of Islam who taught the Unity of God (*Tawḥīd*). He died in the year 632 CE.

mujtahīd one who performs *Ijtihād*.

Muslim a follower of Islam.

nafs "self"; living entity, soul, soul, spirit, mind, animate being, human being, person, self humankind, life essence, human origin, and humanity.

al-nafs al-ammārah a human being's inner self that incites evil thought and action.

al-nafs al-lawwāmah a human being's inner conscience of his/her weaknesses and failures.

al-nafs al-muṭma'innah a human being's inner self that has achieved tranquility and peace.

nushūz a woman's disobedience to her husband.

pesantren an Islamic educational institution in Indonesia.

qiyās one of the methods of *Ijtihād*, strictly speaking, analogical reasoning, or deduction.

Qur'ān the Muslim holy book revealed to Prophet Muḥammad.

Ramaḍān the nineth lunar month, during which Muslims fast every day from dawn to dusk.

Sharī'ah "the revealed law." It literally denotes the way or path to a water hole.

Ṣūfism the mystical expression of Islam, whose adherents promote repentance, renouncement of worldly delights, deprivation of food and sex as a preparation for the Day of Judgment, and experience of proximity with God.

ṣūrah the image of human form and its perfect properties.

'ulamā' religious scholars with a thorough knowledge of the Islamic sciences.

al-unsā the female; the Arabic term to denote the biological phenomenon that is a woman.

uṣūl al-fiqh the theoretical understanding of the science of jurisprudence.

Notes

Introduction

1 Muslim women do not uniformly refer to their interests, endeavors, and struggles for gender justice as feminist movements, for the term "feminism" is loaded with Western connotations. However, as Cooke indicates, there is no better word that captures women's social and political activisms in the Muslim world, except the word "feminism." See Miriam Cooke (2001) *Women Claim Islam*, New York: Routledge, pp. ix–x.

2 Womanists refer to those women who share a similar interest with feminists in that they seek to transform women's personal, social, and political responsibilities and empower them in the private and public spheres. Roald, for instance, believes in the empowerment of women, but she does not label herself as a feminist since Muslim feminist works often disregard the male perspectives that are favorable for women. See, Anne Sofie Roald (2001) *Women in Islam: The Western Experience*, London, New York: Routledge, p. xi.

3 The following works are well-known for a fair treatment of gender issues in Muslim scholarship. See, Qasim Amin (1992) *The Liberation of Women and The New Women*, Cairo, Egypt: The American University in Cairo Press; Munawar Ahmad Anees (1989) *Islam and Biological Futures: Ethics, Gender, and Technology*, London and New York: Mansell; Asgharali Engineer (1992) *The Rights of Women in Islam*, New York: St Martin's Press; and Farid Esack (2001) "Islam and gender Justice: Beyond Simplistic Apologia," in John C. Raines and Daniel C. Maguire (eds), *What Men Owe to Women*, Albany, NY: State University of New York Press, pp. 187–210.

4 See Chandra Talpade Mohanty (1991) "Under Western Eyes: Feminist Scholarship and Colonial Discourse," in Chandra Talpade Mohanty, Ann Russo, and Lourdes Torres (eds), *Third World Women and The Politics of Feminism*, Bloomington and Indianapolis: Indiana University Press, IN, p. 62.

5 See Ann Ferguson (1997) "Moral responsibility and social change: a new theory of self," *Hypatia*, Summer, 12:3, p. 124.

6 Hans Wehr (2000) *A Dictionary of Modern Written Arabic*, J. Milton Cowan (ed.) Beirut: Librairie du Liban, p. 985.

7 See Q.S. 4:1, 6:98, 7:189, and 39:6.

8 E.E. Carvely (1943) "Doctrines of the Soul (*Nafs and Rūḥ*) in Islam," *Muslim World*, 33:254.

9 Michael E. Marmura (1987) "Soul: Islamic Concepts," in Mircea Eliade (ed.) *Encyclopedia of Religion*, New York: Macmillan Publishing Company, p. 461.

10 'Abdur Raḥman I. Doi (1989) *Woman in Shari'ah*, London: Ta-Ha Publishers Ltd, p. 3.

11 Abdur Rahman al-Sheha (2000) *Women in the Shade of Islam*, Riyadh: Islamic Educational Center, p. 4.

12 See introductory remarks of the editors to (1999) "What is Women's Studies," in Amy Kesselman, Lily D. McNair, Nancy Schniedewind (eds) (1999) *Women: Images and Realities*, Mountain View, California: Mayfield Publishing Company, p. 9.

13 Ibid., p. 109.

14 Allan G. Johnson (2000) "Patriarchy, the System: An It, Not a He, a Them, or an Us," in *Women's Lives: Multicultural Perspectives*, in Gwyn Kirk and Margo Okazawa-Rey (eds), New York: McGraw Hill, pp. 29–30.
15 Roald, *Women in Islam*, p. 78.
16 Ibid.
17 Riddell has an elaborate account of the transmission of Islamic teachings and thoughts from the Middle East and South Asia to Malay-Indonesian regions during the past seven centuries and up to present times and Indonesian Muslim responses to the Islamic thought. See Peter G. Riddell (2001) *Islam and Malay-Indonesian World: Transmission and Responses*, Honolulu, HI: University of Hawai'i Press.
18 An excellent introduction that addresses the insiders and outsiders' controversies can be found in Russell T. McCutcheon (ed.) (1999) *The Insider/Outsider Problem in the Study of Religion: A Reader*, London and New York: Cassell.
19 Clifford Geertz (1960) *The Religion of Java*, Chicago, IL: University of Chicago Press.
20 See Roald who also raises similar concerns and questions in her work, *Women in Islam*, p. 78.
21 Hideko Iwai (1985) *Islamic Society and Women in Islam*, Japan: The Institute of Middle Eastern Studies, International University of Japan, pp. 6–7.
22 See McCutcheon, *The Insider/Outsider Problem in the Study of Religion*, p. 6.
23 Al-Qur'ān, Ar-Ra'd, 13:15. Muhammad Asad (trans.) (1980) *The Message of the Qur'ān*, Gibraltar: Dār al-Andalus, p. 361.
24 Maurice Bucaille (1978) *The Bible, the Quran and Science: the Holy Scriptures Examined in the Light of Modern Knowledge*, Indianapolis: American Trust Publications. Ibrahim B. Syed (1987) "Islamization of Attitude and Practice in Embryology," in M.A.K. Lodhi (ed.) *Islamization of Attitudes and Practices in Science and Technology*, Virginia: The International Institute of Islamic Thought, p. 119.
25 See S. Waqar Ahmed Husaini (1980) *Islamic Environmental Systems Engineering*, London: The MacMillan Press, p. 3. See also al-Qur'an Al-Baqara, 2:3. Asad, *The Message of the Qur'ān*, p. 4.
26 Fazlur Rahman (1995) *Islamic Methodology in History*, Pakistan: Islamic Research Institute, (3rd reprint), p. 14.
27 Murata (1992) *The Tao of Islam*. A sourcebook of Gender Relationships in Islamic Thought, Albany, NY: State University of New York Press, pp. 2–3.
28 Fazlur Rahman (1979) *Islam*, Chicago, IL and London: University of Chicago Press, pp. 100–1.
29 Shāh Walī Allāh (1996) *The Conclusive Argument from God*, in Marcia K. Hermansen (trans.), Leiden, New York: E.J. Brill, pp. 275 and 449.
30 Wael B. Hallaq (1984), "Was the gate of ijtihad closed," *International Journal of Middle East Studies* 16, 3.
31 Fazlur Rahman (1984) Islam and Modernity: Transformation of an Intellectual Tradition, Chicago, IL and London: The University of Chicago Press, p. 18.
32 Hallaq has a lengthy discussion of the context in which the *gate* of *ijtihād* was closed. He argues that the *ijtihād* was closed neither in theory nor in practice. Ibid., pp. 3–41.
33 Rahman discusses the earlier reform movements in Muslim world in his work, *Islam and Modernity*, pp. 214–34.
34 Rahman, *Islam and Modernity*, p. 8.
35 Majid Fakhry (1983) *A History of Islamic Philosophy*, New York: Columbia University Press; Seyyed Hossein Nasr and Oliver Leaman (eds) (1996) *History of Islamic Philosophy*, Part I and II, London and New York: Routledge; and Oliver Leaman (1999) *A Brief Introduction to Islamic Philosophy*, United Kingdom: Polity Press.
36 Carol C. Gould (1980) "The Woman Question: Philosophy of Liberation and The Liberation of Philosophy," in Carol C. Gould and Marx W. Wartofsky (eds), *Women and Philosophy: Toward a Theory of Liberation*, New York: A Perigee Book, p. 5.

37 Ibid., p. 8.
38 Ibid., p. 9.
39 Ibid., p. 26.
40 Ibid.
41 Ibid., p. 27.
42 Ibid., p. 28.
43 Ibid.
44 Beverly Clack (1999) *Misogyny in the Western Philosophical Tradition*, New York: Routledge, pp. 6–7.
45 Well-known to the Western readers as Avicenna, Ibn Sīnā's full name was Abū 'Ālī al-Ḥusayn b. 'Abd Allāh b. Ḥasan b. 'Ālī b. Sīnā (980–1037). He is considered the "most celebrated Muslim philosopher and has even been called the *princeps philosophorum* (the great master). His works are numerous and voluminous. G.C. Anawati estimates Ibn Sīnā's writings to be about 276 separate works; see his *Mu'allafāt Ibn Sīnā* (1955) Cairo: Dār al-Ma'ārif. Discussion of Ibn Sīnā's bibliography and its extent can be read in W.E. Gohlman (1974) *The Life of Ibn Sina*, Albany, NY: State University of New York Press, pp. 13–15 and 91–111.
46 Islamic Philosophy, often called *falsafa* and *ḥikma*, originates from Greek philosophy. According to Nasr, it shares a remarkable similar definition to Greeks as follows:

1 Philosophy *(al-falsafa)* is the knowledge of all existing things qua existents *(ashyā' al-mawjūda bi māhiya mawijūda)*.
2 Philosophy is knowledge of divine and human matters.
3 Philosophy is taking refuge in death, that is, love of death.
4 Philosophy is becoming God-like to the extent of human ability.
5 Philosophy is the art *(ṣinā'a)* of arts and the science *('ilm)* of science.
6 Philosophy is the predilection for *ḥikma* [wisdom].

See Seyyed Hossein Nasr, "The Meaning and Concept of Philosophy in Islam," in Nasr and Leaman (eds), *History of Islamic Philosophy*, Part I, pp. 21–22.
47 See Marshall G.S. Hodgson (1977) *The Venture of Islam: Conscience and History in a World Civilization*, vol. 1, Chicago, IL and London: The University of Chicago Press, p. 412.
48 Ibid., pp. 412–3.
49 Ira M. Lapidus (1988) *A History of Islamic Societies*, Cambridge: Cambridge University Press, pp. 93–4.
50 Hodgson, *The Venture of Islam*, vol. 1, p. 419.
51 Edward W. Said (1997) *Covering Islam*, revised edition, New York: Vintage Books, p. 61.
52 F.E. Peters, "The Greek and Syriac Background," in Nasr and Leaman (eds), *History of Islamic Philosophy*, Part I, pp. 41–42.
53 Seyyed Hossein Nasr, "The Qur'ān and Ḥadīth as Source and Inspiration of Islamic Philosophy," in ibid., p. 29.
54 Lapidus, *A History of Islamic Societies*, p. 95.
55 Nasr, "The Qur'ān and Ḥadīth as Source and Inspiration of Islamic Philosophy," in Nasr and Leaman (eds), *History of Islamic Philosophy*, p. 35.
56 Amina Wadud Muhsin distinguishes three configurations of Islam: primary, intellectual, and cultural. Primary Islam refers to the Qur'ān and the tradition of the Prophet. Intellectual Islam arises out of the primary teachings of Islam, such as *sharī'a* (law), ethics, exegesis, logic, philosophy, and aesthetics. Cultural Islam refers to the way in Muslim people from diverse cultures attempt to respond to both the primary and intellectual dimensions of Islam. See Amina Wadud Muhsin (2000) "Alternative Qur'anic Interpretation and the Status of Muslim Women," in Gisela Webb (ed.) *Windows of Faith: Muslim Women Scholar-Activists in North America*, Syracuse, NY: Syracuse University Press (2000), p. 4.

1 Gender thinking and the system it produces

1 Ernst Renan (2000) "Muhammad and the Origin of Islam," in Ibn Warraq (ed. Anmd trans.), *The Quest for the Historical Muhammad*, Amherst, NY: Prometheus Books, p. 157.
2 Khaled Abou El Fadl (2001) *Speaking in God's Name: Islamic Law, Authority, and Women*, Oxford: Oneworld (1996) p. 12.
3 Nimat Hafez Barazangi (1996) "Vicegerency and Gender Justice in Islam," in Nimat Hafez Barazangi, M. Raquibuz Zaman and Omar Afzal (eds), *Islamic Identity and the Struggle for Justice*, Tampa University Press of Florida, pp. 81–2.
4 Asma Barlas (2002) *"Believing Women" in Islam: Unreading Patriarchal Interpretations of the Qur'ān*, Austin, TX: University of Texas Press.
5 Ibid., p. 3.
6 Farid Esack, "Islam and Gender Justice," p. 192.
7 Asad, *The Message of the Qur'ān*, p. 645.
8 Ibid., p. 65.
9 What constitutes the "sapiential tradition" is the works that commonly belong to the theoretical Ṣufism and philosophy and are written with both philosophical and Sufic insights. Those Sufi-philosophers are Ibn 'Arabī, Suhrawardī al-Maqtūl and Mullā Ṣadrā. See Sachiko Murata (1992) *The Tao of Islam: A Sourcebook of Gender Relationships in Islamic Thought*, Albany, NY: State University of New York Press, p. 3.
10 God, the Cosmos and human beings are the common themes of theology, mysticism, and Sufism. Murata speaks of these three themes according to those intellectual traditions. She indicates that she discusses the notion of gender within the "sapiential tradition," but she also argues the issue of gender relationship is essentially theological in its broadest sense. For this reason, theological perspectives on the interconnectedness of the three realities cannot be left out. See ibid., pp. 3 and 18.
11 Ibid., p. 23.
12 Ibid., pp. 69–73.
13 Ibid., pp. 18–19.
14 Khaled Abou El Fadl, *Speaking in God's Name*, p. 10.
15 Ibid.
16 Asghar Ali Engineer (2001) "Islam, Women, and Gender Justice," in John C. Raines and Daniel C. Maguire (eds), *What Men Owe to Women*, Albany, NY: State University of New York Press, p. 112.
17 Fatima Mernissi (1991) *The Veil and the Male Elite: A Feminist Interpretation of Women's Rights in Islam*, trans. Mary Jo Lakeland, New York: Addison-Wesley Publishing Company Inc., p. 43.
18 El Fadl, *Speaking in God's Name*, p. 4.
19 Walther and Tucker portray the lives of Muslim women in Islamic history. See Wiebke Walther (1993) *Women in Islam*, Princeton and New York: Markus Wiener Publishing; and Judith E. Tucker (1993) *Gender and Islamic History*, Washington, DC: American Historical Association.
20 Luce Irigaray (1996) *I Love to You: Sketch of a Possible Felicity in History*, trans. Alison Martin, New York and London: Routledge, p. 47 ff.
21 Michel Foucault (1990) *History of Sexuality*, vol. 1, *An Introduction*, trans. Robert Hurly, New York: Vintage Books, pp. 24–6.
22 Judith Butler (1993) *Bodies That Matter*, New York: Routledge, p. 2.
23 Umar has a vivid explanation of the way in which '*al-dhakar*' and '*al-unsā*'' is used in the Qur'ān. See Nasaruddin Umar (1999) *Argumen Kesetraan Jender: Perspectif al-Qur'ân* [*Argument for Gender Equality: Qur'ânic Perspective*], Jakarta: Paramadina, p. 164.
24 Al-'Allāmah al-Rāghib al-Iṣfahānī, *Mufradāt Alfāẓ al-Qur'ān* (ed.) Ṣafwān 'Adnān Dawdī, Beirut, al-Daār al-Shāmīya, n.d., p. 93. See also Umar, *Argumen Kesetraan Jender*, p. 165.
25 See Asad's translation of Āl 'Imrān, 3:36. Asad, *The Message of the Qur'ān*, p. 71.

26 This is a common translation found in the Indonesian version of the Qur'ān. Umar uses the translation "a male is not the same as a female." See, Umar (1957) *Argumen Kesetaraan Jender*, p. 165. See Zainuddin Hamidy, *Tafsir Qurän*, Jakarta: Penerbit Widjaya.

27 'Abū 'Alī al-Faḍl b. al-Ḥasan al-Ṭabarsī (1971) *Majmū' al-Bayān fī Tafsīr al-Qur'ān*, vol. 2, Beirut, Lebanon: Dār Maktabat al-Ḥayat, p. 66.

28 Ibid.

29 Al-Zamakhsharī in *al-Kashshāf 'an Ḥaqā'iq Ghawāmiḍ al-Tanzīl* holds the view that the male child for whom the 'Imrān family prayed would never have been equal to Mary in excellence and devotion. See al-Zamakhsharī, vol. 1, p. 425.

30 Al-Ṭabrasī, *Majmū' al-Bayān fī Tafsīr al-Qur'ān*, p. 66.

31 Stephen David Ross (1998) *The Gift of Touch*, Albany, NY: SUNY Press, p. 252.

32 The following *ḥadith* is often reiterated to show women's deficiency in reason and religion.

> Once Allah's Apostle went out to the Muṣallā (to offer the prayer) of 'Id al-Aḍḥā or al-Fiṭr prayer. Then he passed by the women and said, "O women! Give alms, as I have seen that the majority of the dwellers of Hell-fire were you (women)." They asked, "Why is it so, O Allah's Apostle?" He replied, "You curse frequently and are ungrateful to your husbands. I have not seen anyone more deficient in intelligence and religion than you. A cautions, sensible man could be led astray by some of you." The women asked, "O Allah's Apostle! What is deficient in our intelligence and religion?" He said, "Is not the evidence of two women equal to the witness of one man?" They replied in the affirmative. He said, "This is the deficiency in her intelligence. Isn't it true that a woman can neither pray nor fast during her menses?" The women replied in the affirmative. He said, "This is the deficiency in her religion."
>
> (Narrated by Abū Sa'īd al-Khuḍrī, *Ṣaḥīḥ al-Bukhārī*, 1.301)

Even though, it is not our purpose to examine the soundness of this *ḥadīth*, it is important to note that *Ṣaḥīḥ al-Bukkhārī* is considered one of sources of the Musilm legal system. According to the four Sunnite schools (*madhāhib*), any *ḥadiṭh* written therein is considered sound (*ṣaḥīḥ*) and is therefore dependable.

33 Jone Johnson Lewis, "Women Prime Ministers and Presidents: 20th Century Global Women Political Leaders." Online available: http://womenshistory.about.com/library/weekly/aa010128a.html (accessed March 8, 2005).

34 Narrated by Abū Bakr in *Sahīh al-Bukharī*, 5.709. See CD *Alim*.

35 Fatima Mernissi (1991) *Women and Islam: An Historical and Theological Inquiry*, trans. Mary Jo Lakeland, UK: Backwell, pp. 3–5.

36 Mernissi, *The Veil and the Male Elite*, pp. 60–1.

37 D.A. Spellberg (1994) *Politics, Gender, and the Islamic Past: The Legacy of 'Ā'isha bint Abi Bakr*, New York: Columbia University Press, pp. 119–21.

38 Haifaa A. Jawad (1998) *The Rights of Women in Islam: An Authentic Approach*, New York: St Martin's Press, Inc., p. 89.

39 Ibid., pp. 138–9.

40 Butler, *Bodies That Matter*, pp. 107–8.

41 Mernissi, *Women and Islam*, pp. 3–5.

42 Ibid.

43 For a lengthy discussion of the reasons for which women are forbidden to engage in public affairs and to become leaders can be found in Jawad, *The Rights of Women in Islam*, pp. 89–96.

44 Ibid., p. 13.

45 Marianne Ferguson (1995) *Women and Religion*, Upper Saddle River, NJ: Prentice Hall, pp. 100–2.

46 Nawal El Saadawi (1980) *The Hidden Face of Eve: women in the Arab world*, Boston, MA: Beacon Press, p. 12.

47 The unwelcome feeling and hostility toward the birth of a female body have their root in the pre-Islamic period. As is known, the birth of girls was considered a disgrace and an embarrassment. See Malik Ram Baveja (1981) *Women in Islam*, New York: Advent Books, pp. 1–2.
48 Spellberg, *Politics, Gender, and the Islamic Past*, p. 62.
49 This attitude is commonly believed to be part of Southeast Asian tradition in which women often enjoy a privileged status. See Shelly Errington (1990) "Recasting Sex, Gender, and Power: A Theoretical and Regional Overview," in Jane Monnig Atkinson and Shelly Errington (eds) *Power and Difference: Gender in Island Southeast Asia*, California: Stanford University of California, pp. 1–58.
50 Leanne Merrett-Balkos (1998) "Just Add Water: Remaking Women through Childbirth, Anganen, Southern Highlands, Papua New Guinea," in Kalpana Ram and Margaret Jolly (ed.) *Maternities and Modernities: Colonial and Postcolonial Experiences in Asia and the Pacific*, Cambridge: Cambridge, UK; New York: Cambridge University Press, p. 223.
51 Errington, "Recasting Sex, Gender, and Power: A Theoretical and Regional Overview," pp. 22.
52 Ibid.
53 Judith Butler (1990) *Gender Trouble*, London and New York: Routledge, p. 6.
54 Jane English (1977) *Sex Equality*, Englewood Cliffs, NJ: Prentice-Hall, p. 72.
55 Luce Irigaray (2001) *Democracy Begins between Two*, trans. Kirsteen Anderson, New York: Routledge, p. 125.
56 Ibid., p. 122.
57 Ibid., p. 129.
58 Ibn Sīnā (1963) "Avicenna: Healing: Metaphysics," trans. Michael E. Marmura, in Ralph Lerner and Muhsin Mahdi (ed.) *Medieval Political Philosophy*, Ithaca, NY: Ithaca University Press, p. 106.
59 Aristotle (1984) *Physics*, Chapter 9 of Book I (192a21–3), trans. R.P. Hardie and R.K. Gaye, in Jonathan Barnes, (ed.) *The Complete Works of Aristotle: The Revised Oxford Translation*, vol. 1, Princeton NJ: Princeton University Press, p. 328.
60 Aristotle (1984) *Politics*, Book II, trans. B. Jowett, in Jonathan Barnes, (ed.) *The Complete Works of Aristotle: The Revised Oxford Translation*, vol. 2, Princeton, NJ: Princeton University Press, 1260a9–16.
61 See E.O. Wilson (1978) *On Human Nature*, Cambridge: Harvard University Press, p. 125.
62 Ibid.
63 Anees, *Islam and Biological Futures*, p. 8.
64 John T. Noonan, Jr (2000) "An Almost Absolute Value in History," in Ronald Munson (ed.) *Intervention and Reflection: Basic Issues in Medical Ethics*, United States: Wadsworth, sixth edition, p. 84.
65 Ronald Munson (2000) "Social Context: The Holy Grail of Biology: the human genome project," in Ronald Munson (ed.) *Intervention and Reflection: Basic Issues in Medical Ethics*, United States: Wadsworth, sixth edition, p. 559.
66 Noonan, "An Almost Absolute Value in History," p. 84.
67 Fatima Mernissi, *Beyond the Veil: Male-Female Dynamics in a Modern Muslim Society*, New York: Schenkman Publishing Company, 1975, pp. 3–13. See also Bullock's accounts and critics of Mernissi's "the Muslim social order" in her work. Katherine Helen Bullock, *Rethinking Muslim Women and The Veil: Challenging Historical & Modern Stereotypes*, London: The International Institute of Islamic Thought, 2002.
68 Mernissi, *Beyond the Veil*, p. 13.
69 Ibid.
70 Deborah L. Black (1996) "Al-Fārābī," in *History of Islamic Philosophy*, Part 1, edited by Seyyed Hossein Nasr and Oliver Leamen, London and New York: Routledge, p. 187.
71 Hodgson, *The Venture of Islam*, vol. 2, p. 171.
72 Ibn Sīnā, "Avicenna: Healing: Metaphysics," p. 104.
73 Ibn Sīnā conceived of the city in the same manner as did Plato; the latter divided the city's residents into three groups: artisans, guardians, and administrators. This composition is

analogous to the human soul: appetite, spirit, and intellect. Each of these has its own virtue: sobriety for the appetite and artisans; bravery for the spirit and guardians; and wisdom for the intellect and rulers. If these groups could perform their virtues, the creation of a just city would result, just as the virtue of each person could create a just person (Book IV, 427d–433e). See Plato (1961) "Republic," trans. Paul Shorey in Edith Hamilton and Huntington Cairns (eds) *The Collected Dialogue of Plato*, Princeton, NJ: Princeton University Press.

74 Ibn Sīnā, "Avicenna: Healing: Metaphysics," p. 105.
75 Lapidus, *A History of Islamic Society*, p. 29.
76 Aristotle, *Politics*, 1259b3–4, p. 1998
77 Ibid., 1260a24–25, p. 1999.
78 Ibid., 1254b14–15, p. 1990.
79 Plato, *Republic*, V, 451d4–10, p. 690.
80 Ibid., 451e1–2.
81 Ibid., 453e2–6, p. 692.
82 Ibid., 454d7–11, p. 693.
83 Ibid., 455d8–9, p. 694.
84 Ibn Sīnā, "Avicenna: Healing: Metaphysics," p. 105.
85 Aristotle, *Politics*, 1261a10–15, 2001.
86 Ibid., 1261a16.
87 Ibid., 1260b40.
88 Ibid., 1261b24–25, p. 2002.
89 Prudence Allen (1985) *The Concept of Women: The Aristotelian Revolution, 750 BC–AD 1250*, Montreal London: Eden Press, p. 86.
90 Ibid., p. 87.
91 Aristotle, *Politics*, 1262b5–17, p. 2003.
92 Ibid., 1262b20–21.
93 Ibid., 1263a37–39, 2004–5.
94 Ibid., 1263b6–14, p. 2006.
95 Ibid., Book II, 1264b1–5, p. 2006.
96 Ibn Sīnā, "Avicenna: Healing: Metaphysics," p. 105.
97 Azizah Y. al-Hibri (2000) "An Introduction to Muslim Women's Rights," in Gisela Webb (ed.) *Windows of Faith: Muslim Women Scholar-Activists in North America*, Syracuse, NY: Syracuse University Press, p. 57.
98 Maysam J. al- Faruqi (2000) "Women's Self-Identity in the Qur'ān and Islamic Law," in Gisela Webb (ed.) *Windows of Faith: Muslim Women Scholar-Activists in North America*, Syracuse, NY: Syracuse University Press, p. 83.
99 Sayyid Abul A'lā Mawdūdi (1989) *Toward Understanding the Qur'ān*, vol. 2, Delhi: Markazi Maktaba Islami, p. 35.
100 Ibn Hajar Al-Asqalani (1996) *Bulugh Al-Marâm*, Saudi Arabia: Dar-us-Salam Publications, p. 374.
101 Ibn Sīnā, "Avicenna: Healing: Metaphysics," p. 105.
102 Ibid., p. 106
103 Al-Faruqi, "Women's Self-Identity in the Qur'ānic and Islamic Law," p. 93.
104 Ibn Sīnā, "Avicenna: Healing: Metaphysics," p. 106.
105 Aristotle, *Politics*, 1253b5–10, p. 1988.
106 Ibid., 1255b19–21, p. 1992.
107 Ibid., 1252b1, p. 1987.
108 Ibid., 1254a20–24, p. 1990.
109 Ibid., 1260a13, p. 1999.
110 Ibid., p. 106.
111 Ibid., p. 168.
112 See the Qur'ānic, an-Nisā', 4:95. Asad, *The Message of the Qur'ānic*, p. 123.
113 Ahmed, *Women and Gender in Islam*, p. 53.

114 See al-Jawzī, *Kitāb Aḥkām al-Nisā'*, p. 69.
115 Ibid., p. 76.
116 Ibid., pp. 68, 72, and 73.
117 Ibid., pp. 136–46.
118 Ibid., p. 133.
119 Ibid., p. 156.
120 Ibid., p. 178.
121 Ibid., pp. 170–1.
122 Ali A. Mazrui (1999) "Islamic Paradoxes," in *Muslim Democrat*, vol. 1, No. 2 (September), 5.
123 See Jamāl al-Dīn al-Jawzī (1996) *Kitāb Aḥkām al-Nisā'*, Beirut: Dār al-Fikr, pp. 104–5. This book not only mentions where the ahādīth come from, but also explains the narrators of the ahādīth.
124 Raga' El-Nimr (1996) "Women in Islamic Law," in Mai Yamani (ed.) *Feminism and Islam*. New York: New York University Press, p. 94.
125 Valentine M. Moghadam (1993) *Modernizing Women: Women and Social Change in the Middle East*, Boulder and London: Lynne Rienner Publishers, pp. 3–4.
126 Nadia H. Youssef (1978) "The Status and Fertility Pattern of Muslim Women," in Lois Beck and Nikkie Keddie (eds), *Muslim Women in the Muslim World*, Cambridge, MA: Harvard University Press, p. 78.
127 For Malaysia, see Maila Stivens (1998) "Sex, Gender and the Making of the New Malay Middle Class," in Krisna Shen and Maila Stivens (eds), *Gender and Power in Affluent Asia*, London: Routledge, pp. 89–126 and Maila Stevens (2000) "Becoming Modern in Malaysia: Women at the End of the Twentieth Century," in Louise Edwards and Mina Roces (eds), *Women in Asia: Tradition, Modernity, and Globalization*, Ann Arbor: The University of Michigan Press, pp. 16–38; for Indonesia see Kathryn Robinson (2000) "Indonesian Women: From *Orde Baru* to *Reformasi*," in Louise Edwards and Mina Roces (eds), *Women in Asia: Tradition, Modernity, and Globalization*, Ann Arbor: The University of Michigan Press, pp. 139–69; (1998) and Krisna Sen (1998) "Indonesian Women at Work: Reframing Subject," in Krisna Shen and Maila Stivens (eds), *Gender and Power in Affluent Asia*, London: Routledge, pp. 35–62.
128 For China, see Barbara L.K. Pillsburry (1978) "Being Female in a Muslim Minority in China," in Lois Beck and Nikkie Keddie (eds), *Muslim Women in the Muslim World*, Cambridge, MA: Harvard University Press, pp. 651–73 and for Australia, see Samina Yasmin, "Muslim Women as Citizens in Australia: Perth as a Case Study," Yvonne Yazbeck Haddah and Jane I. Smith (eds) (2002) *Muslim Minorities in the West: Visible and Invisible*, Walnut Creek, CA; Lanham, MD: AltaMira Press, pp. 217–32 and Santi Rozario (1998) "On being Australian and Muslim: Muslim women as defenders of Islamic heritage," *Women's Studies International Forum*, vol. 21. No. 6, 649–61.
129 Zillah Eisenstein (1998) *Global Obscenities: Patriarchy, Capitalism, and the Lure of Cyberfantasy*, New York and London: New York University Press, p. 135.
130 Muḥammad b. 'Abdul-Aziz al-Musnad (1996) *Islamic Fatawa regarding Women*, trans. Jamaal al-Din Zarabozo, Saudi Arabia: Darussalam, p. 310.
131 Ibid., p. 310.
132 Ibid., p. 314.
133 Baveja, *Woman in Islam*, p. 27.

2 The creation theories as the bases for ontological self and inclusive humanity

1 See for example, Abū al-Qāsim Maḥmūd bin 'Umar al-Zamakhsharī (1966) *al-Kashshāf 'an Ḥaqā'iq al-Tanzīl wa 'Uyūn al-Aqāwīl fi Wujūh al-Ta'wīl*, 4 vols, Cairo: Maṭba'at Muṣṭafā al-Bābī al-Ḥalabī, 'Abd Allāh b. 'Umar al-Bayḍāwī (1911), *Anwār al-Tanzīl fi*

Asrār al-Ta'wīl, Beirut: Dār al-Jīl, and Fakhr al-Dīn al-Rāzī (n.d.), *al-Tafsīr al-Kabīr*, 32 vols, Cairo: 'Abd al-Raḥmān Muḥammad.

2 See Ibn Sīnā (1973) *A Treatise on the 'Canon of Medicine' of Avicenna, Incorporating a Translation of the First Book*, trans. O. Cameron Gruner, New York: AMS Press. See also, Ibn Rushd (1987), *Kitāb al-Kulliyyāt fī al-Ṭibb*, ed. J.M. Fórneas Basteiro and C. Alvarez de Morales, Madrid: Escuela de Estudios Árabes de Granada.

3 Baldick argues that mysticism in Islam (Ṣufism) is derived from Christian, Christian-Jewish, and Gnostic elements. From Eastern Christianity as well as Nestorian Christianity, the Sufis took over the practice of wearing wool. The word "sufi" etymologically derives from the Arabic word for wool (*ṣūf*) which refers the cloth worn by eastern Christian monks. Some Sufi doctrines, such as the idea of the "friend of God" (*walī Allāh*) and "remembrance of God" (*dhikr Allāh*) are taken from Christian teachings. Another striking influence from "Jewish Christianity" is the idea of "the poor" (Arabic *faqīr*, Persian *darwīsh*). These terms become very important in early Islamic mysticism. The influence of the Neoplatonist school of Greek philosophy is another of the Christian contributions to mysticism. As a matter of fact, Christians played a large role in transmitting Greek philosophy to Muslims through their translations of Greek works into Arabic. Thus, some Sufi doctrines, such as the idea of contemplation, the ascending soul, and the love of God were borrowed from the Neoplatonist school. There are also influences from Central Asian shamanism, such as the Sufi dance, and from Gnosticism, such as the imagery of light and darkness, which was followed by certain Sufis. Other minor influences on Islamic mysticism can be identified as coming from Hinduism and Buddhism. See Julian Baldick, *Mystical Islam: An Introduction to Ṣūfism*, New York: New York University Press, 1989, p. 15. Quite contrary to Baldick's approach, Schimmel's extensive studies on the mystical tradition in Islam illustrate that *Ṣūfism* is something inherent within Islamic teaching and arises out of Muslims' attempt to embody the inner teaching (*ḥaqiqa*) of Islam. See, Annemarie Schimmel (1975) *Mystical Dimensions of Islam*, Chapel Hill: University of North Caroline Press, pp. 12–22.

4 Al-Ghazālī, for instance, links the creation of human beings to God's Power over humankind. See Al-Ghazālī (n.d.) *Iḥyā' 'Ulūm al-Dīn*, trans. al-Haj Maulana Fazal-ul-Karim, Book 4, Lahore: Kazi Publications, pp. 463–8.

5 Al-Alousï, for instance, has incorporated the issue of creation of human beings into the general framework of creation. He traces all possible sources that deal with the creation from the Qur'ānic, ḥadīth, and kalām traditions. See, Husâm Muhî Eldîn al-Alousï (1965) *The Problem of Creation in Islamic Thought: Quran, Ḥadīth, Commentaries, and Kalām*, Baghdad: The National Printing and Publishing Co. Quite different from al-Alousï, Haas exclusively refers to the Qur'ān in discussing the idea of the creation of man. See, Samuel S. Haas (1941) "The 'Creation of Man' in the Qur'ān," *Muslim World*, vol. 31.30 (July), 268–73. O'Shaughnessy also discusses the idea of creation in light of the Qur'ānic verses and examines how each Qur'ānic terminology on the creation of human beings works within the universal message of Islam. See, Thomas J. O'Shaughnessy (1985) *Creation and the Teaching of the Qur'ān*, Rome: Biblical Institute Press.

6 Anne Sofie Roald (1998) "Feminist Reinterpretation of Islamic Sources: Muslim Feminist Theology in The Light of the Christian Tradition of Feminist Thought," in Karin Ask and Marit Tjomsland (eds), *Women and Islamization: Contemporary Dimensions of Discourse on Gender Relations*, New York: Berg, pp. 17–44.

7 For further reading, see Riffat Hassan (1999) "Feminism and Islam," in Arvind Sharma and Katherine K. Young (eds), *Feminism and World Religions*, Albany, NY: State University of New York Press, pp. 248–78; and Hassan (1999) "The Issue of Woman–Man Equality in the Islamic Tradition," in Kristen E. Kvam, Linda S. Schearing and Valarie H. Ziegler (eds), *Eve and Adam: Jewish, Christian and Muslim Readings on Genesis and Gender*, Indiana: Indiana Press University, pp. 464–76. See also Amina Wadud-Muhsin's (1992) writings in *Qur'ān and Women*, Kuala Lumpur: Fajar Bakti Sdn; and (2000) "Alternative Qur'ānic Interpretation and

The Status of Muslim Women," in Gisela Webb (ed.) *Windows of Faith: Muslim Women Scholar-Activists in North America*, Syracuse, NY: Syracuse University Press, pp. 3–21.

8 Hassan, "The Issue of Woman–Man Equality in the Islamic Tradition," p. 466.

9 Wadud-Muhsin, *Qur'ān and Women*, p. 15.

10 Barlas, *"Believing Women" in Islam*, p. 134.

11 Esack, "Islam and Gender Justice," p. 191.

12 Asad's translation of Q.S. al-Baqarah, 2: 30–4, *The Message of the Qur'ān*, pp. 8–9.

13 Ali's translation (38:71–77) in CD *Alim*.

14 Ali's translation of Al-Ḥijr, 15: 26–34 in CD *Alim*.

15 Fakhr al-Dīn al-Rāzī, *al-Tafsīr al-Kabīr*, vol. 1, p. 159. See also al-Isrā', 17:70. Asad, *The Message of the Qur'ān*, p. 429.

16 'A'ishah 'Abd al-Raḥmān (Bint al-Shāṭi') (1978) *al-Qur'ān wa Qaḍāyā al-Insān*, 2nd ed., Beirut: Dār al-'Ilm li al-Malāyīn, pp. 31–3.

17 The Qur'ān often makes use the plural term *malāika*, rather than its singular form *malak*, which means, "messenger." The term *malak* is also equivalent to the Hebrew *mal'ak* and the Greek *Angelos*. See Sachiko Murata and William C. Chittick (1994) *The Vision of Islam*, St Paul, Minnesota: Paragon House, p. 84.

18 Al-Rāzī, *al-Tafsīr al-Kabīr*. vol. 1, pp. 163–4.

19 See Asad, *The Message of The Qur'ān*, p. 76; and Hassan, "The Issue of Woman–Man Equality in the Islamic Tradition," p. 467.

20 Ibid., note 47.

21 Ibid.

22 Hassan, "The Issue of Woman–Man Equality in the Islamic Tradition," p. 467.

23 Bint al-Shāṭi', *al-Qur'ān wa Qaḍāyā al-Insān*, p. 36.

24 Al-Rāzī, *al-Tafsīr al-Kabīr*, vol. 1, p. 175.

25 See Asad's discussion of the verses al-Baqara, 2:30, Al-An'ām, 6:165, 'An-Naml, 27:62 and Al-Fāṭir, 35:39 in his work, *The Message of the Qur'ān*, pp. 8, 201, 584, and 671.

26 See Asad's interpretation of al-Furqān, 25:7, *The Message of the Qur'ān*, p. 550 and see also Bint al-Shāṭi', *al-Qur'ān wa Qaḍāyā al-Insān*, p. 15.

27 See also Rahman's discussion on the human's moral dualism in his work, *Islam*, p. 35.

28 O'Shaughnessy, *Creation and the Teaching of the Qur'ān*, p. 17.

29 Ibid.

30 Genesis (1984) 1:26ff and 2:7ff, 3:1–24 in *Holy Bible* in the King James Version, Nashville, Camden, New York,. See Q.S. al-Baqarah, 2:30 and 38:71ff

31 See Q.S. al-Baqarah, 2:31–34 and Genesis 2:19–20.

32 See Q.S. al-Baqarah, 2:35 and Genesis 2:8.

33 See Q.S. al-Baqarah, 2:35 and Genesis 2:17.

34 See Q.S. al-Baqarah, 2:36; Al-Alousī, *The Problem of Creation in Islamic Thought*, p. 137. See also Haas, "The 'Creation of Man' in the Qur'ān," 270; and Genesis 3:1–24.

35 Al-Alousī, *The Problem of Creation in Islamic Thought*, p. 136 and Haas, "The 'Creation of Man' in the Qur'ān," 271.

36 See Arthur Jeffery (1938) *The Foreign Vocabulary of the Qur'ān*, Baroda: Oriental Institute, p. 76.

37 See Q.S al-Ḥajj, 22:5 where the Qur'ān clearly indicates God's power over the procreation of human beings in general and His Power to resurrect them from dust.

38 R.J. Zwi Werblowsky and Geoffrey Wigoder (1997) *The Oxford Dictionary of the Jewish Religion*, New York and Oxford: Oxford University Press, pp. 15–16.

39 Ibid., p. 16.

40 Asad's translation, *The Message of the Qur'ān*, Q.S. al-'Alaq, 96:1–5, p. 963.

41 Bint al-Shāṭi', *al-Qur'ān wa Qaḍāyā al-Insān*, p. 19.

42 Jane I. Smith and Yvonne Y. Haddad (1982) "Eve: Islamic Image of Woman," in Azizah al-Hibri (ed.) *Women and Islam*, Oxford, New York: Pergamon Press, p. 136.

43 Kristen E. Kvam, *et al.*, for instance, record the interpretation of the creation of Eve and Adam in Islam in their book, *Eve and Adam*, which provides a comprehensive analysis of how in the Christian and Jewish traditions Eve was created.

44 Al-Ṭabarī, whose full name is Abū Ja'far Muḥammad b. Jarīr al-Ṭabarī, was born in Āmul during the 'Abbāsid period. His date of birth is not exactly known, it was probably between the end of the year 224 (838–39) and 225 (839–40). In search of knowledge, al-Ṭabarī traveled to al-Rayy, Baghdad—the center of Islamic learning, al-Baṣrah, al-Kūfah, Wāsit, Ira, Syria, Palestine, Beirut, Egypt, Mecca, and Ḥijāz. However, the only place to which he subsequently returned from long journey had been Baghdad and remained to live there to the end of his life, in 310/923. For al-Ṭabarī's bibliography and his works, see Jane Dammen McAuliffe (1991) *Qur'ānic Christians: An Analysis of Classical and Modern Exegesis*, Cambridge: Cambridge University Press, pp. 38–45 and Abū Ja'far Muḥammad b. Jarīr al-Ṭabarī (1989) *The History of al-Ṭabarī (Ta'rīkh al-Rusul wa al-Mulūk)*, vol. 1, General Introduction and From the Creation to the Flood, translated and annotated by Franz Rosenthal, Albany, NY: State university of New York, pp. 5–134.

45 The translation was quoted from *The Commentary on the Qur'ān*, abridged, translated, and annotated by J. Cooper, Oxford, Oxford University Press, 1987, pp. 245–6. A similar account can also be read in al-Ṭabarī, *The History of al-Ṭabarī*, pp. 273–4.

46 Al-Zamakhsharī, *al-Kashshāf 'an Ḥaqā'iq Ghawāmiḍ al-Tanzīl*, vol. 1, p. 274.

47 Muḥammad b. 'Abd Allāh al-Kisā'ī (1978) *The Tales of the Prophets of al-Kisā'ī*, trans. W.M. Thackson, Boston, MA: Twayne Publishers, pp. 31–3.

48 Genesis 2:21–23 states the following:

> So the Lord God caused a deep sleep to fall upon the man, and he slept; then he took one of his ribs and closed up its place with flesh. And the rib that the Lord God had taken from the man he made into a woman and brought her to man. Then, the man said. "This at last is bone of my bones and flesh of my flesh; this one shall be called Women, for out of Man this one was taken."

49 See *Holy Bible* in the King James Version.

50 Mary J. Evans (1983) *Woman in the Bible*, Exeter: The Paternoster Press, p. 14.

51 Carol Meyers (1988) *Discovering Eve: Ancient Israelite Women in Context*, New York, Oxford: Oxford University Press, p. 79.

52 Evans, *Woman in the Bible*, p. 15.

53 Ibid., 15.

54 Phyllis Bird (1974) "Images of Women in the Old Testament," in Rosemary Radford Ruether (ed.) *Religion and Sexism: Images of Woman in the Jewish and Christian Traditions*, New York: Simon and Schuster, p. 73.

55 Evans, *Woman in the Bible*, p. 16.

56 See *Holy Bible* in the King James Version.

57 Evans, *Woman in the Bible*, p. 17.

58 Robert Alter (1996) *Genesis: Translation and Commentary*, London, New York: W.W. Norton & Company, p. 9.

59 Bird, "Images of Women in the Old Testament," p. 73.

60 Ibid.

61 Alter, *Genesis: Translation and Commentary*, p. 5.

62 The word [*'ādām*], is supplied by Haas in his "The 'Creation of Man' in the Qur'ān," 270 where he interprets it to mean man. *King James Version* also uses the generic "man."

63 Bird, "Images of Women in the Old Testament," p. 72.

64 Claus Westermann (1984), *Genesis I-II: A Commentary*, Minneapolis: Augsburg, pp. 148–55. See also Kvam *et al.*, *Eve and Adam*, p. 24.

65 Bird, "Images of Women in the Old Testament," p. 72.

66 Kvam *et al.*, *Eve and Adam*, p. 25.

67 Bird, "Images of Women in the Old Testament," p. 72.

68 Al-Iṣfahānī, *Mufradāt Alfāẓ al-Qur'ān*, pp. 497–8.

69 Bird, "Images of Women in the Old Testament," p. 72.

70 Hassan, "Feminism and Islam," p. 255.

71 *Ṣaḥīḥ al-Bukhārī Ḥadīth*, 4.548, narrated by Abū Hurayra in CD *Alim*.
72 *Ṣaḥīḥ al-Bukhārī Ḥadīth*, 7.114, narrated by Abū Hurayra in CD *Alim*.
73 Hassan, "The Issue of Woman–Man Equality in the Islamic Tradition," pp. 464–5.
74 Hassan, "Feminism and Islam," p. 254.
75 Al-Ṭabarī, *The History of al-Ṭabarī*, p. 277.
76 Smith and Haddad, "Eve," p. 139.
77 Ibid., p. 278.
78 Al-Hibri, "An Introduction to Muslim Women's Rights," p. 53.
79 Barbara Freyer Stowasser (1994) *Women in the Qur'ān, Traditions, and Interpretation*, Oxford and New York: Oxford University Press, p. 27.
80 Smith and Haddad, "Eve," p. 138. See also King James Version, Genesis 3.1–6 and Evans, *Women in the Bible*, p. 18.
81 Alter, *Genesis*, 12 and Evans, *Women in the Bible*, p. 18.
82 Ibid., p. 18.
83 Anwar Hekmat (1997) *Women and The Koran: The Status of Women in Islam*, New York: Promotheus Books, p. 10.
84 Ibid., p. 9.
85 Ergun Mehmet Caner and Emir Fethi Caner (2002) *Unveiling Islam: An Insider's Look at Muslim Life and Belief*, Grand Rapids, MI: Kregel Publications, p. 133.
86 Said, *Covering Islam*, p. 57.
87 Ibid.
88 Ibid., pp. 45 and 66.
89 Q.S. al-Ḥijr, 15: 26–34.
90 Q.S. Āl 'Imrān, 3:59.
91 Q.S. al-Kahf, 18:37.
92 Q.S. al-Kahf, 18:37.
93 Al-Alousī, *The Problem of Creation in Islamic Thought*, p. 13.
94 Although these terms seem to be synonymous, it does not mean that they have the same exact meanings. A female Muslim exegete, such as 'Ā'isha 'Abd al Raḥmān (Bint al-Shāṭī') objects to the idea that there are many synonyms in the Qur'ān. She admits that there are words that have similar meanings and seem to be identical with one another. However, each word in the Qur'ān is unique and therefore irreplaceable by any other word due to different connotation. Bint al-Shāṭī' gives some examples for such terms as *ru'yā* and *ḥilm, ānas* and *abṣar, ḥalaf* and *qasam, ḥushū'* and *khashya*. In her part, these terms seem synonymous, but in fact are not. For more discussion, see, for instance, 'Ā'isha 'Abd al-Raḥmān (Bint al-Shāṭi') (1987), *al-I'jāz al-Bayānī li al-Qur'ān wa Masā'il Ibn al-Azraq: Dirāsah Qur'āniyyah Lughawiyyah wa Bayāniyyah*, 2nd ed., Cairo: Dār al-Ma'ārif, especially pp. 207–38.
95 See, for example, Q.S. 2:29, 26:166, 30:21, 2:228, 7:185, 10:5, 6:16, 61:48, 29:44, 30:8; 45:22, 4:1, 5:18, 20:4, 16:73, 3:11, 7:54, 9:36, 10:3, 6:101, 24:45, and 16:4.
96 Q.S. 25:61, 21:30, 77:26, 78:20–11, etc.
97 Q.S. 50:6, 51:47, etc.
98 Q.S. 13:2, 55:7, 88:18, etc.
99 Q.S. 13:3, 50:7 and 15:19.
100 Q.S. 91:6.
101 Q.S. 7:11 and 3:6.
102 Q.S. 59:24.
103 Asad, *The Message of the Qur'ān*, p. 854.
104 A deep understanding of how the word "*khalq*" is used in Islamic tradition, see R. Arnaldez, "Khalḳ" in *Encyclopaedia of Islam*, CD-ROM edition v. 1.0.
105 Al-Iṣfahānī, *Mufradāt Alfāẓ al-Qur'ān*, p. 256.
106 Ibn Manẓūr, *Lisān al-'Arab*, vol. 10, Beirut: Dār Beyrut, 1956, p. 85.
107 Al-Zabīdī, *Tāj al-'Arūs*, vol. 25, Kuwait: al-Turāth al 'Arabī, 1989, p. 252.

108 Leaman, *A Brief Introduction to Islamic Philosophy*, pp. 24–5.
109 See also Asad's translation, *The Message of the Qur'ān*, p. 681.
110 Al-Ghazālī (1997) *The Incoherence of Philosophers (Tahāfut al-Falāsifa)*, trans. Michael E. Marmura, Provo, Utah: Brigham Young University Press, p. 31.
111 Ash'arism was established by Abū al-Ḥasan al-Ash'arī (260–324/874–935) who was the member of Mu'tazilite circle in Basra. He abandoned the Mu'tazilites after his disagreement over the doctrine of the optimum—the imaginary story of the way God would punish, reward, and neither punish nor reward of three individuals: a believer, an unbeliever, and a child, respectively—with his teacher, Abū 'Ali al-Jubbā'ī (d. 303/915). See Eric L. Ormsby (1984) *Theodicy in Islamic Thought: The Dispute over al-Ghazālī's Best of All Possible Worlds*, Princeton, NJ: Princeton University Press, pp. 16–17 and 23. See also, W. Montgomery Watt (1985) *Islamic Philosophy and Theology*, Edinburgh: Edinburgh University Press, 1985, pp. 64–8.
112 This dialectical theology was originated in Basra by its founder Wāṣil ibn 'Aṭā' (d. 131/748) and 'Amr ibn 'Ubayd (d. 144/761) who were the members of the ascetic al-Ḥasan al-Baṣrī (110/728). Ormsby, *Theodicy in Islamic Thought*, 16–17 and 19 and Watt, *Islamic Philosophy and Theology*, pp. 46–55.
113 Ormsby, *Theodicy in Islamic Thought*, p. 18.
114 Ibid., p. 24.
115 Ibn Sīnā (1986) *Tis' Rasā'il fi al-Ḥikmah wa al-Ṭabī'iyyāt*, ed. Ḥasan 'Aṣī, Beirut: Dār al-Qābis, pp. 106–8; see also Asad's translation, *The Message of the Qur'ān*, pp. 681 and 447.
116 Asad's translation, *The Message of the Qur'ān*, p. 447.
117 See the Qur'ān, 96:2, 22:5, 23:14, 75:38, etc.
118 Ibid., 86:6, 25:54–56, 77:20, etc.
119 Ibid., 75:37–39.
120 Ibid., 80:17–19, 75:37, 76:2, etc.
121 Ibid., 15:26, 28, 33, and 55:14.
122 Ibid., 38:71, 3:49, 5:110, 6:2, etc.
123 Ibid., 3:59, 18:37, 22:5, etc.
124 Ibid., 19:9 and 67.
125 Al-Bayḍāwī, *Anwār al-Tanzīl fi Asrār al-Ta'wīl*, p. 403.
126 Al-Zamakhsharī, *al-Kashshāf 'an Ḥaqā'iq Ghawāmiḍ al-Tanzīl*, vol. 2, p. 504.
127 See A. Yusuf Ali's translation of al-Insān, 91:1 in his work, *The Holy Qur'ān: Text, Translation and Commentary*, Brentwood, MD: Amana Corp, 1983.
128 Asad, *The Message of the Qur'ān*, p. 458.
129 Ibid., 465.
130 Al-Alousi', *The Problem of Creation in Islamic Thought*, p. 21.
131 Richard Bell (1958) *Introduction to the Qur'ān*, Edinburgh: University Press, p. 101.
132 Al-Alousi', *The Problem of Creation in Islamic Thought*, pp. 86–7.
133 The term "out of clay" or "dust," according to Asad, is used to indicate "man's lowly biological origins as well as the fact that his body is composed of various organic and inorganic substances—existing in other combinations or other elementary forms—on or in the earth. See Muhammad Asad's translation of the Qur'ān, *The Message of The Qur'ān*, note 24, p. 385.
134 Ibn Sīnā (1959) *al-Shifā': al-Ilāhīyāt* 2, ed. G. Anawātī, A.F. Awānī, M. Khuḍayrī, and S. Zāyid, revised edition, Cairo: al-Hay'a al-'Āmma li Shu'ūn al-Maṭābi' al-Amīrīya, Book 6, Chapter 2, p. 266.
135 See, for instance, ibid., p. 267.
136 See Q.S. al-Nisā', 4:1.
137 Wadud-Muhsin, *Qur'ān and Women*, pp. 15–28.
138 See Asad's *The Message of the Qur'ān*, note 1, p. 100.
139 'Abd Allāh b. 'Umar al-Bayḍāwī was born in al-Bayḍa and died in Tabrīz (d. 685 or 710), He echoes the themes of traditionalism in that he translates the Qur'ān by relying on

the Qur'ānic texts and the prophetic sayings (*aḥadīth*). For instance, even though his commentary of the Qur'ān, *Anwār al-Tanzīl wa Asrār al-Ta'wīl* follows al-Zamakhsharī's *al-Kashshāf 'an Ḥaqā'iq al-Tanzīl wa 'Uyūn al-Aqāwīl fi Wujūh al-Ta'wīl*, the former eliminates the the latter's Mu'tazilite's rational approach to the Qur'ān. See, George C. Decesa (1999) *The Qur'ānic Concept of Umma and its Function in Philippine Muslim Society*, Roma: Editrice Pontificia Università Gregoriana, pp. 220–7. See also McAuliffe, *Qur'ānic Christians*, p. 53.

140 Abū al-Qāsim Maḥmūd bin 'Umar al-Zamakhsharī was born in 467/1075 in Khwārazm and died in 538/1144 in Jurjāniyyah, Zamakhsarī. His commentary of the Qur'ān, *al-Kashshāf 'an Ḥaqā'iq al-Tanzīl wa 'Uyūn al-Aqāwīl fi Wujūh al-Ta'wīl*, shifted a new direction in the Qur'ānic scholarship. Al-Zamakhsharī imbued his work with individual reasoning, which was indebted to his Mu'tazilite background. Because his work combined the individual reasoning and the Qur'ānic texts and the prophetic sayings (*aḥadīth*), his commentary of the Qur'ān is categorized as *tafsīr bi al-ra'y*— the interpretation of the Qur'ān which heavily depended on personal reasoning and judgment. See McAuliffe, *Qur'ānic Christians*, pp. 49–54.

141 Al-Bayḍāwī, *Anwār al-Tanzīl wa Asrār al-Ta'wīl*, p. 101. See also, al-Zamakhsharī, *al-Kashshāf 'an Ḥaqā'iq Ghawāmiḍ al-Tanzīl*, vol. 1, p. 492.

142 Wadud-Muhsin, *Qur'ān and Woman*, p. 19.

143 Muḥammad 'Abduh (1970) *Tafsīr al-Qur'ān al-Ḥakīm*. 2nd edn, vol. 4, Beirut: Dār al-Ma'rifah, p. 323

144 Asad, *The Message of the Qur'ān*, note 1, p. 100.

145 Wadud-Muhsin, *Qur'ān and Woman*, p. 19.

146 Ibid., 21.

147 See Chilla Bulbeck (1998) *Re-orienting Western Feminism*, Cambridge: Cambridge University Press, pp. 44–52

148 Susan J. Brison (1997) "Outliving Oneself: Trauma, Memory, and Personal Identity," in Diana Tietjens Meyers (ed.) *Feminist Rethinks the Self*, Colorado, Westview Press, p. 14.

149 Ibn Sīnā, *al-Shifā': al-Ilāhīyāt 2*, Book 5, Chapter 7, p. 237.

150 Marmura (1984) "Ibn Sīnā's Flying Man, in Context," *The Monist*, 69: 390.

151 Ibid., 391.

152 Ibid.

153 Brison, "Outliving Oneself: Trauma, Memory, and Personal Identity," p. 15.

154 Julius R. Weinberg (1966) *A Short History of Medieval Philosophy*, Princeton and New Jersey: Princeton University Press, pp. 112–13.

3 The transmission of generative self and women's contribution to conception

1 See Asad's translation of *al-Najm*, 53: 45–6. Asad, *The Message of the Qur'ān*, p. 816. (45) and that it is He who creates the two kinds of the male and the female—(46) out of a (mere) drop of sperm as it is poured forth.

2 Mohammed Ali Albar has also examined the order of the stages of human development. See Mohammed Ali Albar (1989) *Human Development as Revealed in the Holy Qur'ān and Hadith (The Creation of Man between the Medicine and the Qur'ān)*, Jeddah: Saudi Publishing and Distributing House, p. 58.

3 Toshihiko Izutsu (1964) *God and Man in the Koran: Semantics of the Koranic Weltanschauung*, Tokyo: The Keio Institute of Cultural and Linguistic Studies, p. 120.

4 Asad's Translation of al-An'ām, 6:2 in *The Message of The Qur'ān*, p. 171.

5 Ziauddin Sardar (1984) "Introduction: Islamic and Western Approaches to Science" in Ziauddin Sardar (ed.) The *Touch of Midas: Science, Values, and Environment in Islam and the West*, Manchester: University Press, pp. 3–4.

6 See Pervez Hoodhboy (1991) *Islam and Science: Religious Orthodoxy and the Battle for Rationality*, London: Zed Books, p. 8.

7 M. Husain Sadar (1984) "Science and Islam: Is There a Conlfict?," in Ziauddin Sardar (ed.) *The Touch of Midas: Science, Values, and Environment in Islam and the West*, Manchester: University Press, pp. 20–1.
8 Basim Musallam (1990) "The Human Embryo in Arabic Scientific and Religious Thought," in G.R. Dunstan (ed.) *The Human Embryo: Aristotle and The Arabic and European Traditions*, Great Britain: University of Exeter Press, p. 41.
9 Hippocrates (1981) "On Generation," in *The Hipporatic Treatises: "On Generation," "On the Nature of the Child," and "Diseases IV"*, A Commentary by Iain M. Lonie, Berlin, New York: Walter de Gruyter, 7.1–2 to 8.1, 4.
10 Aristotle (1984) *Generation of Animals*, trans. A. Platt, in Jonathan Barnes, *The Complete Works of Aristotle*, Princeton, NJ: Princeton University Press, Book 1, Chapter 19, pp. 1111–218.
11 Galen (1992) *On Semen*, Edition, Translation, and Commentary by Philip de Lacy, Germany: Akademie Verlag, I.7,4–6, p. 87. See also Musallam, "The Human Embryo in Arabic Scientific and Religious Thought," p. 32.
12 Ibn Sīnā (1970) *al-Ḥayawān*, section 8 of *al-Ṭabi'īyāt of al-Shifā'* (eds) 'Abd al-Ḥalīm Muntaṣir, Sa'īd *Zāyd*, and 'Abd Allah Ismā'īl, Cairo n.p., p. 145.
13 Ibid., p. 399.
14 Allen demonstrates the extent to which Ibn Sīnā's theory of generation adopted Aristotelian tradition. See her work, *The Concept of Women*, pp. 340–4.
15 Ibn Sīnā, *A Treatise on the "Canon of Medicine" of Avicenna, Incorporating a Translation of the First Book*, p. 99.
16 Allen, *The Concept of Women*, p. 344.
17 Aristotle (1984) *Physics*, trans. R.P. Hardie and R.K. Gaye, in Jonathan Barnes (ed.) *The Complete Works of Aristotle*, Princeton, NJ: Princeton University Press, Book II, 193a27–193b6, p. 330.
18 Anthony Preus (1997) *Notes on Greek Philosophy from Thales to Aristotle*, Binghamton: Global Publications, p. 145.
19 Aristotle, *Generation of Animals*, 738b19–25, p. 1146.
20 Allen, *The Concept of Women*, p. 91.
21 Ibn Sīnā (1973) *The Metaphysics of Avicenna: A Critical translation – commentary and analysis of the fundamental argument in Avicenna's Metaphysica in the* Dānish Nāma-i 'alā'ī (The Book of Scientific Knowledge), London: Routledge and Kegan Paul, p. 37.
22 Aristotle (1984) *Metaphysics*, trans. W.D. Ross, in Jonathan Barnes, (ed.) *The Complete Works of Aristotle: The Revised Oxford Translation*, vol. 2, Princeton, NJ: Princeton University Press, I.5 986a20–23, p. 1559.
23 Aristotle, *Generation of Animals*, 765b9–18, p. 1184.
24 Allen, *The Concept of Women*, p. 95. See also Hippocrates (1931) *Hippocrates*, trans. W.H.S. Jones, London and New York: William Heinemann Ltd. and G.P. Putnam's Sons, vol. 4, pp. xxxv and 281.
25 Nancy Tuana (1994) "Aristotle and the Politics of Reproduction" in Bat-Ami Bar On (ed.) *Engendering Origins: Critical Feminist Readings in Plato and Aristotle*, Albany, NY: State University of New York Press, p. 198.
26 Aristotle, *Generation of Animals*, 728a16–22, p, 1130.
27 Ibid., 727a3–4, p. 1128.
28 Ibid., 735a31–32, p. 1141.
29 Ibid., 735b5–6.
30 Ibid., 735b34–35, p. 1142.
31 Ibid., 726a30–11, p. 1128.
32 Ibid., 728a16–20, p. 1130.
33 Ibid., 727a3–4, p. 1128.
34 Ibid., 727a5–9, p. 1128–9.
35 Tuana, "Aristotle and the Politics of Reproduction," p. 198.

36 Tuana, "Aristotle and the Politics of Reproduction," p. 199. See also Aristotle, *Generation of Animals*, 727b34–36, p. 1130.
37 Ibid., 724a17. In Barnes' translation, he only mentions "semen." Differently, Preus, as does Aristotle, uses the word "*sperma*" as applicable to male semen and female menstrual fluid. See Anthony Preus (1975) *Science and Philosophy in Aristotle's Biological Works*, New York: Georg Olms Verlag Hildesheim, p. 54.
38 Aristotle, *Generation of Animals*, 729a21–22, p. 1132.
39 Preus, *Science and Philosophy in Aristotle's Biological Works*, p. 56.
40 Ibn Sīnā, *al-Ḥayawān*, p. 396.
41 Ibn Sīnā, *A Treatise on the "Canon of Medicine" of Avicenna, Incorporating a Translation of the First Book*, p. 99.
42 Aristotle, *Generation of Animals*, 729a12–14, p. 1132.
43 Ibid., 114.
44 Aristotle, *Generation of Animals*, 729b12–18, p. 1132.
45 Preus, *Science and Philosophy in Aristotle's Biological Works*, p. 59.
46 Aristotle, *Generation of Animals*, 730b10–21, p. 1134.
47 Ibid.
48 Ibid., 728a18–19, p. 1130.
49 Ibid., 734b35, p. 1140.
50 Ibn Sīnā, *al-Ḥayawān*, p. 146
51 Aristotle, *Generation of Animals*, Book 1. 21, 729b1–20, pp. 1132–3.
52 Ibn Sīnā, *al-Ḥayawān*, p. 172.
53 Ibn Sīnā, *A Treatise on the "Canon of Medicine" of Avicenna, Incorporating a Translation of the First Book*, Book 1, Part 1, no. 125, p. 99.
54 Aristotle, *Generation of Animals*, 729a21–22, p. 1132.
55 Ibn Sīnā *A Treatise on the "Canon of Medicine" of Avicenna, Incorporating a Translation of the First Book*, Book 1, Part 1, p. 123.
56 Ibid., Book I, Part I, no.145, 114; Aristotle, *Generation of Animals*, 735a–26, p. 1141 and see also Preus' discussion on wheather semen has the soul in his book, *Science and Philosophy in Aristotle's Biological Work*, pp. 73–4.
57 Preus, *Science and Philosophy in Aristotle's Biological Work*, pp. 83–4.
58 Aristotle, *Generation of Animals*, 736b5–8, p. 1141.
59 Ibid., 736b2–26, pp. 1141–2.
60 Aristotle, *Generation of Animals*, 736b27–28, p. 1143.
61 Ibid., 737a7–12, p. 1144.
62 Ibn Sīnā, *A Treatise on the "Canon of Medicine" of Avicenna, Incorporating a Translation of the First Book*, Book 1, Part 1, p. 167.
63 Ibn Sīnā (1952) *Avicenna's Psychology: An English Translation of Kitāb al-Najāt, Book 11, Chapter IV*, trans. Fazlur Rahman. London: Oxford University Press, p. 56.
64 Ibid., p. 24.
65 Ibid., pp. 59–60.
66 Asad's translation of Q.S. al-Qiyāma, 75:37–39, p. 914.
67 Aristotle, *Generation of Animals*, 716a6–13 and 731b19–20, pp. 1112 and 1135.
68 Kathleen C. Cook (1996) "Sexual Inequality in Aristotle's Theories of Reproduction and Inheritance," in Julie K. Ward (ed.) *Feminism and Ancient Philosophy*, New York and London: Routledge, p. 53.
69 Ibid., pp. 53–4.
70 Preus, *Science and Philosophy in Aristotle's Biological Works*, p. 48.
71 Daryl McGowan Tress (1996) "The Metaphysical Science of Aristotle's Generation of Animals and Its Feminist Critique" in Julie K. Ward (ed.) *Feminism and Ancient Philosophy*, New York and London: Routledge, p. 50. See also Aristotle, *Generation of Animals*, 715b5–16, p. 1112.
72 Ibid., pp. 34–5, and 50.
73 Aristotle, Metaphysics, 1044a34–b1, p. 1649. See also Preus, *Science and Philosophy in Aristotle's Biological Works*, p. 48.

74 Tress, "The Metaphysical Science of Aristotle's Generation of Animals and Its Feminist Critique," pp. 32–3.

75 Ibn Sīnā, *A Treatise on the "Canon of Medicine" of Avicenna, Incorporating a Translation of the First Book*, Book 1, Part 1, no. 56. See also Asad's translation of al-Ḥijr, 15:29 "... breathed into him My spirit (*rūḥī*)." See, Asad, *The Message of the Qur'ān*, p. 386.

76 Ibn Rushd (1986) *Ibn Rushd's Metaphysics: A Translation of Ibn Rushd's Commentary on Aristotle's Metaphysics, Book Lām*, trans. Charles Genequand, Leiden: E.J. Brill, p. 137.

77 Ibid., p. 129.

78 Ibn Rushd (1999) *Kitāb al-Kullīyyāt fī al-Ṭibb: ma' Mu'jam bi al-Muṣṭalaḥāt al-Ṭibbīyah al-'Arabīya*, ed. Muḥammad 'Abīd Jābirī, Beirut: Markaz Dirāsat al-Waḥda al-'Arabīya, p. 72.

79 Ibid.

80 Averroes (1984) *Commentaria Averrois in Galenum*, ed. Concepcion Vazquez Benito, Madrid: Instituto Hispano-Arabe de Cultura, p. 56.

81 Al-Ghazali, *Iḥyā' 'Ulūm al-Dīn*, vol. 2, p. 45.

82 Ibn Qayyim al-Jawziyyah (d. 1350) whose real name was Shams al-Dīn Abū 'Abd Allāh Muḥammad b. Abī Bakr, was a Ḥanbalī theologian. He attempted to reconcile between Islamic teachings and Greek philosophy as can be seen in his work *Tuḥfat al-Mawdūd bi Aḥkām al-Mawlūd*, Cairo: al-Maktabah al-Qayyimah (n.d.) and *al-Tibyān fī Aqsām al-Qur'ān*, Cairo: Dār al-Ṭibā'a al-Muḥammadīya (n.d.). See also Musallam, "The Human Embryo in Arabic Scientific and Religious Thought," pp. 32–46.

83 Ibn Qayyim al-Jawziyyah, *Tuḥfat al-Mawdūd bi Aḥkām al-Mawlūd*, p. 191.

84 Hippocrates, *The Hippocratic Treatises*, p. 1.

85 Ibn Qayyīm al-Jawziyyah (n.d.) *al-Tibyān fī Aqsām al-Qur'ān*, Cairo: Dār al-Ṭibā'a al-Muḥammadiyyah, pp. 210–11.

86 Ibid., p. 210.

87 Musallam, "The Human Embryo in Arabic Scientific and Religious Thought," p. 36 and Ibn Qayyim al-Jawziyyah, *al-Tibyān fī Aqsām al-Qur'ān*, p. 210.

88 Narrated by Zaynab b. Umm Salama, *Ṣaḥīḥ al-Bukhārī Ḥadīth*, 8.113 in CD *Alim*.

89 Ibid., p. 211.

90 See Asad's interpretation of al-Ṭāriq, 86:6–7, *The Message of the Qur'ān*, p. 944.

91 Narrated by Anas, *Ṣaḥīḥ al-Bukhārī*, 4.546 in CD *Alim*.

92 Hippocrates, "On Generation", 8.1, 4. A relevant passage is to be found in Ibn Qayyim al-Jawziyyah, *Tuḥfat al-Mawdūd bi Aḥkām al-Mawlūd*, p. 220.

93 Ibid.

94 Ibn Qayyim al-Jawziyyah, *al-Tibyān fī Aqsām al-Qur'ān*, p. 211.

95 Aristotle, *Generation of Animals*, Book IV, 3, 768a22, p. 1189.

96 Harvey whose full name was William Harvey and who was well-known with his theory of the circulation of the blood was born in 1578. His interest in embryology was greatly influenced by one of his teachers at the University of Padua, Fabricius Aquapendente, whom he called as his informant. For the account of William Harvey's life, his career, and his writings, see *The Works of William Harvey, M.D.* Translated from the Latin with A life of the Author by Robert Willis (1965) New York and London: Johnson Reprint Corporation. See also Keith L. Moore and T.V.N. Persaud (1993), *The Developing Human: Clinically Oriented Embryology*, Canada: W.B. Saunders Company, p. 8.

97 Willis, *The Works of William Harvey*, pp. 270–1 and 307–9.

98 A.H. Sturtevant (1967) "Mendel and the Gene Theory," in *Heritage from Mendel*, eds R. Alexander Brink and E. Derek Styles, Madison, Milwaukee, and London: The University of Wisconsin Press, p. 11.

99 Gregor Mendel (1902) "Experiments in Plant-Hybridization," in W. Bateson (with a translation of Mendel's Original papers on Hybridization), *Mendel's Principle of Heredity: A Defence*, Cambridge: Cambridge University Press, p. 40.

100 M. Demerec (1967) "Properties of Genes," in R. Alexander Brink and E. Derek Styles (ed.) *Heritage from Mendel*, Madison, Milwaukee, and London: The University of Wisconsin Press, p. 58 and Mendel, "Experiments in Plant-Hybridization," p. 42.

101 Demerec (2000) "Properties of Genes," pp. 58–9. See also Eileen P. Flynn, *Issues in Health Care Ethics*, New Jersey: Prentice Hall, Upper Saddle River, p. 85.
102 C.P. Oliver (1967) "Dogma and the Early Development of Genetics," in R. Alexander Brink and E. Derek Styles (eds), *Heritage from Mendel*, Madison, Milwaukee, and London: The University of Wisconsin Press, 1967, p. 58 and Mendel, "Experiments in Plant-Hybridization," p. 4.
103 Ibid., p. 5.
104 Moore and Persaud, *The Developing Human*, p. 14.
105 Ibid., p. 4.
106 W.J. Hamilton and H.W. Mossman (1972) *Human Embryology: Prenatal Development of Form and Function*, Cambridge: W. Heffer & Sons LTD and Baltimore: The Williams & Wilkins Company, pp. 32–3.
107 Ibid., p. 35.
108 Ibn Qayyim al-Jawziyyah, *Tuḥfat al-Mawdūd bi Aḥkām al-Mawlud*, p. 191.
109 See also Q.S. al-Sajdah, 32:8.
110 Quotations are taken from *The Hippocratic Treatises*, "On The Nature of the Child," passages 14.1, 7. See also the relevant passages at Ibn Qayyim al-Jawziyyah's *Tuḥfat al-Mawdūd bi Aḥkām al-Mawlūd*, p. 193 and Musallam, "The Human Embryo in Arabic Scientific and Religious Thought," p. 41.
111 Quotation is a translation of Musallam in his work, "The Human Embryo in Arabic Scientific and Religious Thought." The Arabic version can be read in Ibn Qayyim's *Tuḥfat al-Mawdūd bi Aḥkām al-Mawlūd*, p. 194. The relevant passages can be found in Hippocratic writing, "On the Nature of the Child," 14.2.
112 See Asad's translation of Q.S. al-Zumar, 39:6. See also Ibn Qayyim's *Tuḥfat al-Mawdūd bi Aḥkām al-Mawlūd*, p. 193.
113 Ibid.
114 Asad interprets the darkness as referring to the successive stages of embryonic development, such as sperm, germ-cell, and embryonic lump. See al-Ḥajj, 22:5 in Asad's translation, *The Message of the Qur'ān*, note 4, p. 505.
115 Keith L. Moore, "A scientist's interpretation of reference to embryology in the Qur'ān," p. 15.
116 Albar, *Human Development as Revealed in the Holy Qur'ān and Hadith*, p. 63.
117 See the translation of the verse al-Mu'inūn (23:12–14) in Asad's *The Message of the Qur'ān*. p. 520, T.B. Irving (1998) *The Qur'ān (The Noble Reading)*, Tehran, Iran: Suhrawardī Research & Publication Center, p. 342; A. Yusuf Ali's and M. Pickthall's translation in CD *The Alim*.
118 Rohi Baalbaki (1994) *Al-Mawrid: a modern Arabic-English dictionary*, Beirut, Lebanon: Dar El-Ilm Lilmalayin, p. 189 and Wehr, *A Dictionary of Modern Written Arabic*, p. 60.
119 Faruq Sherif (1985) *A Guide to the Contents of the Qur'ān*, London: Ithaca Press, 47.
120 Asad, *The Message of the Qur'ān*, note 4, p. 963.
121 Ibid., note 4, p. 520.
122 The Qur'ān indicates that God created every human out of dust. See Asad's interpretation of al-Ḥajj, 22:5.
123 *The Holy Bible*, New York: Thomas Nelson Publishers, 1984).
124 See the interpretation of al-Qiyāma 75:36–37. The verse 36 uses the word '*al-insān*' when it addresses its audiences. However, Irving and Asad translate *al-insān* as man.
Irving's translation: "Was he [*al-insān*, human] not once a drop of ejected semen?"
Asad's translation: "Was he [*al-insān*, human] not once a [mere] drop of semen that had been spilt?"
125 O'Shaughnessy, Creation and the Teaching of the Qur'ān, p. 13.
126 See Irving's translation of (*al-Najm*, 53:45–46) in his work, *The Qur'ān (The Noble Reading)*, 528.
127 Rabia Terri Harris (2000) "Reading the Signs: Unfolding Truth and the Transformation of Authority," in Gisela Webb (ed.) *Windows of Faith: Muslim Women Scholar-Activists in North America*, Syracuse, NY: Syracuse University Press, 182.

128 Moore, "A Scientist's Interpretation of Reference to Embryology in The Qur'ān," p. 15.
129 Asad, *The Message of the Qur'ān*, p. 915.
130 Ibid.
131 Mohammed Ali Albar has also examined the order of the stages of human development. See his work, *Human Development as Revealed in the Holy Qur'ān and Ḥadith*, p. 25.
132 Abduh, *Tafsīr Juz' 'Amma*, p. 62.
133 Ibid., p. 63.
134 Syed, "Islamization of Attitude and Practice in Embryology," p. 125.
135 Moore, "A Scientist's Interpretation of Reference to Embryology in the Qur'ān," pp. 15–16.
136 Ibid.
137 Ali's Translation, Iqrā', 96:1–2 in CD *Alim*.
138 Albar, *Human Development as Revealed in the Holy Qur'ān and Hadith*, p. 63.
139 Muḥammad 'Abduh (1967) *Tafsīr Juz' 'Amma*, Cairo: Maktabah wa Maṭba'at Muḥammad 'Alī Shabīh wa Ālā'ih, p. 122.
140 Richard Bell (1968) *The Origin of Islam in Its Christian Environment*, Edinburgh: Frank Cass & Co. Ltd, p. 77.
141 Asad, *The Message of the Qur'ān*, p. 963.
142 Albar, *Human Development as Revealed in the Holy Qur'ān and Ḥadīth*, p. 72.
143 Bradley M. Patten, *Human Embryology*, Philadelphia, Toronto: The Blakiston Company, 1947, p. 85.
144 Ibid., p. 92
145 Moore, "A Scientist's Interpretation of Reference to Embryology in The Qur'ān," pp. 15–16.
146 Ibid.
147 Moore and Persaud, *The Developing Human*, pp. 89–91.
148 Moore, "A Scientist's Interpretation of Reference to Embryology in The Qur'ān," pp. 15–16.
149 Al-Zabīdī, *Tāj al-'Arūs*, vol. 25, p. 251.
150 See Q.S. al-Ṭīn, 95: 4.
151 Al-Zabīdī (1989) *Tāj al-'Arūs*, vol. 25, Kuwait: al-Turāth al-'Arabī, p. 251.
152 Aristotle, *Generation of Animals*, Book I, Chapter 21, 729b13–14, p. 1132.
153 Ibid., 729b15–17, p. 1132.
154 Ibid., 730a26–29, p. 1133.
155 Ibid., 730b11–120, p. 1134.
156 Preus, *Aristotle's Biological Works*, p. 59
157 Aristotle, *Generation of Animals*, Book I, Chapter 22, 730b21–24, p. 1134. See also Preus, *Aristotle's Biological Works*, p. 62.
158 Ibid., p. 63.
159 Keith Moore (2001) "The miracle and challenge of the Qur'ān," *Weekly Mirror International* (Wednesday, May 23).
160 Haas, "The 'Creation of Man' in the Qur'ān," p. 269.
161 Michael C. Brannigan and Judith A. Bross (2001) *Healthcare Ethics in a Diverse Society*, Mountain View, CA: Mayfield Publishing Company, p. 175.
162 Ibid.
163 Ibid.
164 Rispler-Chim has a lengthy discussion of abortion in Islam. See Vardit Rispler-Chaim (1993) *Islamic Medical Ethics*, Leiden, New York: E.J. Brill, pp. 7–18.
165 Ibid., p. 10.
166 Ibid., p. 11.
167 Ibn Qayyim al-Jawziyyah, *Tuḥfat al-Mawdūd bi Aḥkām al-Mawlūd*, p. 193.
168 Adriana, *et al.* (1998) *Hak-Hak Reproduksi Perempuan Yang Terpasung*, Jakarta: Pustaka Sinar Harapan, p. 118.
169 Rispler-Chaim, *Islamic Medical Ethics*, p. 12.
170 Munson, *Intervention and Reflection: Basic Issues in Medical Ethics*, 660–2.
171 Brannigan and Boss, *Healthcare Ethics in a Diverse Society*, p. 276.

172 The issue of surrogate motherhood is very controversial. Charlesworth, for instance, argues that it would impossible for a woman to autonomously and freely choose to be a surrogate mother. Even if woman chooses to bear a child for other woman or couple, it shows that assisted reproduction benefits male dominance. See Max Charlesworth (1995) "Whose body: Feminists views on reproductive technology," in Paul A. Komersaroff (ed.) *Trouble Bodies: Critical Perspectives on Postmodernism, Medical Ethics, and the Body*, Durham and London: Duke University Press, p. 129.

4 The embodiment of masculinity and femiminity: the making of material self

1 Hassan, "Feminism in Islam," p. 250.
2 Butler, *Bodies That Matter*, p. 2.
3 Murata, *The Tao of Islam*, p. 56.
4 The story of Joseph is to be found in a long single *sūrah* which also conveys his name, Joseph (Yūsuf). It is the 12th *sūrah* of the Qur'ān; Stowasser (1995) *Women in the Qur'ān, Traditions, and Interpretation*, p. 50; H.A.R. Gibb and J.H. Kramers, *Shorter Encyclopaedia of Islam*, Leiden and New York: E. J. Brill, pp. 646–8; Hakim Nuruddin Abdurrahman Jami (1980) *Yusuf and Zulaikha: An Allegorical Interpretation*, trans. David Pendlebury, London: The Octagon Press. For the Jewish account of Joseph, see Moses Aberbach (1971–2) "Joseph," in *Encyclopaedia Judaica*, New York: Macmillan, vol. 1, pp. 202–11. For the Biblical account, see Lee Humphreys (1988) *Joseph and His Family: A Literary Study*, Columbia, South Carolina: University of South Carolina Press.
5 Stowasser, *Women in the Qur'ān, Traditions, and Interpretation*, p. 50.
6 Ibid.
7 Ibid.
8 Fatima Mernissi (1987) *Beyond the Veil*, revised edition, Bloomington and Indianapolis: Indiana University Press, p. 41.
9 Al-Ṭabarī (1987) *The History of Ṭabarī (Ta'rīkh al-Rusul wa al-Mulūk)*, vol. 2, *Prophets and Patriarchs*, translated and annotated by William M. Brinner, Albany, NY: State University of New York Press, p. 154. Relevant stories are to be found in Genesis 37–50.
10 Ibid., p. 154. See also Bouhdiba, *Sexuality in Islam*, p. 23.
11 Humphreys, *Joseph and His Family*, p. 71.
12 Jami, *Yusuf and Zulaikha*, pp. 50–1.
13 Bouhdiba, *Sexuality in Islam*, p. 23.
14 See al-Kisā'ī's commentary on Q. S. Yūsuf, 12:24 in, *The Tales of the Prophets of al-Kisā'ī*, pp. 174–5.
15 Ibid., p. 175.
16 Al-Ṭabarī, *The History of Ṭabarī (Ta'rīkh al-Rusul wa al-Mulūk)*, p. 156.
17 Jami, *Yusuf and Zulaikha*, p. 88.
18 According to Ibn Isḥāq's account, the witness was a counselor who made use of his intellect. See Gordon Daniel Newby (1989) *The Making of the Last Prophet*, Columbia, South Carolina: South Carolina Press, p. 105.
19 Al-Ṭabarī, *The History of Ṭabarī (Ta'rīkh al-Rusul wa al-Mulūk)*, p. 157.
20 See Asad's translation of Qur'ān Yūsuf, 12:28, pp. 340–1.
21 Amin, *The Liberation of Women and The New Women*, p. 30.
22 Bouhdiba, *Sexuality in Islam*, p. 25.
23 Al-Zamakhsharī, *al-Kashshāf 'an Ḥaqā'iq Ghawāmiḍ al-Tanzīl*, vol. 2, p. 315. See also al-Bayḍāwī, *Anwār al-Tanzīl fi Asrār al-Ta'wīl*, p. 312.
24 Al-Zamakhsharī, *al-Kashshāf 'an Ḥaqā'iq Ghawāmiḍ al-Tanzīl*, vol. 2, p. 315.
25 Al-Bayḍāwī, *Anwār al-Tanzīl fi Asrār al-Ta'wīl*, p. 312. See also Stowasser, *Women in the Qur'ān, Traditions, and Interpretation*, p. 53
26 Ibid., p. 52.

27 Al-Ṭabarī, *The History of Ṭabarī (Ta'rīkh al-Rusul wa al-Mulūk)*, p. 156.
28 Bouhdiba, *Sexuality in Islam*, p. 26.
29 Jami, *Yusuf and Zulaikha*, p. 128.
30 Ibn Ḥajar (1997) *Fatḥ al-Bārī*, vol. 7, Riyāḍ: Maktabat Dār al-Salām, p. 168.
31 Peter Heath (1992) *Allegory and Philosophy in Avicenna (Ibn Sînâ)*, Philadelphia: University of Pennsylvania Press, p. 211.
32 For further explanation of Ibn Sīnā's theory of imagination, one may read Rahman's (1952) *Avicenna's Psychology: An English Translation of Kitāb al-Najāt, Book 11, Chapter IV*, London: Oxford University Press. The quotation is taken from Heath's *Allegory and Philosophy in Avicenna (Ibn Sînâ)*, p. 211.
33 Ibid., Book III, p. 104.
34 The quotation is taken from *Ṣaḥīḥ Muslim Ḥadīth*, Ḥadīth No. 6.604, narrated by Usamah ibn Zayd b. Harith and Sa'īd b. Zayd ibn Amr b. Nawfal, in CD *Alim*.
35 Ibid., Ḥadīth 6.606, narrated by Abū Sa'īd al-Khuḍrī, in CD *Alim*.
36 Sayyid Qutb, born at the district of Asyut, is one of the modern Islamic thinkers who advocates Islam as a revolutionary religion. He is the most important ideologue of the Islamic revivalist movement, Muslim Brotherhood to which he joined in 1953. He perceives Islam as a political solution to the Muslim's backwardness and social and political problem. He was labeled as a fundamentalist because of his thought against anything Western. See Lamia Rustum Shahedah (2000) "Women in the Discourse of Sayyid Qutb," *Arab Studies Quarterly*, vol. 22, no. 3 (Summer), 45.
37 Look at the section of "Matrimonials" in *Islamic Horizons*, March/April, 1426/2005 as an example in which parents or relatives describe their prospective in laws.
38 Carol Delaney (1991) *The Seed and the Soil*, California: University of California, p. 26.
39 Ibid., p. 3.
40 Islamic ethics shares a kind of de-ontological ethics. It focuses on the concept of good will, which is good in itself. The good will manifests itself in acting from a sense of duty. Acting done from duty demonstrates a submission and respect to the moral law. As the moral law lies on the principle of volition in which the actions have been done, it commands people to do what is universally valid. Therefore, de-ontological ethics is a view that places emphasis on what actions ought to be done regardless of their consequences. See Immanuel Kant (1993) *Grounding for the Metaphysics of Morals*, trans. James W. Ellington, Indianapolis/Cambridge: Hackett Publishing Company, Inc., pp. 7–17.
41 Mernissi, *The Veil and the Male Elite*, p. 74.
42 Ross, *The Gift of Touch*, p. 252.
43 Foucault, *History of Sexuality*, vol. 1, pp. 92–3.
44 Ibid., p. 93.
45 Michel Foucault (1997) *Power/Knowledge: Selected Interviews & Other Writings*, ed. Colin Gordon, New York: Pantheon Books, p. 98.
46 See V.R. and L. Bevan Jones, *Woman in Islam*, Westport, CT: Hyperion Press, Inc., 1941, pp. 4–9 and Ahmed, *Women and Gender in Islam*, p. 44.
47 Hekmat, *Women and The Koran*, p. 122.
48 Lama Abu-Odeh (1996) "Crime of Honour and the Construction of Gender in Arab Societies," in May Yamani (ed.) *Feminism and Islam: Legal and Literary Perspectives*, New York: New York University Press, pp. 141–88.
49 Georges Contenau, *Everyday life in Babylon and Assyria*, London, Edward Arnold (Publishers) Ltd, 1969, p. 15.
50 Ibid., pp. 16–17, and 117.
51 Roald has an excellent discussion on the contemporary discourse on the veiling. See her work, *Women in Islam*, pp. 154–294.
52 Mernissi, *The Veil and the Male Elite*, p. 85.
53 Fadwa El Guindi (1999) *Veil: modesty, privacy, and resistance*, Oxford, New York: Berg, p. 157.

54 There are various meanings of the veil (*ḥijāb*) in Islam. For the meaning of *ḥijāb* and its significance in early Islam, see Stowasser, *Women in the Qur'ān, Traditions, and Interpretations*, pp. 90–4. See also Mernissi, *The Veil and the Male Elite*, pp. 85–101.

55 Fakhr al-Dīn al-Rāzī (n.d.) *al-Tafsīr al-Kabīr li al-Imām al-Fakhr al-Rāzī*, vol. 25, Cairo: 'Iltizām 'Abd al-Raḥmān Muḥammad, p. 226.

56 Al-Zamakhsharī, *al-Kashshāf 'an ḥaqā'iq Ghawāmiḍ al-Tanzīl*, vol. 3, p. 437.

57 Al-Bayḍāwī, *Anwār al-Tanzīl fi Asrār al-Ta'wīl*, p. 562.

58 Examples of the *aḥadīth* dealing with the veil are:

'Umar bin al-Khattab used to say to Allah's Apostle "Let your wives be veiled." But he did not do so. The wives of the Prophet used to go out to answer the call of nature at night only at Al-Manasi.' Once Sauda, the daughter of Zam'a went out and she was a tall woman. 'Umar bin al-Khattab saw her while he was in a gathering, and said, "I have recognized you, O Sauda!" He ('Umar) said so as he was anxious for some Divine orders regarding the veil (the veiling of women.) So Allah revealed the Verse of veiling. [Al-Hijab; a complete body cover excluding the eyes].

Narrated by 'Ā'ishā, *Saḥīh al-Bukhārī*, Ḥadīth 8.257

'Umar bin al-Khattab asked the permission of Allah's Apostle to see him while some Quraishi women were sitting with him, talking to him and asking him for more expenses, raising their voices above the voice of Allah's Apostle.

When 'Umar asked for the permission to enter, the women quickly put on their veils. Allah's Apostle allowed him to enter and 'Umar came in while Allah's Apostle was smiling, 'Umar said "O Allah's Apostle! May Allah always keep you smiling." The Prophet said, "These women who have been here, roused my wonder, for as soon as they heard your voice, they quickly put on their veils." 'Umar said, "O Allah's Apostle! You have more right to be feared by them than I." Then 'Umar addressed the women saying, "O enemies of yourselves! You fear me more than you do Allah's Apostle?" They said, "Yes, for you are harsher and sterner than Allah's Apostle." Then Allah's Apostle said, "O Ibn al-Khattab! By Him in Whose Hands my life is! Never does Satan find you going on a way, but he takes another way other than yours."

Narrated by Ibn Abbās, *Ṣaḥīh al-Bukhārī*, Ḥadīth, 7.119

59 Mernissi, *The Veil and the Male Elite*, p. 162.

60 Al-Bayḍāwī, *Anwār al-Tanzīl fi Asrār al-Ta'wīl*, p. 561 and al-Rāzī, *al-Tafsīr al-Kabīr*, vol. 25, p. 223.

61 Asad, *The Message of the Qur'ān*, n. 69, p. 650.

62 Mernissi, *The Veil and the Male Elite*, p. 180.

63 Stowasser, *Women in the Qur'ān, Traditions, and Interpretation*, p. 91.

64 See Amin's *The Liberation of Women and The New Women*, p. 58, in which he writes:

". . . if a woman's seclusion were lifted, she might love some else besides her husband. This fear leads them to shove their wives behind bolted doors, thinking that this will alleviate their concerns and suspicions."

See also Ahmed's criticism of Amin's methods of his writing in *Women and Gender in Islam*, pp. 144–68.

65 See Asad's translation of al-Aḥzāb, 33:45 in *The Message of the Qur'ān*, p. 647.

66 Al-Rāzī, *al-Tafsīr al-Kabīr*, vol. 25, p. 223.

67 Translation of al-Aḥzāb, 33:32 is taken from Asad's *The Message of the Qur'ān*, p. 644.

68 Ibid., note 38, p. 539.

69 The ḥadīth narrates as follows:

Asma', daughter of Abu Bakr, entered upon the Apostle of Allah (peace be upon him) wearing thin clothes. The Apostle of Allah (peace be upon him) turned his attention from her. He said: O Asma', when a woman reaches the age of menstruation, it does not suit her that she displays her parts of body except this and this, and he pointed to her face and hands.

Narrated by 'Ā'ishah, *Sunan of Abū Dawūd*, Ḥadīth 4092

70 Al-Rāzī, *al-Tafsīr al-Kabīr*, vol. 23, p. 204.

71 El Guindi, *Veil*, p. 149.
72 Fatmagül Berktay (1998) *Women and Religion*, trans. Belma Ötü -Baskett. Montréal, New York: Black Rose Books, p. 65. See also, El Guindi, *Veil*, pp. 13–22.
73 Mernissi, *The Veil and the Male Elite*, pp. 87–95.
74 Ahmed, *Women and Gender in Islam*, p. 55.
75 Ibid., p. 15.
76 Ibid., p. 54.
77 Ibid., p. 55.
78 Ibid.
79 Barlas, *"Believing Women" in Islam*, pp. 54–8.
80 *Ibid.*, p. 56.
81 Nil fer G le (1996) *The Forbidden Modern*, Ann Arbor, The University of Michigan Press, pp. 2, 3, 4, and 95.
82 Ibid., p. 110.
83 Ibid., pp. 93 and 95.
84 Ibid., p. 109.
85 Ibid., pp. 108–9.
86 Ibid., p. 4.
87 See Zahra Kamalkhani (1998) *Women's Islam: Religious Practice Among Women in Today's Iran*, London and New York: Kegan Paul International, pp. 143–53 and Physicians for Human Rights, The Taliban War on Women: A Health and Human Rights Crisis in Afghanistan, Boston and Washington, 1998.
88 Hekmat, *Women and The Koran*, p. 183.
89 Ibid.
90 Fakhr al-Dīn al-Rāzī, *al-Tafsīr al-Kabīr*, vol. 23, pp. 204–5.
91 Lama Abu-Odeh, "Crimes of Honour and the Construction of Gender in Arab Societies," p. 178.
92 El Saadawi, *The Hidden Face of Eve: women in the Arab world*, p. 25.
93 Ibid., pp. 7–8.
94 Jawad, *The Rights of Women in Islam*, p. 54 and Efua Dorkenoo, *Cutting the Rose, Female Genital Mutilation: the practice and its prevention*, London: Minority Rights Publication, 1995, pp. 5–8.
95 Jawad, *The Rights of Women in Islam*, p. 53.
96 Ibid., p. 55.
97 Vardit Rispler-Chaim (1993) *Islamic Medical Ethics in the Twentieth Century*, Leiden: E. J. Brill, p. 86.
98 Jawad, *The Rights of Women in Islam*, p. 55.
99 Amna Abdel Rahman Hassan (2000) "Recent Research Findings on FGM in Sudan-July 2000," *Women's International Networks News*; 26,4 (Autumn), 26.
100 Ibid. See "African Immigrants to South Africa Bring FGM along," *Daily Mail & Guardian*, Johannesburg, S.A. (September 10, 1999).
101 *The New York Times*, has series of stories of Fauziya Kasinga who fled her homeland of Togo to avoid genital mutilation. See, "U.S. Hearing to Decide Rights of Women Who Flee Genital Mutilation" (May 2, 1996), "A Refugee's Body Is Intact but Her Family Is Torn" (September 11, 1996), and "Woman's Plea for Asylum Puts Tribal Ritual on Trial" (April 15, 1996).
102 El Saadawi, *The Hidden Face of Eve: women in the Arab world*, p. 13.
103 Anees, *Islam and Biological Futures*, p. 52.
104 Al-Jawzī, *Kitāb Aḥkām al-Nisā'*, pp. 28–9.
105 Anees, *Islam and Biological Futures*, p. 59.
106 "But Have Some Art with You": An Interview with Nawal El Saadawi in *Literature and Medicine* 14.1 (1995), p. 65.
107 Ibid.

108 Center for Reproductive Law and Policy, "Female Genital Mutilation: A Matter of Human Rights: An Advocate's Guide to Action," in *Women's International Networks News*; 26,4 (Autumn 2000), 31.
109 The Centre for Development and Population Activities (2000) "Egypt: Ending Female Genital Cutting: A USAID funded Program Promoting a 'Positive Deviance' Approach," in *Women's International Networks News* (Autumn) 26, 4, 30.
110 Doi, *Woman in Shari'ah*, p. 3.
111 Al-Musnad, *Islamic Fatawa regarding women*, p. 339.
112 Many Islamist movements in the Muslim world, like Pakistan, Algeria, Egypt, and Turkey advocate the ideal role of a woman as wife and/or mother. For Pakistan, see Khawaz Mumtaz (1994) "Identity Politics and Women: 'Fundamentalism' and Women in Pakistan," in Valentine M. Moghadam (ed.) *Identity Politics and Women, Cultural Reassertions and Feminisms in International Perspective*, Boulder: Westview Press, pp. 228–2. For Algeria, see Cherifa Bouatta (1994) "The Social Representation of Women in Algeria's Islamist Movement," in Valentine M. Moghadam (ed.) *Identity Politics and Women, Cultural Reassertions and Feminisms in International Perspective*, Boulder: Westview Press, pp. 183–201. For Egypt, see Margot Badran (1994) "Gender Activism: Feminists and Islamists in Egypt," in Valentine M. Moghadam (ed.) *Identity Politics and Women, Cultural Reassertions and Feminisms in International Perspective*, Boulder: Westview Press, pp. 202–27. For Turkey, see Binnaz Toprak (1994) "Women and Fundamentalism: The Case of Turkey," in Valentine M. Moghadam (ed.) *Identity Politics and Women, Cultural Reassertions and Feminisms in International Perspective*, Boulder: Westview Press, pp. 293–306.

5 The performance of the self: engendering dependency and pleasures

1 Butler, *Gender Trouble* p. 25.
2 Esack, "Islam and Gender Justice: Beyond Simplistic Apologia," p. 187.
3 Rosenberger discusses the dynamics of the self among the Japanese women in the 90s. Women have been required to retain Japanese national identity in the midst of western ideas of individuality and independence. The multiplicity of the self are: the essential self referring to the stable self, the interactional self referring to the public opinion of the self; the centrifugal self referring to the individuality of the affluent housewives; the societal self referring to the individual relations to people; the compassionate self referring to the women's responsibility to the elderly; the motherly (empathetic) self referring to the women's care for the family, sons, husbands and daughters; and the spontaneous self referring to the self-indulgence and the true self. See Nancy Rosenberger (2001), *Gambling with Virtue*, Hawai'i: University of Hawai'i Press,.
4 See the Qur'ān, al-Fātiḥah, 1:5, "Thee (alone) we worship; Thee alone we ask for help."
5 Ibid., p. 460.
6 Ibid., p. 462.
7 Ibid., p. 464.
8 See Q.S. al-Nisā', 4:1:

> O mankind! Be conscious of your Sustainer, who has created you out of one living entity [*nafs wāḥida*], and out of it created its mate, and out of the two spread abroad a multitude of men and women. And conscious of God, in whose name you demand [your rights] from one another, and of these ties of kinship. Verily, God is ever watchful over you.
>
> (Asad, *The Message of the Qur'ān*, p. 100)

9 Dimitri Gutas (1988) *Avicenna and The Aristotelian Tradition: Introduction to Reading Avicenna's Philosophical Works*, Leiden and New York: E. J. Brill, p. 85.
10 Aristotle (1908) *The Works of Aristotle, De Anima*, vol. 2, translated by J.A. Smith under Ross' editorship, Book 2, 1, London: Oxford University Press, 412a.

11 Rahman, *Ibn Sīnā's Psychology*, pp. 72–3.
12 Peter Heath, *Allegory and Philosophy in Avicenna*, p. 55.
13 Rahman, *Ibn Sīnā's Psychology*, p. 21.
14 Gutas, *Ibn Sīnā and the Aristotelian Tradition*, p. 85.
15 Rahman, *Ibn Sīnā's Psychology*, p. 1.
16 Ibid., p. 25.
17 Ibid., p. 24.
18 Ibid., p. 25.
19 Heath, *Allegory and Philosophy in Avicenna*, p. 61.
20 Ibid., p. 62.
21 A.J. Arberry (1951) *Avicenna on Theology*, London: John Murray, p. 51.
22 Heath, *Allegory and Philosophy in Avicenna*, pp. 62–3.
23 Ibid.
24 Rahman, *Ibn Sīnā's Psychology*, p. 25.
25 Heath, *Allegory and Philosophy in Avicenna*, p. 63.
26 Ibid., 64.
27 Seyyed Hossein Nasr (1966) *Three Muslim Sages: Avicenna, Suhrawardī and Ibn 'Arabī*, Delmar, New York: Caravan Books, p. 39.
28 Heath, *Allegory and Philosophy in Avicenna*, p. 63.
29 Ibid., p. 63.
30 Nasr, *Three Muslim Sages*, pp. 39–40.
31 Ibn Sīnā, "Avicenna: Healing: Metaphysics," p. 106.
32 Al-Musnad, *Islamic Fatawa regarding Women*, p. 306.
33 Brison, "Outliving Oneself: Trauma, Memory, and Personal Identity," p. 14.
34 John Walbridge (1999) "Selfhood/personhood in Islamic Philosophy," in Eliot Deutsch and Ron Bontekoe (eds), *A Companion to World Philosophies*, Malden, MA: Blackwell, p. 472.
35 Ibid., p. 30.
36 Lapidus, *A History of Islamic Society*, p. 29.
37 Irigaray, *Democracy Begins between Two*, p. 96.
38 Honor rape in Pakistan is not only done to punish one member of the family, but also among the contending tribes. See Shahla Haeri (1999) "Woman's Body, Nation's Honor: Rape in Pakistan," in Asma Afsaruddin (ed.) *Hermeneutics and Honor: female "public" space in Islamic/ate societies*, Cambridge, MA: Harvard University Press, pp. 55–69.
39 *People*, March 7, 2005, pp. 199–222.
40 Ibid., 120.
41 The quote is taken from *The Qur'ān: Arabic text with corresponding English meanings* in Ṣaḥīh International (ed.) (1997), Saudi Arabia: Abulqasim Publishing House, p. 34,
42 *Women's International Network News*, 28:3 (Summer 2002), 29.
43 The Prophet saw praised Allāh, extolled Him, and said, "Yet, I pray and sleep: I fast and break my fast; and I marry women. He who is displeased with my Sunna (practices) is not my follower." See al-Asqalani, *Bulūgh Al-Marâm*, p. 342.
44 Ṣāliḥ Aḥmad al-Shāmī (1995) *al-Jāmi' bayn al-Ṣaḥīḥayn li al-Imāmayn al-Bukhārī wa Muslim*, Damascus: Dār al-Qalam; Beirut: Dār al-Shāmiyyah, p. 51. Translation is taken from Asad, *The Message of Islam*, p. 109.
45 Barlas, *"Believing Women" in Islam*, p. 188.
46 Mernissi, *The Veil and the Male Elite*, pp. 153–60.
47 Naṣir al-Dīn al-Ṭūsī (1964) *The Nasirean Ethics*, trans. G.M. Wickens, London: George Allen & Unwin LTD, p. 161.
48 Al-Ghazālī, *Iḥyā' 'Ulūm al-Dīn*, Book 2, p. 50.
49 Anantanand Rambachan (2001) "A Hindu Perspective" in John C. Raines and Daniel C. Maguire (eds), *What Men Owe to Women*, Albany, NY: State University of New York, p. 19.
50 Ibid., p. 21.

51 Denise Lardner Carmody (1991) *Religious Woman: Contemporary Reflections on Eastern Texts* Crossroad, New York: The Crossroad Publishing Company, p. 84.
52 Tavivat Puntarigvivat (2001) "A Thai Buddhist Perspective," in John C. Raines and Daniel C. Maguire (eds), *What Men Owe to Women*, Albany, NY: State University of New York, p. 219.
53 Carmody, *Religious Woman*, p. 90.
54 Ali A. Mazrui (1998) "Male and Female as an Islamic Dialectic: the legacy of Ayesha", part of a lecture delivered at Oxford University and sponsored by the Oxford Centre for Islamic Studies, Oxford, England, October.
55 Spellberg, *Politics, Gender, and the Islamic Past*, p. 68.
56 Ibid., p. 71.
57 Ibid., p. 61.
58 Ibid., p. 63.
59 Ibid., pp. 62–3.
60 Abu-Odeh, "Crime of Honour and the Construction of Gender in Arab Societies," pp. 141–88. International Network for the Rights of Female Victims of Violence in Pakistan has over the period of time constantly provided reports on violence against women, including honor killing. See the list serve: the Rights of Female Victims of Violence in Pakistan List inrfvvp@listserv.louisville.edu. (accessed April 15, 2004).
61 UN WIRE "Pakistan: Violence against Women Increases Despite President's Condemnation," News Release by the International Secretariat of Amnesty International, (May 10, 2002) in *Women's International Network News* 28:3 (Summer 2002), 20.
62 Lapidus, *A History of Islamic Societies*, p. 38.
63 Wadud-Muhsin, *Qur'ān and Women*, p. 29
64 Marlyn Friedman (1997) "Autonomy and Social Relationship: Rethinking the Feminist Critique," in Diana Tietjens Meyers (ed.) *Feminist Rethinks the Self*, Colorado, Westview Press, p. 46.
65 Winnie Tomm (1995) "A Religious Philosophy of Self," in Mornt Joy and Eva K. Neumaier-Dargyay (eds), *Gender, Genre, and Religion: Feminist Reflections*, Canada: Wilfrid Laurier University Press, p. 239.
66 Wadud-Muhsin, *Qur'ān and Woman*, p. 22.
67 Ibid.
68 Khawhaz Mumtaz reports that the role of women as the reproducers has become the main agenda of the fundamentalist women in Pakistan. See for detail, "Identity Politics and Women," pp. 228–42.
69 Anita L. Allen (1997) "Forgetting Yourself," in Diana Tietjens Meyers (ed.) *Feminist Rethinks the Self*, Colorado, Westview Press, p. 104.
70 Foucault, *History of Sexuality*, vol. 1, p. 56.
71 Ibid. See also Bulbeck, *Re-orienting Western Feminism*, p. 130.
72 Ibid., p. 57.
73 Al-Ghazālī, *Iḥyā' 'Ulūm al-Dīn*, Book 3, p. 102.
74 Ibid., Book 2, p. 26.
75 Ibid., Book 3, p. 102.
76 Ibid., Book 4, p. 312.
77 Ibid.
78 Ibid., p. 313.
79 Al-Ghazālī (1998) *The Niche of Lights* (*Mishkāt al-Anwār*), A parallel English-Arabic text translated, introduced, and annotated by David Buchman, Provo, Utah: Brigham Young University Press, p. 16. See also Hermann Landolt (1991) "Ghazālī and Religionswissenschaft," in *Asiatische Studien* 45, no. 1: 22–3 and 60. In this analytical study of *The Niche of Lights* (*Mishkāt al-Anwār*), Landolt argues that the nature of "philosophy of religion" of the "veils-section" is not compatible with the major points written in the *Iḥyā'* and certainly not with the major part of the *The Niche of Lights* (*Mishkāt al-Anwār*).
80 Ibid., p. 61.

81 Al-Ghazālī, *The Incoherence of Philosophers (Tahafut al-Falāsifa)*, p. 90.
82 Landolt, "Ghazālī and Religionswissenschaft," 63.
83 Abū 'Alī al-Ḥusayn Ibn Sīnā, *Tis' Rasā'il fī al-Ḥikmah wa al-Ṭabī'iyyāt*, ed. Ḥasan 'Aṣī, Beirut: Dār Qābis, 1986, p. 106.
84 Abū 'Alī al-Ḥusayn Ibn Sīnā, *al-Ishārāt wa al-Tanbīhāt*. With a Commentary by Naṣīr al-Dīn al-Ṭūsī, vol. 3, ed. Sulaymān Dunyā, Cairo: Dār al-Ma'ārif, 1958, p. 483.
85 Asad's translation of Fuṣṣilat, 41:53 in *The Message of the Qur'ān*, p. 738. Emphasis is mine.
86 Landolt notes that Ibn Sīnā's attempt to prove the existence of God from existence itself follows the line of Neoplatonic tradition. See Landolt, "Ghāzālī and Religionswissenschaft," 51.
87 Ibn Sīnā, *al-Ishārāt wa al-Tanbīhāt*, vol. 3, p. 483. See also Landolt, "Ghazālī and Religionswissenschaft," 51.
88 This quotation is taken from Landolt, "Ghazālī and Religionswissenschaft," 63. It corresponds to al-Ghazālī, *Iḥyā' 'Ulūm al-Dīn*, Book 4, p. 238.
89 Ibn Sīnā, *al-Ishārāt wa al-Tanbīhāt*, vol. 3, pp. 482–3.
90 See Abū 'Alī al-Ḥusayn Ibn Sīnā (1996) *al-Ishārāt wa al-Tanbīhāt*, vol. 4, pp. 818–27. See also Shams Inati, *Ibn Sīnā and Mysticism: Remarks and Admonitions. Part Four*, London and New York: Kegan Paul International, p. 85.
91 Ibn Sīnā (1996) *al-Ishārāt wa al-Tanbīhāt*, vol. 4, pp. 828–35. See also Shams Inati, *Ibn Sīnā and Mysticism: Remarks and Admonitions.* Part Four, London and New York: Kegan Paul International, pp. 86–8.
92 Quotation is taken from Inati's *Ibn Sīnā and Mysticism*, pp. 87–8.
93 Ibn Sīnā, *al-Ishārāt wa al-Tanbīhāt*, vol. 4, Tenth Class, Chapter Twenty Four, p. 891 and Inati, *Ibn Sīnā and Mysticism*, pp. 103–4. See also al-Ghazālī, *Iḥyā' 'Ulūm al-Dīn*, Book 4, p. 238.
94 Ibid.
95 Schimmel, *Mystical Dimensions of Islam*, pp. 66–7 and 354.
96 Ḥusayn ibn Manṣūr al-Ḥallāj (1974) *The Tawasin of Mansur al-Hallaj*, trans. Aisha Abd Ar-Rahman At-Tarjumuna, Berkeley and London: Diwan Press, p. 46. See also Schimmel, *Mystical Dimensions of Islam*, p. 66.
97 Al-Ḥallāj, *The Tawasin of Mansur al-Hallaj*, p. 46.
98 Louis Massignon (1997) *Essay on the Origins of the Technical Language of Islamic Philosophy*, trans. Benjamin Clark, Notre Dame, Indiana: University of Notre Dame Press, pp. 191 and 209.
99 Al-Ghazālī, *Iḥyā 'Ulūm al-Dīn*, Book 4, pp. 238–9.
100 Foucault, *History of Sexuality*, pp. 57–8.
101 Scholars like Katz and Penner argue that there is no such pure experience which is unmediated through language of their tradition. See Steven T. Katz (1992) "The 'Conservative' Character of Mystical Experience," in Steven T. Katz (ed.) *Mysticism and Religious Tradition*, Oxford: Oxford University Press, p. 4; and see also Hans H. Penner, "The Mystical Illusion," in ibid., p. 89.
102 An excellent and concise account on *mi'rāj* can be found in the works of Gerhard Böwering, "Mi'râj" in *Encyclopedia of Religion*, vol. 9, 552–6. Annemarie Shimmel discusses the issue of *mi'rāj* and its subsequent influences in Islamic society in her book, *And Muḥammad Is His Messenger: The Veneration of The Prophet in Islamic Piety*, Chapel Hill: University of North Carolina Press, 1985. Peter Heath analyzes Ibn Sīnā's interpretation of the Prophet's "Night Journey" (*al-isrā'*) and "Ascension" (*mi'rāj*) in his excellent work, *Allegory and Philosophy in Avicenna.*
103 See Asad's translation of al-Isrā' 17:1, p. 417.
104 This approach is in accordance with the parable of Moses and the Sage in verses 60–82 of *al-Kahf* (Qur'ān, *Sūrat* 18) that characterizes the mystic quest. Asad notes that the allegorical meaning of these verses lies in the explanation of the "two seas" which represent two sources of knowledge. One of these sources is "observation and intellectual coordination of outward phenomena (*ilm al-ẓāhir*), whereas, the other consists of intuitive and mystic

insight (*ilm al-bāṭin*), which becomes Moses' quest. See Asad's note on the interpretation of 18:60 in his work, *The Message of the Qur'ān*, pp. 448–9.

105 Geo Widengren (1955) *Muhammad, the Apostle of God, and His Ascension*, Uppala & Wiesbaden: Lundequistka & Harrassowitz, pp. 96–114.

106 Schimmel, *Mystical Dimensions of Islam*, p. 24.

107 In a larger picture, this claim is in line with Irigaray who says that the question of sexual difference is one of the most important issues of the age. See Luce Irigaray (1993) *An Ethics of Sexual Difference*, trans. Carolyn Burke and Gillian C. Gill, Ithaca, NY: Cornell University, p. 5. See also, Stephen David Ross (1995) *Plenishment in the Earth: An Ethics of Inclusion*, Albany, NY: State University of New York Press, p. 11; and Irigaray, *I Love to You*, p. 43 ff.

108 See the examples of different women's movements in the Muslim world in Valentine M. Moghadam, ed., *Identity Politics and Women, Cultural Reassertions and Feminisms in International Perspective*, Boulder: Westview Press, 1994.

Bibliography

'Abd al-Raḥmān, 'Ā'ishah (1987) *Al-I'jāz al-Bayānī li al-Qur'ān wa Masā'il Ibn al-Azraq: Dirāsah Qur'āniyyah Lughawiyyah wa Bayāniyyah*, 2nd ed., Cairo, Egypt: Dār al-Ma'ārif.

'Abduh, Muḥammad (1967) *Tafsīr Juz' 'Amma*, Cairo, Egypt: Maktabah wa Maṭba'at Muḥammad 'Alī Shabīh wa Ālā'ih.

—— (1970) *Tafsīr al-Qur'ān al-Ḥakīm*, 2nd ed., Beirut: Dār al-Ma'rifah, n.d.

Aberbach, Moses (1971–72) "Joseph," *Encyclopaedia Judaica*, vol. 1, New York: Macmillan, pp. 202–11.

Abu-Odeh, Lama (1996) "Crime of Honour and the Construction of Gender in Arab Societies," in May Yamani (ed.) *Feminism and Islam: Legal and Literary Perspectives*, New York: New York University Press, pp. 141–88.

Affifi, A.E. (1938) *The Mystical Philosophy of Muhyid Din-Ibnul Arabi*, Lahore: S.H. Muhammad Ashraf.

Ahmed, Leila (1992) *Women and Gender in Islam: Historical Roots of a Modern Debate*, New Haven and London: Yale University Press.

Albar, Mohammed Ali (1989) *Human Development As Revealed in the Holy Qur'an and Hadith: The Creation of Man between the Medicine and the Qur'an*, Jeddah: Saudi Publishing and Distributing House.

Ali, Yusuf (1983) The Holy Qur'ān: Text, Translation and Commentary, Brentwood, MD: Amana Corp.

Allen, Anita L. (1997) "Forgetting Yourself," in Diana Tietjens Meyers (ed.) *Feminist Rethinks the Self*, Colorado, Westview Press, pp. 104–23.

Allen, Prudence (1985) *The Concept of Women: The Aristotelian Revolution, 750* BC–AD *1250*, Montreal, London: Eden Press.

al-Alousï, Husâm Muhî Eldîn (1965) *The Problem of Creation in Islamic Thought: Quran, hadith, Commentaries, and Kalam*, Baghdad: The National Printing and Publishing Co.

Alter, Robert (1996) *Genesis: Translation and Commentary*, London, New York: W.W. Norton & Company.

Amin, Qasim (1992) *The Liberation of Women and The New Women*, Cairo, Egypt, The American University in Cairo Press.

Anawati, Georges Chehata (1955) *Mu'allafāt Ibn Sīnā*. Cairo, Egypt: Dār al-Ma'ārif.

Anees, Munawar Ahmad (1989) *Islam and Biological Futures: Ethics, Gender, and Technology*, London and New York: Mansell.

Arberry, Arthur John (1951) *Avicenna on Theology*, London: John Murray.

Aristotle (1984) *Generation of Animals*, trans. A. Platt, in Jonathan Barnes (ed.) *The Complete Works of Aristotle: the revised oxford translation*, vol. 1, Princeton, N J: Princeton University Press, pp. 1111–218.

Aristotle (1984) *Metaphysics*, trans. W.D. Ross, in Jonathan Barnes, (ed.) *The Complete Works of Aristotle: the revised oxford translation*, vol. 2, Princeton, NJ: Princeton University Press, pp. 1552–728.

—— (1984) *Politics*, Book 2, trans. B. Jowett, in Jonathan Barnes, (ed.) *The Complete Works of Aristotle: The Revised Oxford Translation*, vol. 2, Princeton, NJ: Princeton University Press, pp. 1986–2129.

—— (1984) *Physics*, trans. R.P. Hardie and R.K. Gaye, in Jonathan Barnes (ed.) *The Complete Works of Aristotle*, Princeton, NJ: Princeton University Press, Book 2, pp. 315–446.

Arnaldez, Roger (1999) "Khalḳ," in *Encyclopaedia of Islam*, CD-ROM Edition V. 1.0.

Asad, Muhammad (1980) *The Message of the Qur'ān*, Gibraltar: Dar al-Andalus.

al-'Asqalani, Ibn Hajar (1996) *Bulugh Al-Marām*, Saudi Arabia: Dar-us-Salam Publications.

Averroes (1984) *Commentaria Averrois in Galenum*, Concepcion Vazquez Benito (ed.) Madrid: Instituto Hispano-Arabe de Cultura.

Baalbaki, Rohi (1994) *Al-Mawrid: a modern Arabic–English dictionary*, Beirut, Lebanon: Dar El-Ilm Lilmalayin.

Badran, Margot (1994) "Gender Activism: Feminists and Islamists in Egypt," in Valentine M. Moghadam (ed.) *Identity Politics and Women, Cultural Reassertions and Feminisms in International Perspective*, Boulder, CO: Westview Press, pp. 202–27.

Baldick, Julian (1989) *Mystical Islam: An Introduction to Sufism*, New York: New York University Press.

Barlas, Asma (2002) *"Believing Women" in Islam: Unreading Patriarchal Interpretations of the Qur'ān*, Austin, TX: University of Texas Press.

Baveja, Malik Ram (1981) *Women in Islam*, New York: Advent Books.

al-Bayḍāwī, 'Abd Allah b. 'Umar (1911) *Anwār al-Tanzīl fi Asrār al-Ta'wīl*, Beirut: Dār al-Jīl.

Bell, Richard (1958) *Introduction to the Qur'ān*, Edinburgh: University Press.

—— (1968) *The Origin of Islam in its Christian Environment*, Edinburgh: Frank Cass & Co. Ltd.

Berktay, Fatmagül (1998) *Women and Religion*, trans. Belma Ötü -Baskett, Montréal, New York, Black Rose Books.

Bird, Phyllis (1974) "Images of Women in the Old Testament," in Rosemary Radford Ruether (ed.) *Religion and Sexism: Images of Woman in the Jewish and Christian Traditions*, New York: Simon and Schuster, pp. 41–88.

Black, Deborah L. (1996) "Al-Fārābī," in Seyyed Hossein Nasr and Oliver Leaman (eds) *History of Islamic Philosophy*, part 1, London and New York: Routledge, pp. 178–97.

Blum, Louise A. (2001) *You're Not from Around Here, Are You: a lesbian in small-town America (living out: gay and lesbian autobiographies)*, Madison, WI: University of Wisconsin Press.

Bouatta, Cherifa (1994) "The Social Representation of Women in Algeria's Islamist Movement," in Valentine M. Moghadam (ed.) *Identity Politics and Women, Cultural Reassertions and Feminisms in International Perspective*, Boulder, CO: Westview Press, pp.183–201.

Bouhdiba, Abdelwahab (1998) *Sexuality in Islam*, trans. Alan Sheridan, London: Saqi Books.

Böwering, Gerhard (1987) "Mi'râj," in Mircea Eliade (ed.) *Encyclopedia of Religion*, vol. 9, New York: Macmillan Publishing Company, pp. 552–6.

Brannigan, Michael C. and Judith A. Boss (2001) *Healthcare Ethics in a Diverse Society*, Mountain View, CA: Mayfield Publishing Company.

Brison, Susan J. (1997) "Outliving Oneself: Trauma, Memory, and Personal Identity," in Diana Tietjens Meyers (ed.) *Feminist Rethinks the Self*, Colorado: Westview Press, pp. 12–39.

Bucaille, Maurice (1978) *The Bible, the Quran and Science: the holy scriptures examined in the light of modern knowledge*, Indianapolis, IN: American Trust Publications.

Bukhārī and Muslim (1995) *al-Jāmi' bayn al-Ṣaḥīḥayn li al-Imāmayn al-Bukhārī wa Muslim*, Ṣāliḥ Aḥmad al-Shāmī (ed.) Damascus: Dār al-Qalam; Beirut: Dār al-Shāmiyyah.

Bullock, Katherine Helen (2002) *Rethinking Muslim Women and The Veil: Challenging Historical & Modern Stereotypes*, London: The International Institute of Islamic Thought.

Burckhardt, Titus (1995) *Introduction to Sufism*, trans. D.M. Matheson, 3rd edition, London: Thorsons.

Butler, Judith (1990) *Gender Trouble*, London and New York: Routledge.

—— (1993) *Bodies That Matter*, New York: Routledge.

Carmody, Denise Lardner (1991) *Religious Woman: Contemporary Reflections on Eastern Texts*, Crossroad, New York: The Crossroad Publishing Company.

Carvely, E.E. (1943) "Doctrines of the soul *(nafs* and *rūḥ)* in Islam," *Muslim World*, 33: 254–61.

Center for Reproductive Law and Policy (2000) "Female Genital Mutilation: A Matter of Human Rights: An Advocate's Guide to Action," *Women's International Networks News* (Autumn) 26, 4: 31.

Charlesworth, Max (1995) "Whose body? Feminists Views on Reproductive Technology," in Paul A. Komersaroff (ed.) *Trouble Bodies: Critical Perspectives on Postmodernism, Medical Ethics, and the Body*, Durham and London: Duke University Press, pp. 125–39.

Chittick, William C. (1989) *Ibn Arabi's Metaphysics of Knowledge: The Sufi Path of Knowledge*, Albany, NY: State University of New York Press.

—— (1996) "Ibn 'Arabī," in Seyyed Hossein Nasr and Oliver Leaman (eds, NY) *History of Islamic Philosophy*, part 1, London and New York: Routledge, pp. 497–509.

Contenau, Georges (1969) *Everyday life in Babylon and Assyria*, London: Edward Arnold (Publishers) Ltd.

Cook, Kathleen C. (1996) "Sexual Inequality in Aristotle's Theories of Reproduction and Inheritance," in Julie K. Ward (ed.) *Feminism and Ancient Philosophy*, New York and London: Routledge, pp. 51–67.

Cooke, Miriam (2001) *Women Claim Islam*, New York: Routledge.

Corbin, Henry (1964) *History of Islamic Philosophy*, London and New York: Kegan Paul international.

Daily Mail and Guardian (1999) "African Immigrants to South Africa Bring FGM along," Johannesburg, S.A (September 10).

Davidson, Laurie and Laura Kramer Gordon (1979) *The Sociology of Gender*, Chicago, IL: Rand McNally College Publishing Company.

Delaney, Carol (1991) *The Seed and the Soil*, California: University of California.

Demerec, Milislav (1967) "Properties of Genes," in R. Alexander Brink and E. Derek Styles (eds) *Heritage from Mendel*, Madison, Milwaukee, and London: The University of Wisconsin Press, pp. 49–61.

Doi, 'Abdur Raḥman I. (1989) *Woman in Shari'ah*, London: Ta-Ha Publishers Ltd.

Dorkenoo, Efua (1995) *Cutting the Rose, Female Genital Mutilation: the practice and its prevention*, London: Minority Rights Publication.

Durán, Khalid (2002) *Children of Abraham: an introduction to Islam for Jews*, New Jersey: Ktav Publishing House.

El Fadl, Khaled Abou (2001) *Speaking in God's Name: Islamic law, authority, and women*, Oxford: Oneworld.

El Guindi, Fadwa (1999) *Veil: modesty, privacy, and resistance*, Oxford, NY: Berg.

El Saadawi, Nawal (1980) *The Hidden Face of Eve: women in the Arab world*, Boston, MA: Beacon Press.

Engineer, Asgharali (2001) "Islam, Women, and Gender Justice," in John C. Raines and Daniel C. Maguire (eds) *What Men Owe to Women*, Albany, NY: State University of New York, pp. 109–28.

—— (1992) *The Rights of Women in Islam*. New York: St Martin's Press, 1992.

English, Jane (1997) *Sex Equality*, Englewood Cliffs, NJ: Prentice-Hall.

Errington, Shelly (1990) "Recasting Sex, Gender, and Power: A Theoretical and Regional Overview." in Jane Monnig Atkinson and Shelly Errington (eds) *Power and Difference: Gender in Island Southeast Asia*, California: Stanford University of California pp. 1–58.

Esack, Farid (2001) "Islam and Gender Justice," in John C. Raines and Daniel C. Maguire (eds) *What Men Owe to Women*, Albany, NY: State University of New York Press, pp. 187–210.

al-Faruqi, Maysam J. (2000) "Women's Self-Identity in the Qur'an and Islamic Law," in Gisela Webb (ed.) *Windows of Faith: Muslim Women Scholar-Activists in North America*, Syracuse, NY: Syracuse University Press, pp. 72–101.

Fatna Aït Sabbah (1984) *Woman in the Muslim Consciousness*, trans. Mary Jo Lakeland, New York: Pergamon Press.

Feillard, Andrée (1996) "A Glimpse into Debates on Women and Islam in Indonesia Today: The Viewpoints of Some Women Leaders," paper presented at International Conference on Islam and the 21st Century, Leiden, June 3–7, pp. 1–26.

Ferguson, Ann (1997) "Moral responsibility and social change: a new theory of self," *Hypatia*, (Summer) 12, 3:116–39.

Flynn, Eileen Patricia (2000) *Issues in Health Care Ethics*, New Jersey: Prentice Hall, Upper Saddle River.

Foucault, Michel (1977) *Power/Knowledge: Selected Interviews & Other Writings*, Colin Gordon (ed.) New York: Pantheon Books.

—— (1990) *History of Sexuality. Volume 1: An Introduction*, trans. Robert Hurly, New York: Vintage Books.

Friedman, Marlyn (1997) "Autonomy and Social Relationship: Rethinking the Feminist Critique," in Diana Tietjens Meyers (ed.) *Feminist Rethinks the Self*, Colorado: Westview Press, pp. 40–61.

Galen (1992) *On Semen*, edition, translation, and commentary by Philip de Lacy, Germany: Akademie Verlag.

al-Ghazālī (1997) *The Incoherence of Philosophers (Tahafut al-Falasifah)*, trans. Michael E. Marmura, Provo, Utah: Brigham Young University Press.

—— (1998) *The Niche of Lights* (*Mishkāt al-Anwār*): A parallel English-Arabic text translated, introduced, and annotated by David Buchman, Provo, Utah: Brigham Young University Press.

—— (n.d.) *Iḥyā 'Ulūm al-Dīn*, trans. al-Haj Maulana Fazal-ul-Karim, Lahore: Kazi Publications.

Gibb, Hamilton Alexander Rosskeen and Johannes Hendrik Kramers (1995) *Shorter Encyclopaedia of Islam*, Leiden and New York: E. J. Brill, pp. 646–8.

Glassé, Cyril (1989) *The Concise Encyclopedia of Islam*, San Francisco, CA: Harper and Row Publishers, Inc.

Gohlman, William E. (1974) *The Life of Ibn Sina*, Albany, NY: State University of New York Press.

Göle, Nilüfer (1996) *The Forbidden Modern*, Ann Arbor, MI: The University of Michigan Press.

Gould, Carol C. (1980) "The Woman Question: Philosophy of Liberation and The Liberation of Philosophy," in Carol C. Gould and Marx W. Wartofsky (eds) *Women and Philosophy: Toward a Theory of Liberation*, New York: A Perigee Book, pp. 5–44.

Gutas, Dimitri (1988) *Avicenna and The Aristotelian Tradition: Introduction to Reading Avicenna's Philosophical Works*, Leiden and New York: E. J. Brill.

Haas, Samuel S. (1941) "The 'Creation of Man' in the Qur'ān," *Muslim World*, 31, 30: 268–73.

al-Ḥallāj, Ḥusayn b. Manṣūr (1974) *The Tawasin of Mansur al-Hallaj*, trans. Aisha Abd Ar-Rahman At-Tarjumuna, Berkeley, CA and London: Diwan Press.

Hallaq, Wael. B. (1984) "Was the gate of *ijtihad* closed," *International Journal of Middle East Studies*, 16: 3–41.

Hamidy, Zainuddin (1957) *Tafsir Qurän*, Jakarta: Penerbit Widjaya.

Hamilton, William John and Harland Winfield Mossman (1972) *Human Embryology: Prenatal Development of Form and Function*, Cambridge and Baltimore: W. Heffer & Sons Ltd and The Williams & Wilkins Company.

Harris, Rabia Terri (2000) "Reading the Signs: Unfolding Truth and the Transformation of Authority," in Gisela Webb (ed.) *Windows of Faith: Muslim Women Scholar-Activists in North America*, Syracuse, NY: Syracuse University Press, pp. 172–94.

Hassan Amna Abdel Rahman (2000) "Recent Research Findings on FGM in Sudan-July 2000," *Women's International Networks News*, 26, 4: 26–7.

Hassan, Riffat (1999) "The Issue of Woman-Man Equality in the Islamic Tradition," in Kristen E. Kvam, Linda S. Schearing and Valarie H. Ziegler (eds) *Eve and Adam: Jewish, Christian and Muslim Readings on Genesis and Gender*, Bloomington, IN and Indianapolis, IN: Indiana University Press, pp. 464–76.

—— (1999) "Feminism and Islam," in Arvind Sharma and Katherine K. Young (eds) *Feminism and World Religions*, Albany, NY: State University of New York Press, pp. 248–278

Heath, Peter (1992) *Allegory and Philosophy in Avicenna (Ibn Sînâ)*, Philadelphia, PA: University of Pennsylvania Press.

Hekmat, Anwar (1997) *Women and The Koran: The Status of Women in Islam*, New York: Promotheus Books.

al-Hibri, Azizah Y. (2000) "An Introduction to Muslim Women's Rights," in Gisela Webb (ed.) *Windows of Faith: Muslim Women Scholar-Activists in North America*, Syracuse, NY: Syracuse University Press, pp. 51–71.

Hippocrates (1931) *Hippocrates*, trans. W.H.S. Jones, London and New York: William Heinemann Ltd. and G.P. Putnam's Sons.

—— (1981) "On Generation," in *The Hipporatic Treatises: "On Generation," "On the Nature of the Child," and 'Diseases IV'*, Iain M. Lonie (ed.) Berlin, New York: Walter de Gruyter.

Hodgson, Marshall G.S. (1974) *The Venture of Islam: Conscience and History in a World Civilization*, vols 1 and 2, Chicago, IL and London: The University of Chicago Press.

Holy Bible King James Version (1984) Nashville, IN Camden, New York.

Hoodhboy, Pervez (1991) *Islam and Science: Religious Orthodoxy and the Battle for Rationality*, London: Zed Books.

Humphreys, Lee (1988) *Joseph and His Family: A Literary Study*, Columbia, SC: University of South Carolina Press.

Husaini, S. Waqar Ahmed (1980) *Islamic Environmental Systems Engineering*, London: the MacMillan Press.

Iacopino, Vincent (1998) *The Taliban War on Women: a Health and Human Rights Crisis in Afghanistan*, Boston, MA and Washington, DC: Physicians for Human Rights.

Ibn Ḥajar (1997) *Fatḥ al-Bārī*, Riyadh: Maktabat Dār al-Salām.

Ibn al-Manẓūr (1956) *Lisān al-'Arab*, Beirut: Dār Bayrūt.

Ibn Qayyim al-Jawziyyah (n.d). *Tuḥfat al-Mawdūd bi Aḥkām al-Mawlūd*. Cairo, Egypt: al-Maktaba al-Qāyima.

—— (n.d.) *Al-Tibyān fī Aqsām al-Qur'ān*, Cairo: Dār al-Ṭibā'ah al-Muḥammadiyyah.

Ibn Rushd (1984) *Talḥiṣāt ibn Rushd ilā Jālīnūs*, Madrid: al-Majlis al-A 'lā li al-Buḥūth al-'Ilmiyyah.

—— (1986) *Ibn Rushd's Metaphysics: a translation of Ibn Rushd's commentary on Aristotle' Metaphysics, Book Lām*, trans. Charles Genequand, Leiden: E.J. Brill.

Ibn Rushd (1987) *Kitāb al-Kulliyyāt fī al-Ṭibb*, J. M. Fórneas Basteiro and C. Alvarez de Morales (ed.) Madrid: Escuela de Estudios Árabes de Granada.

Ibn Sīnā, Abū 'Alī al-Ḥusayn (1952) *Avicenna's Psychology: An English Translation of Kitāb al-Najāt, Book 11, Chapter IV*, trans. Fazlur Rahman, London: Oxford University Press.

—— (1958) *Al-Ishārāt wa al-Tanbīhāt*, With a Commentary by Naṣīr al-Dīn al-Ṭusī, 4 vols, Sulaymān Dunyā (ed.) Cairo, Egypt: Dār al-Ma'ārif.

—— (1963) "Avicenna: Healing: Metaphysics," trans. Michael E. Marmura, in Ralph Lerner and Muhsin Mahdi (eds) *Medieval Political Philosophy*, Ithaca, NY: Ithaca University Press, pp. 98–111.

—— (1970) *Al-Ḥayawān*, section 8 of *al-Ṭabī'iyyāt of al-Shifā'*, 'Abd al-Ḥalīm Muntaṣir, Sa 'īd Zāyid, and 'Abdullah Ismā'īl (eds) Cairo, Egypt: n.p.

—— (1973) *A Treatise on the "Canon of Medicine" of Avicenna, incorporating a translation of the first book*, trans. O. Cameron Gruner, New York: AMS Press.

—— (1986) *Tis' Rasā'il fi al-Ḥikmah wa al-Ṭabī'iyyāt*, Ḥasan 'Aṣī (ed.) Beirut: Dār Qābis.

Inati, Shams (1996) *Ibn Sīnā and Mysticism: Remarks and Admonitions. Part Four*, London and New York: Kegan Paul International.

Iqbal, Muhammad (1962) *The Reconstruction of Religious Thought in Islam*, Lahore: Shaikh Muhammad Ashraf.

Irigaray, Luce (1993) *An Ethics of Sexual Difference*, trans. Carolyn Burke and Gillian C. Gill, Ithaca, NY: Cornell University.

—— (1996) *I Love to You: Sketch of a Possible Felicity in History*, trans. Alison Martin, New York and London: Routledge.

—— (2001) *Democracy Begins Between Two*, trans. Kirsteen Anderson, New York: Routledge.

Irving, Thomas B. (1998) *The Qur'ān (The Noble Reading)*, Tehran, Iran: Suhrawardī Research & Publication Center.

al-Iṣfahānī, al-'Allāmah al-Rāghib (n.d.) *Mufradāt Alfāẓ al-Qur'ān*, Ṣafwān 'Adnān Dawdī (ed.) Beirut, al-Dār al-Shāmiyyah.

Islamic Horizons, March/April, 1426/2005.

Iwai, Hideko (1985) *Islamic Society and Women in Islam*, Japan: The Institute of Middle Eastern Studies, International University of Japan.

Izutsu, Toshihiko (1964) *God and Man in the Koran: Semantics of the Koranic Weltanschauung*, Tokyo: The Keio Institute of Cultural and Linguistic Studies.

Jami, Hakim Nuruddin Abdurrahman (1980) *Yusuf and Zulaikha: An Allegorical Interpretation*, trans. David Pendlebury, London: The Octagon Press.

Jawad, Haifaa A. (1998) *The Rights of Women in Islam*, New York: St Martin's Press, Inc.

al-Jawzī, Jamāl al-Dīn (1996) *Kitāb Aḥkām al-Nisā'*, Beirut: Dār al-Fikr.

Jeffery, Arthur (1938) *The Foreign Vocabulary of the Qur'ān*, Baroda: Oriental Institute.

Johnson, Allan G. (2000) "Patriarchy, the System: An It, Not a He, a Them, or an Us," in Gwyn Kirk and Margo Okazawa-Rey (eds) *Women's Lives: Multicultural Perspectives*, New York: McGraw Hill, pp. 24–34.

Jonathan Barnes (ed) (1984) *The Complete Works of Aristotle*, Princeton, NJ: Princeton University Press.

Jone Johnson Lewis, "Women Prime Ministers and Presidents: 20th Century Global Women Political Leaders," online, available http://womenshistory.about.com/library/weekly/aa010128a.htm (access Tuesday, March 8, 2005)

Jones, V.R. and L. Bevan (1941) *Woman in Islam*, Westport, CT: Hyperion Press inc.

Kamalkhani, Zahra (1998) *Women's Islam: Religious Practice Among Women in Today's Iran*, London and New York: Kegan Paul International.

Kant, Immanuel (1993) *Grounding for the Metaphysics of Morals*, trans. James W. Ellington, Indianapolis/Cambridge: Hackett Publishing Company, Inc.

Katz, Steven T. (1992) "The 'Conservative' Character of Mystical Experience," in *Mysticism and Religious Tradition*, Oxford: Oxford University Press, pp. 3–60.

—— (1992) "The 'Conservative' Character of Mystical Experience," in Steven T. Katz (ed.) *Mysticism and Religious Tradition*, Oxford: Oxford University Press, pp. 3–60.

Kesselman, Amy, Lily D. McNair, Nancy Schniedewind (eds) (1999) "What is Women's Studies," in *Women: Images and Realities*, Mountain View, California: Mayfield Publishing Company, pp. 7–13.

al-Kisā'ī, Muḥammad b. 'Abd Allāh (1978) *The Tales of the Prophets of al-Kisā'ī*; trans. W.M. Thackson, Boston, MA: Twayne Publishers.

Knappert, Jan (1993) "Mi'rāj," in C.E. Bosworth E. Van Donzel, W.P. Heirinchs and Ch. Pellat (eds) *Encyclopaedia of Islam*, Leiden, New York: E.J. Brill, pp. 97–103.

Landolt, Hermann (1991) "Ghazālī and Religionswissenschaft," *Asiatische Studien* 45, 1: 19–72.

Lapidus, Ira M. (1988) *A History of Islamic Society*, Cambridge: Cambridge University Press.

Leaman, Oliver (1999) *A Brief Introduction to Islamic Philosophy*, Great Britain: Polity Press.

McAuliffe, Jane Dammen (1991) *Qur'ānic Christians: An Analysis of Classical and Modern Exegesis*, Cambridge: Cambridge University Press.

McCutcheon, Russell T. (1999) *The Insider/Outsider Problem in the Study of Religion: A Reader*, London and New York: Cassell.

Marmura, Michael E. (1987) "Soul: Islamic Concepts," in Mircea Eliade (ed.) *Encyclopedia of Religion*, New York: Macmillan Publishing Company, pp. 460–5.

—— (1984) "Avicenna's 'Flying Man' in Context," *The Monist*, 69: 383–95.

Massignon, Louis (1997) *Essay on the Origins of the Technical Language of Islamic Philosophy*, trans. Benjamin Clark, Notre Dame, Indiana: University of Notre Dame Press.

Mawdūdi, Sayyid Abul A'lā (1989) *Toward Understanding the Qur'ān*, vol. 2, Delhi: Markazi Maktaba Islami.

Mazrui, Ali Amin (1998) "Male and Female as an Islamic Dialectic: the legacy of Ayesha," part of a lecture delivered at Oxford University and sponsored by the Oxford Centre for Islamic Studies, Oxford, England, October.

Mendel, Gregor (1902) "Experiments in Plant-Hybridization," in *Mendel's Principle of Heredity: A Defence*, with a Translation of Mendel's Original papers on Hybridization, W. Bateson, Cambridge: Cambridge University Press, pp. 40–95.

Mernissi, Fatima (1975) *Beyond the Veil: Male-Female Dynamics in a Modern Muslim Society*, New York: Schenkman Publishing Company.

—— (1991) *The Veil and the Male Elite: A Feminist Interpretation of Women's Rights in Islam*, trans. Mary Jo Lakeland, New York: Addison-Wesley Publishing Company inc.

—— (1991) *Women and Islam: An Historical and Theological Inquiry*, trans. Mary Jo Lakeland, UK: Blackwell.

Merrett-Balkos, Leanne (1998) "Just Add Water: Remaking Women through Childbirth, Anganen, Southern Highlands, Papua New Guinea," in Kalpana Ram and Margaret Jolly (eds) *Maternities and Modernities: Colonial and Postcolonial Experiences in Asia and the Pacific*, Cambridge: Cambridge, UK; New York: Cambridge University Press, pp. 213–238

Meyers, Carol (1988) *Discovering Eve: Ancient Israelite Women in Context*. New York, Oxford: Oxford University Press.

Mohanty, Chandra Talpade (1991) "Under Western Eyes: Feminist Scholarship and Colonial Discourse," in Chandra Talpade Mohanty, Ann Russo, and Lourdes Torres (eds) *Third World Women and The Politics of Feminism*, Bloomington, IN and Indianapolis, IN: Indiana University Press, pp. 51–80.

Moore, Keith L. (1986) "A scientist's interpretation of reference to embryology in the Qur'an." *The Journal of the Islamic Medical Association* (January–June) 18: pp. 15–6.

Moore, Keith L. (2001) "The miracle and challenge of the Qur'an," in *Weekly Mirror International*, Wednesday, May 23.

Moore, Keith L. and T.V.N. Persaud (1993) *The Developing Human: Clinically Oriented Embryology*, Canada: W.B. Saunders Company.

Morewedge, Parviz (1973) *The Metaphysics of Avicenna: A Critical translation—commentary and analysis of the fundamental argument in Avicenna's Metaphysica in the Dānish Nāma-i 'alā'ī (The Book of Scientific Knowledge)*, London: Routledge and Kegan Paul.

Mumtaz, Khawaz (1994) "Identity Politics and Women: 'Fundamentalism' and Women in Pakistan," in Valentine M. Moghadam (ed.) *Identity Politics and Women, Cultural Reassertions and Feminism in International Perspective*, Boulder, CO: Westview Press, pp. 228–42.

Munson, Ronald (2000) "Social Context: The Holy Grail of Biology: the human genome project," in Ronald Munson (ed.) *Intervention and Reflection: basic issues in Medical Ethics*, United States: Wadsworth, sixth edition, pp. 559–62.

—— (2000) *Intervention and Reflection: Basic Issues in Medical Ethics*, Belmont, CA: Wadsworth.

Murata, Sachiko (1992) *The Tao of Islam: a sourcebook of gender relationships in Islamic thought*, Albany, NY: State University of New York Press.

Musallam, Basim (1990) "The Human Embryo in Arabic Scientific and Religious Thought," in G.R. Dunstan (ed.) *The Human Embryo: Aristotle and The Arabic and European Traditions*, Great Britain: University of Exeter Press, pp. 32–46.

al-Musnad, Muhammad bin Abdul-Aziz (1996) *Islamic Fatawa regarding Women*; trans. Jamaal al-Din Zarabozo, Saudi Arabia: Darussalam.

Nasr, Seyyed Hossein (1966) *Three Muslim Sages: Avicenna, Suhrawardī and Ibn 'Arabī*, Delmar, New York: Caravan Books.

—— (1996) "The Meaning and Concept of Philosophy in Islam," in Seyyed Hossein Nasr and Oliver Leaman (eds) *History of Islamic Philosophy*, part 1, London and New York: Rotledge, pp. 21–6.

—— (1996) "The Qur'ān abd Ḥadīth as source and inspiration of Islamic philosophy," in Seyyed Hossein Nasr and Oliver Leaman (eds) *History of Islamic Philosophy*. Part I. London and New York: Rotledge, pp. 27–39.

Nawal El-Shadawi (1995) "But Have Some Art with You: an Interview with El Saadawi" *Literature and Medicine* 14, 1:53–9.

Newby, Gordon Daniel (1989) *The Making of the Last Prophet*, Columbia, SC: South Carolina Press.

El-Nimr, Raga (1996) "Women in Islamic Law," in Mai Yamani (ed.) *Feminism and Islam*, New York: New York University Press, pp. 87–102.

Noonan, John T. Jr (2000) "An Almost Absolute Value in History," in Ronald Munson (ed.) *Intervention and Reflection: Basic Issues in Medical Ethics*, United States: Wadsworth, sixth edition, pp. 83–96.

Oliver, Clarence Paul (1967) "Dogma and the Early Development of Genetics," in R. Alexander Brink and E. Derek Styles (eds) *Heritage from Mendel*, Madison, Milwaukee, WI and London: The University of Wisconsin Press, pp. 3–10.

Ormsby, Eric L. (1984) *Theodicy in Islamic Thought: The Dispute over al-Ghazālī's Best of All Possible Worlds*, Princeton, NJ: Princeton University Press.

O'Shaughnessy, Thomas J.S.J. (1985) *Creation and the Teaching of the Qur'ān*, Rome: Biblical Institute Press.

Patten, Bradley M. (1947) *Human Embryology*, Philadelphia, Toronto: The Blakiston Company.

Penner, Hans H. (1992) "The Mystical Illusion," in Steven T. Katz (ed.) *Mysticism and Religious Tradition*, Oxford: Oxford University Press, pp. 89–116.

People, March 7, 2005, pp. 199–122.

Peters, F.E. (1996) "The Greek and Syriac Background," in Seyyed Hossein Nasr and Oliver Leaman (eds) *History of Islamic Philosophy*, part 1, London and New York: Routledge, pp. 40–51.

Pillsburry, Barbara L.K. (1978) "Being Female in a Muslim Minority in China," in Lois Beck and Nikkie Keddie (eds), *Muslim Women in the Muslim World*, Cambridge, MA: Harvard University Press, pp. 651–73.

Plato (1961) "Republic," trans. Paul Sorey, in Edith Hamilton and Huntington Cairns (eds) *The Collected Dialogue of Plato*, Princeton, NJ: Princeton University Press.

Preus, Anthony (1975) *Science and Philosophy in Aristotle's Biological Works*, Hildesheim and New York: G. Olms.

—— (1997) *Notes on Greek Philosophy from Thales to Aristotle*, Binghamton: Global Publications.

Puntarigvivat, Tavivat (2001) "A Thai Buddhist Perspective," in John C. Raines and Daniel C. Maguire (eds) *What Men Owe to Women*, Albany, NY: State University of New York, pp. 211–37.

Rahman, Fazlur (1979) *Islam*, Chicago and London: University of Chicago Press.

—— (1984) *Islam and Modernity: Transformation of an Intellectual Tradition*, Chicago and London: The University of Chicago Press.

—— (1995) *Islamic Methodology in History*, Pakistan: Islamic Research Institute.

Rambachan, Anantanand (2001) "A Hindu Perspective," in John C. Raines and Daniel C. Maguire (eds) *What Men Owe to Women*, Albany, NY: State University of New York, pp. 17–39.

Renan, Ernst (2000) "Muhammad and the Origin of Islam," in Ibn Warraq (ed.) *The Quest for the Historical Muhammad*, Amherst, NY: Prometheus Books, pp. 127–66.

Riḍā, Muḥammad Rashīd (1970) *Tasfīr al-Qur'ān al-Ḥakīm*, vol. 4, Beirut: Dār al-Ma'rifah.

Riddell, Peter G. (2001) *Islam and Malay-Indonesian World: Transmission and Responses*, Honolulu, HI: University of Hawai'i Press.

Rispler-Chaim, Vardit (1993) *Islamic Medical Ethics in the Twentieth Century*, Leiden: E.J. Brill.

Roald, Anne Sofie (1998) "Feminist Reinterpretation of Islamic Sources: Muslim feminist theology in the light of the Christian tradition of feminist thought," in Karin Ask and Marit Tjomsland (eds) *Women and Islamization: Contemporary Dimensions of Discourse on Gender Relations*, New York: Berg, pp. 17–44.

—— (2001) *Women in Islam: the Western Experience*, London, New York: Routledge.

Robinson, Kathryn (2000) "Indonesian Women: from *Orde Baru* to *Reformasi*," in Louise Edwards and Mina Roces (eds) *Women in Asia: Tradition, Modernity, and Globalization*, Ann Arbor, MI: The University of Michigan Press, pp. 139–69.

Ross, Stephen David (1995) *Plenishment in the Earth: An Ethics of Inclusion*, Albany, NY: State University of New York Press.

—— (1998) *The Gift of Touch*, Albany, NY: SUNY Press.

Rozario, Santi (1998) "On being Australian and Muslim: Muslim women as defenders of Islamic heritage," *Women's Studies International Forum*, 21, 6: 649–61.

Sadar, M. Husain (1984) "Science and Islam: Is There a Conlfict?" in Ziauddin Sardar (ed.) *The Touch of Midas: Science, Values, and Environment in Islam and the West*, Manchester: University Press, pp. 15–25.

Ṣaḥīh International (ed.) (1997) *The Qur'ān: Arabic text with corresponding English meanings*, Saudi Arabia: Abulqasim Publishing House

Said, Edward W. (1997) *Covering Islam*, revised edition, New York: Vintage Books.

Sardar, Ziauddin (1984) "Introduction: Islamic and Western Approaches to Science," in *The Touch of Midas: Science, Values, and Environment in Islam and the West*, Manchester: University Press, pp. 1–12.

Schimmel, Annemarie (1975) *Mystical Dimensions of Islam*, Chapel Hill: University of North Carolina Press.

—— (1985) *And Muḥammad Is His Messanger: The Veneration of The Prophet in Islamic Piety*, Chapel Hill, NC: University of North Carolina Press.

Sen, Krisna (1998) "Indonesian Women at Work: Reframing Subject," in Krisna Shen and Maila Stivens (ed.) *Gender and Power in Affluent Asia*, London: Routledge, pp. 35–62.

Shāh Walī Allāh (1996) *The Conclusive Argument from God*, trans. Marcia K. Hermansen, Leiden and New York: E.J. Brill.

Shahla Haeri (1999) "Woman's Body, Nation's Honor: Rape in Pakistan," in Asma Afsaruddin (ed.) *Hermeneutics and Honor: female "public" space in Islamiclate societies*, Cambridge, MA: Harvard University Press, pp. 55–69.

Sherif, Faruq (1985) *A Guide to the Contents of the Qur'ān*, London: Ithaca Press.

Smith, Jane I. Smith and Haddad, Yvonne Y. (1982) "Eve: Islamic Image of Woman," in Azizah al-Hibri (ed.) *Women and Islam*, Oxford, New York: Pergamon Press.

Spellberg, D.A. (1994) *Politics, Gender, and the Islamic Past: A Legacy of 'Ā'isha bint Abi Bakr*, New York: Columbia University Press.

Stevens, Maila (2000) "Becoming Modern in Malaysia: Women at the End of the Twentieth Century," in Louise Edwards and Mina Roces (eds) *Women in Asia: Tradition, Modernity, and* Globalization, Ann Arbor, MI: The University of Michigan Press, pp. 16–38.

—— (1998) "Sex, Gender and the Making of the New Malay Middle Class," in Krisna Shen and Maila Stivens (eds) *Gender and Power in Affluent Asia*, London: Routledge, pp. 89–126.

Stowasser, Barbara Freyer (1994) *Women in the Qur'an, Traditions, and Interpretation*. Oxford, New York: Oxford University Press.

Sturtevant, A.H. (1967) "Mendel and the Gene Theory," in R. Alexander Brink and E. Derek Styles (eds), *Heritage from Mendel*, Madison, Milwaukee, and London: The University of Wisconsin Press, pp. 11–15.

Syed, Ibrahim B. (1987) "Islamization of Attitude and Practice in Embriology," in M.A.K. Lodhi (ed.) *Islamization of Attitudes and Practices in Science and Technology*, Virginia: The International Institute of Islamic Thought, pp. 117–29.

al-Ṭabarī, Abū Ja'far Muḥammad b. Jarīr (1987) *The History of Ṭabarī (Ta'rīkh al-Rusul wa al-Mulūk)*, vol. 2, *Prophets and Patriarchs*, translated and annotated by William M. Brinner, Albany, NY: State University of New York Press.

—— (1989) *The History of al-Ṭabarī (Ta'rīkh al-Rusul wa al-Mulūk)*, vol. 1, general introduction and from the creation to the flood, translated and annotated by Franz Rosenthal, Albany, NY: State university of New York.

al-Ṭabarsī, 'Abū 'Alī al-Faḍl b. al-Ḥasan (1971) *Majmū' al-Bayān fī Tafsīr al-Qur'ān*, vol. 2, Beirut, Lebanon: Dār Maktabat al-Ḥayat.

Takeshita, Masataka (1987) *Ibn 'Arabī's Theory of the Perfect Man and its Place in the History of Islamic Thought*, Tokyo: Institute for the Study of Languages and Cultures of Asia and Africa.

The Centre for Development and Population Activities (2000) "Egypt: Ending Female Genital Cutting: A USAID funded Program Promoting a 'Positive Deviance' Approach," *Women's International Networks News* (Autumn) 26, 4: 30.

The Commentary on the Qur'ān (1987) abridged, translated, and annotated by J. Cooper. Oxford, Oxford University Press.

The Holy Bible (1984) New York: Thomas Nelson Publishers.

The New York Times (1996) "A Refugee's Body Is Intact but Her Family Is Torn," September 11.

—— (1996) "U.S. Hearing to Decide Rights of Women Who Flee Genital Mutilation," May 2.

—— (1996) "Woman's Plea for Asylum Puts Tribal Ritual on Trial," April 15.

Tomm, Winnie (1995) "A Religious Philosophy of Self," in Mornt Joy and Eva K. Neumaier Dargyay (eds) *Gender, Genre, and Religion: Feminist Reflections*, Canada: Wilfrid Laurier University Press, pp. 239–55.

Toprak, Binnaz. (1994) "Women and Fundamentalism: The Case of Turkey," in Valentine M. Moghadam (ed.) *Identity Politics and Women, Cultural Reassertions and Feminisms in International Perspective*, Boulder, CO: Westview Press, pp. 293–306.

Tress, Daryl McGowan (1996) "The Metaphysical Science of Aristotle's Generation of Animals and Its Feminist Critique," in Julie K. Ward (ed.) *Feminism and Ancient Philosophy*, New York and London: Routledge, pp. 31–50.

Tuana, Nancy (1994) "Aristotle and the Politics of Reproduction," in Bat-Ami Bar On (ed.) *Engendering Origins: Critical Feminist Readings in Plato and Aristotle*, Albany, NY: State University of New York Press, pp. 189–206.

Tucker, Judith E. (1993) *Gender and Islamic History*, Washington, DC: American Historical Association.

al-Ṭūsī, Naṣir al-Dīn (1964) *The Nasirean Ethics*, trans. G.M. Wickens, London: George Allen & Unwin ltd.

Umar, Nasaruddin (1999) *Argumen Kesetraan Jender: Perspectif al-Qur'ân [Argument for Gender Equality: Qur'ânic Perspective]*, Jakarta: Paramadina.

UN WIRE (2002) "Pakistan: Violence against Women Increases Despite President's Condemnation," News Release by the International Secretariat of Amnesty International, (May 10, 2002) in *Women's International Network News*, (Summer) 28–3:20.

Wadud-Muhsin, Amina (1992) *Qur'ān and Women*, Kuala Lumpur: Fajar Bakti Sdn.

—— (2000) "Alternative Qur'anic Interpretation and the Status of Muslim Women," in Gisela Webb (ed.) *Windows of Faith: Muslim Women Scholar-Activists in North America*, Syracuse, NY: Syracuse University Press, pp. 3–21.

Walbridge, John (1999) "Selfhood/personhood in Islamic Philosophy," in Eliot Deutsch and Ron Bontekoe (eds) *A Companion to World Philosophies*. Malden, MA: Blackwell, pp. 472–83.

Walther, Wiebke (1993) *Women in Islam*, Princeton and New York: Markus Wiener Publishing.

Ward, Julie K. (1996) "Introduction," in Julie K. Ward (ed). *Feminism and Ancient Philosophy*. Routledge: New York and London, pp. I–xxiii.

Watt, William Montgomery (1970) *Bell's Introduction to the Qur'ān*, Edinburgh: Edinburgh University press.

—— (1985) *Islamic Philosophy and Theology*, Edinburgh: Edinburgh University Press.

Wehr, Hans (2000) *A Dictionary of Modern Written Arabic*, in J. Milton Cowan (ed), Beirut: Librairie du Liban.

Weinberg, Julius R. (1966) *A Short History of Medieval Philosophy*, Princeton and New Jersey: Princeton University Press.

Werblowsky, R.J., Zwi and Geoffrey Wigoder (eds) (1997) *The Oxford Dictionary of the Jewish Religion*, New York, Oxford: Oxford University Press, pp. 15–16.

Westermann, Claus (1984) *Genesis I-II: A Commentary*, Minneapolis: Augsburg.

Widengren, Geo (1955) *Muhammad, the Apostle of God, and His Ascension*, Uppala and Wiesbaden: Lundequistka & Harrassowitz.

Wilcox, Lyn (1998) *Women and the Holy Qur'an: A Sufi Perspective*, Riverside, CA.: M.T.O. Shahmaghsoudi Publications.

Willis, Robert (1965) *The Works of William Harvey, M.D*, translated from the Latin with A life of the Author by Robert Willis, New York and London: Johnson Reprint Corporation.

Wilson, Edward Osborne (1978) *On Human Nature*, Cambridge: Harvard University Press.

Women's International Network News (2002) *Women's International Network News*, (Summer) 28–3:29.

Yasmin, Samina (2002) "Muslim Women as Citizens in Australia: Perth as a Case Study," in Yvonne Yazbeck Haddah and Jane I. Smith (eds), *Muslim Minorities in the West: Visible and Invisible*, Walnut Creek, CA and Lanham, MD: AltaMira Press, pp. 217–32.

Youssef, Nadia Hasan (1978) "The Status and Fertility Pattern of Muslim Women," in Lois Beck and Nikkie Keddie (eds) *Muslim Women in the Muslim World*, Cambridge, MA: Harvard University Press, pp. 69–99.

al-Zabīdi (1989) *Tāj al-'Arūs*, Kuwait: al-Turāth al-'Arabī.

al-Zamakhsharī, Abū al-Qāsim Maḥmūd b. 'Umar (1966) *Al-Kashshāf 'an Ḥaqā'iq Ghawāmiḍ al-Tanzīl*, Cairo, Egypt: Maṭba'at Muṣṭafā al-Bābī al-Ḥalabī.

Index

abangan 6
Abbasid 12
'Abduh, Muhammad 66, 88, 89
abortion 91, 92; types of 91
Abrahamic religions 53; similarities 52
Abū Bakr 27–8, 104, 129
Adam 2–3, 14, 18, 22, 45–61, 65–6, 69–71, 86, 95–6, 98, 125, 142–3; angelic and satanic forces of 51; as an archetype of humankind 50–1, 53; creation of 50; expulsion from the Garden 52; intellectual progress of 54; meaning of 53; origin of 47, 51–2, 61, 63–4, 70, 142
adultery 27, 97
Afghanistan 103, 129
agency 28, 111, 122, 130, 133, 140; moral agent 2, 65
Ahmed, Leila 110
Albar, Mohammad Ali 72, 88
alienation 5, 19, 30
alimony 4, 132
Allen, Prudence 77
Alousï, Husām 64
Amin, Ahmad 107
anatomy 57, 65, 69, 76, 88
Anees, Munawwar Ahmad 113
Aphraates 52
approach: insider's approach 7; objective of 7; objectivity of 7; outsider's approach 7
'ārif 134–8
Aristotle 11, 31, 34–6, 38, 75–84, 90, 119
Asad, Muhammad 51, 64, 66, 88, 89
Ash'arite 62–3
Australia 42
authority 5, 8, 14, 19, 23–4, 28, 31, 36, 39–41, 44, 57, 67, 93, 96, 100–1, 104, 115–16, 118, 121, 125–6, 141, 143–4
Baghdad 12
Bali 29
Barlas, Asma 20, 47, 110, 126
Battle of Camel 27
Bayḍāwī 99
Bayt al-Ḥikmah 12
de Beauvoir, Simone 30
Bhutto, Benazir 26
Bibi, Mukhtaran 125
Bible 46, 58; Biblical account 91
Bint al-Shāṭī' ('Ā'ishah bt. 'Abd. al-Raḥmān) 50–1
Bisṭāmī, Abū Yazīd 137
Bouhdiba, Abdelwahab 97
breastfeeding 132
Brison, Susan J. 67, 69
Buddhism 127

China 42
Christianity 110
Çiller, Tansu 26
circumcision 15, 95, 96, 102, 112–14
cleansing 103
colonization 67, 145
conception: beginning of life 91
Confucianism 29, 127
cosmology 74
creation: Biblical account of 56; equality in 3, 14, 20, 46, 56, 61, 65–6, 70, 131, 142, 145; ex-nihilo 61–4; Genesis 52–3, 56, 58, 60, 87, 91; in God's image 56, 57; *ibdā'* 62; intentional 58; Islamic and Judeo-Christian accounts of 52; *khalq* 52, 61–2, 64, 89, 136; misogynist understanding of 58; primary and intentional 58; story of 56, 59; *taṣwīr* 57, 61, 130; women as secondary 60

culture 5, 6, 13, 16, 24, 28–30, 38, 42, 47, 55–6, 67, 69, 73, 102, 108–10, 119, 127, 129–30, 139, 142; Islamic 29, 61, 103, 123

democracy 4, 12, 132, 145
dependency 132; extensional 25, 118, 123–5, 128–30, 139–40, 143; reciprocal 38, 123, 132
Descartes, Rene 11
differentia 68
discrimination 12, 20, 144
divorce 9, 19, 36–8, 103–4, 132, 142
domain: private 106–8; public 12, 17, 20, 38, 40, 44, 69, 71, 93, 104, 107, 118, 125, 141
domination 11, 98, 125
dowry 37

education 9, 34, 36, 41, 43, 71, 103–4, 131, 144–5
egalitarianism 19, 65; ethics of 61; formulation of egalitarian principles 6; male egalitarianist 1, 139; seed of non-egalitarian view 61
Egypt 107, 114
Eisentein, Albert 42
emanation 63–4, 80, 135
embryo 78–9, 84, 86–91, 93
equality 1–2, 5, 9, 16, 20–1, 23, 27–8, 36, 47–8, 56, 61, 65–6, 69–70, 73, 82, 87, 107, 117, 123, 130–2, 139, 145; equal identity 56; human origin 61; and moral responsibility 70, 118
ethics 17, 23, 61, 73, 107, 118; Islamic 122–3, 144
Eve 46, 48, 50, 54–61, 66, 69, 71, 95, 100, 115, 125, 142, 143; as Adam's dependent 55; creation of 46, 48, 54–6, 58, 65–6, 98; crooked rib carries negative traits 58–9, 98, 115; extensional role of 55; intellectual property 55; Judeo-Christian origin of creation theories 55; Muslims' reception of 59; repentance of 55

Fārābī 118
Fāṭimah 138
fall: Adam's and Eve's 59; cause of 60
family 1–4, 11, 14–15, 17, 19–20, 24–5, 28–9, 32–3, 35–8, 41, 43–4, 69, 84, 92–3, 102–4, 106, 112–15, 118, 121–2, 124–32, 139, 140, 143, 145
family planning 92, 102; abortion 91
fanā' 136
fatwā 94, 95; embodiments of 95
female genital mutilation: *See* mutilation; genital
femininity 4–5, 12, 14–15, 23, 40, 60, 89, 93–8, 100–2, 107, 112, 114–16, 139, 140, 143; construction of 23, 94, 114; feminine traits 95–6, 98–9, 107, 114–15; masculine conception of 115
feminism 1, 4, 9, 145
feminists 1, 12, 46–7, 110, 139, 141, 144
fitnah 28, 32
Flying Man 68
Foucault, Michael 103, 133, 137
fruit: forbidden 59

Galen 75, 83
Garden of Eden 58
Geertz, Clifford 6
gender egalitarianism 1, 2, 20, 23, 56, 61
gender justice 17, 132, 139, 144
gender studies: approaches in 5; insider approach to 6; methodology in 6
gender system 1–5, 12, 14–19, 23, 25, 29, 32–3, 44, 71, 117, 123, 133, 140–1, 143–4, 146; contradictory claims of 1; egalitarian 1–2, 12, 14, 17, 21–2, 70, 139, 141, 144–5; hierarchical 1–2, 4–5, 9, 11–12, 14–15, 18–19, 25, 71, 96, 101, 118, 124, 126, 133, 138–42, 145–6; operation of 3; roots of 2, 4
gender thinking 2, 5, 12, 14, 16–17, 25, 33, 43–4, 55–6, 94–5, 126, 140, 142; politics of 56
Ghazālī 62–3, 82, 83, 100, 133, 134–7
globalization 1, 12; global forces 1

Haas, Samuel S. 52, 91
ḥadīth 1–2, 9, 16–17, 19–20, 24–8, 58, 72, 83, 85–6, 94–5, 101, 113, 117–18, 141, 143; misogynistic 58; transmission of 104
Ḥallāj, Ḥusayn b. Manṣūr 137
Ḥanafī 91
Ḥanbalī 91
Hallaq, Wael B. 9
harem 107
Harris, Rabia Terri 88
Hasina Wajed, Sheikh 26
Hassan, Reffat 47, 58–9, 94
Ḥawwā' 46, 54–5, 58–9, 61, 66, 69

Hekmat, Anwar 60, 111
Hellenism 13
hierarchical principles of gender: formulation of 6
ḥijāb 105, 106, 109; and private domain 107
Hijrah 105, 110
Hinduism 127
Hippocrates 75, 83–4, 86; Hippocratic philosophy 75, 77, 83, 86
honor: family 29
Hoodhboy, Pervez 74
human rights 1, 4, 9, 12, 60, 114
humanity 5, 11, 15, 30, 32–3, 46–8, 50–1, 53–4, 57–8, 60, 65–8, 70–1, 87, 89, 125, 139, 140–5; Abrahamic basis for inclusive 58; *bashar* 48–54, 65, 70; clay as origin of 47, 49–51, 53, 59, 61, 63–5, 70, 74, 86–7, 89, 142; constituents of 57, 119, 142; a drop of water as origin of 53; dust as origin of 47, 51–3, 61, 63–6, 70, 86–7, 89, 142; fall of 58–9; gendered view of 58–60; as genus 57, 68; as God's image 57; germ-cells as origin of 53; human genome 32; inclusive 2, 14, 46, 53–4, 57–8, 70, 142–3; *insān* 48–50, 53, 138, 144; irreducibility of 54, 57; *khalīfah* 18, 48–9, 51–4, 65, 69–70; material cause of 53, 61, 63–4, 81; men and women as contraries 76; moral qualities of 16, 57; moral responsibility of 43, 52–3, 58–9, 117, 128; origin of 46–7, 51–2, 61, 66, 74, 75, 86; as a pair 60, 65–6; physical form of 57; properties of 57; self as essence of 119
Humphreys, Lee 97
Ḥunayn (b. Isḥāq) 12

Iblīs 48–2, 54, 59, 137; betrayal of 50; *diabolos* 52
Ibn 'Abbās ('Abd Allāh b. 'Abbās) 54, 99
Ibn Ḥajar (al-'Asqalānī) 100
Ibn Manẓūr 62
Ibn Mas'ūd ('Abd Allāh b. Ibn Mas'ūd) 54
Ibn Qayyim (al-Jawziyyah) 82–4, 86–7, 92
Ibn Rushd 82, 118
Ibn Sīnā 3, 12, 30–1, 33–9, 63, 68–70, 75–6, 78–82, 100, 118–19, 121, 135–7
ijmā' 28
ijtihād 8–9; close of the gate of 8; definition of 8
Indonesia 6, 26, 29, 42, 92
inequality: arguments for 61
infanticide 92; female 16, 103–4, 130, 144
inferiority: argument for women's 56
inheritance 2, 8, 19, 36–8, 104, 124, 142
intellect: acquired 120; active 69, 120; actual 120; material 120
Iran 103, 111, 129; Iranian revolution 111
Iraq 27
'irfān 70, 137
Irigaray, Luce 30, 125
Iṣfahānī 62
Islam: basic message of universal 61; cultural 111; as last link 52; partial 13; particular 13, 102, 126; political 111; total submission 7, 51, 126; universal 13, 20, 23, 142
Isrā' 100, 138; *Isrā'* as spiritual journey 100, 138

Java 29
Jesus 3, 51
jilbāb 108–10
Joseph 15, 95–9
Joseph-Zulaykhā Story 97
Judaism 53, 110
Jundashipur 12

kalām 8, 50, 118
Kant, Immanuel 11
Kashmir 111
Khadījah 17, 138
khalīfah 18, 23, 48–9, 51–4, 57, 59, 65, 69–70, 101, 129, 139, 144, *khalīfah*: human supremacy 18, 48–9, 51–4, 65, 69, 70
khimār 108–9
Khosrau 27
killings: honor 129
Kindī 118
kinship 20, 27–9, 35, 65, 104, 118, 125
Kisā'ī 55, 98

labor division 11–12, 19, 42, 44, 71, 102
legitimacy: religious 1–2, 44, 102, 117, 139–41, 143
liberation 2, 4, 10–11, 20, 115; contextualization of 4; *Liber graduum* 52
love 11, 35–6, 38–9, 47, 66, 97, 124–5, 127, 131–2, 137

macrocosm 7, 8, 22–3, 57, 74, 91, 118, 137, 142
madrasah 6

malā'ikah 48, 50; characteristics of 50; obedience of 50; seniority over Adam 50
Malaysia 29, 42
Mālikī 91
Ma'mūn (Caliph) 12
Marmura, Michael 68
marriage 9, 17, 19, 31, 33–9, 42, 101, 104, 106, 112, 124–6, 128–9, 131; monogamous 114; polygamous 104
Mary 3, 26, 51, 138
masculinity 1, 4–5, 14–15, 23, 30, 44, 60, 93–6, 98, 101–2, 107, 112, 114–16, 128–9, 140, 143; characteristics of 60; construction of 23, 94, 114; masculine traits 114
maṣlaḥah 28, 33
Mecca 138
Medina 52, 107, 110
Megawati Sukarnoputri 26
men: authority of 55; as majority 67
Mernissi, Fatima 24, 27, 32, 106, 110
microcosm 7, 8, 22–3, 74, 91, 118, 132, 137, 142
Middle East 6, 29, 42, 129
Minagkabau 29
minority: religious 67
mi'rāj 100, 138
misogynistic tradition 17, 56
misogyny 59
modernization 145
modesty 102, 105, 110–11, 126, 129
Moore, Keith L. 87–9
morality 1, 12, 16, 19, 22, 39, 94, 102, 105, 108, 112, 117, 125, 128, 131, 139–41, 144–5; double standard in defining 112; feminine chastity 21, 22, 108–11, 114, 128–9; moral agent 2, 65
mosque 107; and Muḥammad's household 107
motherhood 40–2, 93; foster-mothers 132; surrogate 93; mothering 35, 41–2, 73, 131
Mughīrah (Ibn Shu'bah) 27
Muḥammad 3, 22, 24, 27–8, 41, 52–3, 55, 83, 87, 91, 104, 108, 126, 128–9, 138, 144
mujtahid 8
Murata, Sachiko 8, 23
Mu'tazilite 62
mutilation: genital 113–14; types of genital 113; violence and genital 113
mysticism 8, 121
nafs 2–6, 9, 11–17, 19–23, 25, 30, 32–3, 36, 38, 41–4, 46–7, 50–1, 55, 57, 59, 65–72, 81, 94–7, 99–104, 107, 116–19, 122–6, 129–33, 136, 139–46; *ammārah* 3; as human soul 3; *lauwāmah* 3; material self 3, 15, 94–7, 100–2, 105, 115, 117–18, 139; meaning of 3; *muṭma'innah* 3; as origin of humanity 3
narrative: religious 1, 12, 15, 94–5, 101
nationalism 145
Necessary Being 63, 121, 135
Nestorian Church 12
niyyah 54, 83, 99, 118, 123, 145
non-governmental organization (NGO) 114

obedience 19, 30–1, 40, 50–1, 126–8
occassionalism 62
ontology 1, 3, 5, 10, 17, 46–8, 65–8, 94, 117, 132, 139, 141–2, 144
oppression 6, 10, 11–12, 30, 38, 60, 67, 139, 142–3, 146

Papua New Guinea 29
patriarchy: characteristics of 5; definition of 5; patriarchal system 4, 11, 46, 56, 73, 94, 105, 111–12, 114, 116; roots of 4, 56
pesantren 6
Pharaoh 137
philosophy 9, 10–13, 17, 30, 33, 38, 47, 74–6, 80–1, 90, 92; Greek philosophical heritage 12; Islamic 11–13, 62, 92; meaning of 11; Muslim philosopher 11–13, 15, 33, 40, 74–5
Plato 11, 34
pleasure 31, 36, 39, 82, 93, 99, 102, 112, 114, 116, 118, 120, 127, 132–4, 136–40; sexual 113, 134, 137; spiritual 134
pluralism 12, 35, 53, 66–7, 76, 136, 142, 143
post-colonization 1, 9, 145
Potiphar 97–8
power 1, 5, 17, 19, 24, 31–2, 37, 43, 46, 53, 62–4, 67, 73, 76–81, 84, 89–90, 92–5, 97, 99, 102–5, 111, 124–5, 127, 130, 140–1, 143–4
prayer 103, 121, 145
priyayi 6
Pythagorean philosophy 76

qiyās 8
Qur'ān: contents of 7; contextual understanding 47, 105, 110, 117; Qur'ānic vocabulary: Syriac origin 52
Quṭb, Sayyid 101

Rabī'ah al-'Adawiyyah 138
Rahman, Fazlur 119
Rā'īl 97, 98
rape 9, 91, 125
Rāzī, Fakhr al-Dīn 50–1, 106, 109
reproduction 4, 7, 14, 45, 72–5, 77–85, 87–8, 91–2, 115, 119–21, 125, 131, 140, 143; assisted 92; cloning 92; equal roles of male and female in 72; female's passive role 90; *mā'* 83, 86, 88; male element as a formative power 78; male's superiority in 72, 74, 75, 80, 82; men and women as agents 73; men and women as principles of generation 81; men contribute to form, women to matter 76; menstrual blood in 75, 77–9, 82, 84; Menstrual fluid as material cause 81; *muḍghah* 89, 92; *nuṭfah* 63, 81, 83, 86–8, 92; reproductive principles 75; reproductive technology 92, 131; *ṣalṣāl* 47, 49, 61, 63–4, 70, 142; semen as efficient cause 79; semen as principle of motion 78–9, 81; semen in 72, 75–9, 82–4, 86–7, 90; sperm in 63–4, 72–3, 75, 78–88, 90–2; *ṭīn* 47, 51–2, 61, 63–4, 70, 142; *turāb* 47, 61, 63–4, 70, 86–7, 89, 142; women as tilth 72–3
responsibility 2, 20, 22, 33–4, 36–9, 43, 45, 60, 69, 93, 102, 122–4, 130, 132, 142; moral 4, 51, 65, 117, 132, 139, 140
riyāḍah 136
Roald, Anne Sofie 6
rūḥ 3, 50, 52, 92; *See also nafs*

St. Ephrem 52
Salmān al-Fārisī 138
santri 6
Saudi Arabia 3, 13, 16, 42, 103, 129
scarf 110
Scripture: hierarchical reading of 56, 142; non-hierarchical reading of 56
seclusion 39, 42, 60, 103, 105–8, 145
segregation 42, 85, 110
self: concept of 118, 132; construction of 3, 15, 95–6, 124, 130; construction of material 102; embodied 133; equality of 117; generative 32, 71–4, 81, 82, 91, 119, 125, 130; ontological 3, 46, 117, 132, 139, 142; psychological dimension of 119; public perception of 118, 124; *see also nafs*
senses: external 120; internal 120
sexuality 19, 21, 23, 27–9, 32, 37–8, 47, 68, 70, 91, 94, 99, 101, 108, 112, 114, 122, 130, 133, 140–1, 143, 145; *ars erotica* (erotic art) 133; benefits of sexual passion 133; control over 37, 112; *scientia sexualis* (science of sexuality) 133; sexist attitude toward women 121
Shāfi'ī 91
shadhdh al-dharā'i' 28
Sharī'ah 8–9, 13–14, 16, 33, 59, 91; imposition of — on women 8
ṣiddīq 135, 136
Socrates 34–6
soul 3, 14, 20–1, 30–1, 46–7, 57, 65–70, 79–81, 87, 90–1, 118–22, 131–3, 136, 142; animal 120–1; as first entelechy 119; functions of 79; immaterial 69–70; kinds of 119; priority over body 80; rational 79–80, 119–21; vegetative 120–1
Southeast Asia 3, 7, 29
species 30, 33, 68, 77
Spirit 3, 11, 13, 49–50, 52, 66, 92, 95, 117, 144
Stoics 119
Stowasser 96
subordination 11, 19, 38, 59, 60, 111, 133, 140; logic of men's — over women 56; men over women 56
Sudan 113
Ṣūfī 8, 46, 69, 136, 138
Sulamī, Ṣafwān ibn al-Mu'aṭṭal 128
Sulawesi, South 29
Sumatra, North 29
Sunda 29
Sunnah 8
superiority: arguments against 56; gender difference as argument for 57; male 4, 12, 14, 17, 19, 33, 36–8, 40, 55–6, 72, 74, 76, 125, 140, 143; theological assumptions for 58

Ṭabarī 55, 69
taboo 114, 133
tafsīr 20
takhrīj al-manāt 8
Taliban 103, 111, 129
tawḥīd 33, 53, 135–6, 142; Islam's core teaching 53

Tress, Daryl McGowan 81
Truth 23, 74, 99, 108, 135–8
Turkey 26
Ṭūsī 126

'ulamā' 67, 117
ummah 122
universalism 70, 143
uṣūl al-fiqh 8

veil 87, 97, 105–7, 110–11; as an identity 111; as a symbol of political Islam 111
veiling 7, 15, 95–6, 102–6, 109–12, 145; and Assyrian law 105; historical context of 111; meanings of 111; and modesty 105; original functions of 104; and repression 105
violence 9, 43, 112, 126, 144
virginity 15, 95–6, 102–3, 112

Wadud-Muhsin, Amina 47, 65–6, 129
Westermann, Claus 57
westernization 9, 12
Widengren, Geo 138
wife-beating 126
women: characteristics of 131; common misconceptions of 60; education of 104; as identical with body 102; masculine concept of 101–2, 133; as minority 67; mistreatment of 20, 60–1; as object of sexual pleasure 73; oppression of 30, 38, 67; pre-Islamic Arab 103; as privation of men 76; rights and protections of 104; as sexual beings 101; social role of 10, 28; and social tranquility 102; as symbol of imagination faculty 100; womanist 1, 12, 65, 139, 145

Youssef, Nadia H. 42

Zabīdī 62
Zamakhsharī 63, 66, 99
Zulaykhā 15, 95–100, 115; as allegory 99; as negative prototype of women 98, 107; as prototype of female temptation 95–7, 99; as symbol of sexual aggressiveness 97